Relational Mental Health
Beyond Evidence-Based Interventions

Relational Mental Health
Beyond Evidence-Based Interventions

José Guimón
University of Geneva Medical School
Chene-Bourg, Switzerland

KLUWER ACADEMIC / PLENUM PUBLISHERS
NEW YORK, BOSTON, DORDRECHT, LONDON, MOSCOW

Library of Congress Cataloging-in-Publication Data

Guimón, J.
Relational mental health : beyond evidence-based interventions / by José Guimón.
p. cm.
Includes bibliographical references and index.
ISBN 0-306-47857-9—ISBN 0-306-47967-2 (ebk.)
1. Psychiatry. 2. Mental health. 3. Mental illness—Treatment. I. Title.

RC454.G783 2003
616.89—dc22 2003055643

ISBN 0-306-47857-9 (hardbound)
0-306-47967-2 (e-book)

233 Spring Street, New York, New York 10013

http://www.kluweronline.com

10 9 8 7 6 5 4 3 2 1

A C.I.P. record for this book is available from the Library of Congress.

Printed in the United States of America.

This book is dedicated to José, Pablo and Mariana

Contents

Acknowledgements

To Delories Dunn for the translation of most of the material of this book

To Brocher Foundation (Geneva) for the support given to the realization of the manuscript

Foreword

The present volume, authored by one of the most prestigious European psychiatrists, Professor of the Department of Psychiatry of the University of Geneva Medical School, offers a refreshing, actual, broad scope perspective on the profession of psychiatry and its role in the field of mental health. It offers the reader a clearly stated, balanced view of where the field of mental health delivery systems is moving at this time, and the role of psychiatry and the mental health profession at large in this rapidly changing professional area. Its main purpose, excellently achieved, is to provide the psychiatrist, the biological researcher, the psychoanalyst, the mental health practitioner, the educator and the researcher in these areas with a broad overview of the concepts of mental health and mental illness, and the present controversies regarding etiology, psychopathology, treatment, and prevention. Dr. Guimón's text is one of the very rare ones that combines a deep understanding of biological determinants of illness with the psychodynamic concept of personality development, and the contribution of the social sciences to both.

For the American reader, the information about recent developments in psychiatry in Europe, integrated with a thorough understanding of corresponding developments in the United States provides a critical perspective regarding the issues the psychiatric profession is struggling with today. Thus, it helps to transcend the potentially restricted viewpoints determined by any local scene. The fact that a broad historical perspective introduces many areas of contemporary controversies regarding etiology, diagnosis, and treatment also contributes to elevating the level of discourse beyond narrow speculations. Guimón elegantly indicates how the revolution in the neurosciences can be complemented with a contemporary psychodynamic approach derived from psychoanalytic understanding. He appropriately challenges the psychoanalytic profession to reexamine its responsibility toward both the scientific development of its field and its social responsibility in the prevention and treatment of mental illness. While clearly sympathetic to psychoanalytic approaches, Guimón points to both strengths and weaknesses in psychoanalytic contributions, and is critical of psychoanalytic education as well as of frequently narrow perspectives in psychiatric residency training. His critical review of psychodynamic research approaches strengthens this critique.

This book examines lucidly the contributions of transcultural studies in the evaluation of etiology, frequency, and symptoms of mental illness as they are influenced by socio-cultural factors, and explores the integration of this perspective in the clinical management of the main psychopathological constellations. The overview of the treatment of organic mental disorders, the major psychoses, and the personality disorders is enriched by this combination of biological, psychodynamic, and socio-cultural perspectives. The reader will find up to date summaries of the present strategies of treatment that reflect this integration of approaches.

The major emphasis of this volume is on psychosocial modalities of treatment, both in the context of institutional therapeutic programs as well as in the individual treatment of patients. In this context, it provides the reader with detailed information about the present state of group and family interventions, that are taught in a rather perfunctory manner in most texts of psychiatric therapeutics. Guimón provides thoughtful information regarding areas where evidence based treatments may contribute significantly to clinical practice, and areas where this is not the case: he presents an original exploration of the natural limits of evidence based treatments.

Nowadays, there are few comprehensive texts in psychiatry still written by a single author. The field of psychiatry has become so broad and complex that multi-authored textbooks are the order of the day. Guimón's volume shows that an extremely knowledgeable, original, and passionate scholar still may provide a synthesis that enriches the field; stimulates the reader to become concerned with it beyond his or her limited personal sphere of activity; and, in explaining the present in terms of its development from the past, signals new roads and challenges for the future.

Otto F. Kernberg, M.D.*

*Director, Personality Disorders Institute, The New York Presbyterian Hospital, Westchester Division

Professor of Psychiatry, Weill Medical College of Cornell University.

Training and Supervising Analyst, Columbia University Center for Psychoanalytic Training and Research

1

Mental Health

Concepts and Trends

We shall begin by defining a number of mental health concepts, and then address the concept of abnormality, ending with a discussion of the scientific basis of key concepts on which current diagnostic and therapeutic interventions in mental health are based.

MENTAL HEALTH OR PSYCHIATRY?

Mental Health: An Endeavour

The term *mental health* has been progressively gaining ground as an alternative to psychiatry, to underline its preventive aspects—as first recommended by the World Health Organization (WHO)—and the fact that this field requires the participation, not only of psychiatrists, but also other professionals, as well as segments of the general population, legislators, and politicians. Therefore, more than a science or a simple clinical activity, mental health is an endeavour, and a burning issue, involving social and humanitarian commitment.

The mental health field is wider than that of clinical psychiatry, because it also includes the detection of undiagnosed cases in the general population, and prevention in normal subjects, to avoid their contracting psychological disorders. Indeed, in a survey conducted during the Epidemiological Catchment Area (ECA) project (an epidemiological study in the United States), approximately 30% of the general population had, in the previous 6 months, presented a psychiatric disorder as defined by the American Psychiatric Association's *Diagnostic and Statistical Manual*. This prevalence would have been at least 10% higher if substance abuse had also been taken into account. However, it has been estimated that only 2% of the population suffers from a severe psychiatric disorder (e.g., psychosis).

A mere 1% of patients with a mental illness consults a psychiatrist. This means that the rest of the patients are not seen, or, if they are, they mainly visit their general practitioner for somatic disorders. Since general practitioners' detection capacity is probably no higher than 60%, a large proportion of the population with psychiatric problems is never diagnosed adequately.

This situation cannot be improved solely with the indispensable knowledge and abilities of psychiatrists; it also requires the participation of other professionals, such as sociologists, educators, and clergymen, as well as the patients themselves and their families. In addition, public administrators need to get involved in these problems, which affect a considerable proportion of the population, and provide the necessary resources for prevention and rehabilitation programmes. Since, in addition, mental patients encounter major barriers to accessing the services they need, and suffer from stigmatisation on the part of the rest of the population, it is essential that laws be passed to avoid or ease these inequalities (Guimón, 2001).

The term *public mental health* is sometimes used for exclusively official programmes, in contrast with *community mental health*, which not only receives state funding, but also involves the participation of volunteers and private donors. The term *community psychiatry* has been used as a synonym for *community mental health*, but the latter has acquired more strictly care-related connotations.

What Is Psychiatry?

Although the concept and scope of mental health are wider-ranging than those of psychiatry, the former comprises the fundamental bases of the latter. However, the very concept of *psychiatry* has changed over the last few decades (Guimón, 1982, 1986). Indeed, it is a very enlightening exercise to examine the decisive divergences in the definitions proposed by different psychiatrists, conditioned by the passing of time and, above all, by each author's ideological orientation.

Many authors simply avoid defining psychiatry at all; others provide definitions in accordance with the scientific value that they assign to it, and with what they consider to be its proper object of study; for most authors, it is a branch of the *medical sciences*.

Psychodynamically-oriented authors, in their definitions, tend to highlight the concept of *interpersonal relations*. On the other hand, those who are more sociologically-oriented include psychiatry among the *behavioural sciences*, which they define as including anthropology, sociology, and psychology, excluding certain specialities such as physiological psychology, archaeology, technical linguistics and physical anthropology, and adding certain aspects of social geography, psychiatry, economics, political science, and law.

The "Mental Patient"

The *UN Principles for the Protection of Persons with Mental Illness and the Improvement of Mental Health Care* (UN, 1991) define the term *patient* as an individual receiving mental health care, and include all those persons admitted to a mental health programme of any kind.

The *Recommendations on the Situation of the Mentally Ill of the Council of Europe* (EU, 1998) consider that the definition of mental illness 'is extremely difficult', given that criteria are constantly changing and that a whole new range of psychological disorders has appeared, related to the problems of modern life. The Council of Europe also supports the World Psychiatric Association's Hawaii Declaration (WPA 1992) condemning the misuse of psychiatry for the suppression of dissidence, and applauds its decision to establish an international ethical code for psychiatric practice.

The Mental Health "Professionals"

In the 1970s, within the context of the community psychiatry movement, the limits between the different mental health specialities became somewhat blurred. Consequently, over the last three decades, all over the world, psychiatrists have been delegating the practice of psychotherapy to other professionals, especially psychologists, but also social workers, and (above all in hospital settings) to nurses. On the other hand, in some countries, psychologists have been focusing more on biologically-based training, and have tried to acquire the right to prescribe medication. Similarly, a new speciality in clinical psychology, *health psychology*, is being introduced into an important sector of psychophysiological medicine that was traditionally the area of *liaison psychiatrists*. Finally, general practitioners have, increasingly, been acquiring psychiatric training, and some American universities have been trying to create a sub-speciality in psychiatry for internists (Guimón, 1998).

THE CONCEPTS OF NORMAL AND ABNORMAL IN MENTAL HEALTH

Quantitative and Qualitative Criteria

The barriers between normal and abnormal in human behaviour and experience are not easy to establish. Attempts have been made to describe normality in a statistical manner, considering abnormal those traits that stray from the mean. However, there are many limitations to this approach to normality: not all human behaviours and experiences fit into a Gauss-curve distribution; individuals are just as abnormal for falling off the curve due to excess as those who do so because of a defect; there are major cultural variations regarding what is desirable in behavioural terms, and so on.

Qualitative criteria for abnormality have also been proposed, such as the presence of anxiety, unhappiness, guilt, or inefficiency, but the exceptions to these criteria, which limit an approach of this kind are obvious. A more acceptable qualitative criteria for normality would be the acquisition of 'mature' behavioural patterns, characterised by self-sufficiency, the capacity to establish stable emotional relationships, and sufficient adaptability to change.

In an attempt to define abnormal psychological phenomena, based on the work of Jaspers (1946) and his followers, a movement arose that aimed to describe the conscious experiences and observable behaviours of human beings in order to achieve an (objective) explanation or (subjective) understanding of these phenomena. One result was the differentiation between *developments* and *psychic reactions*. Some quantitative anomalies of the psyche have a psychological origin, and are accessible to understanding, as compared with *illnesses*, which were considered to be of somatic origin and would comprise qualitatively incomprehensible anomalies. The latter present in the form of *phases* or *outbreaks* when they are acquired briefly, or in the form of *processes* when they are more persistent.

European and American psychiatric studies prior to World War II tended to adopt the concept of *normality* as defining health. Later, *ideal* and *average* criteria were used, which were also called into question due to their lack of objectivity. The WHO became more interested in the *disabilities* aspect of these disorders.

In any case, one of the basic findings of social research in mental health is the relativity of the concept of *psychological abnormality*.

Normality and Transcultural Psychiatry

The anthropological branch of psychiatry considers that mental alterations, although they may have a biological basis, are frequently due to secondary or compensatory processes, which can be influenced by cultural and social factors. The existence of these factors would explain the differences in the symptoms of these illnesses from one society to another, from one social group to another within the same society, as well as from one historical period to another.

Theoretical sociologists tend to consider psychiatric disorders as a form of social deviation. The patient is considered ill because he has transgressed the local code of norms or social conduct. Although it is true that the cultural response to a behaviour considered deviant can have an influence on whether the patient improves or gets worse, it is abusive to consider the violation of social codes as a *sine qua non* for the existence of a disorder. The cultural context has an influence on how a disorder first presents (*pathoplasty*), and sometimes can set off a disorder or extend its duration, but it is also necessary to invoke biological or constitutional factors, a basic diathesis or individual tendency, to explain the occurrence of many disorders.

The concept of *transcultural psychiatry* comes from the appreciation of differences in the clinical picture of different disorders, according to whether they are observed in one culture or another. Some authors use the concept of *metacultural psychiatry* to designate a diagnostic method useful for any culture, which makes it possible to disregard the aspects unique to the culture of each society. Devereux (1961) used the concept of *ethnopsychiatry* as an equivalent of transcultural psychiatry, although etymologically and historically it had been used to designate the questionable concept of the influence of race on the presentation of clinical pictures.

Whichever term we use, there are three basic concepts involved in the findings of transcultural psychiatry: the relativity of the concept of what is normal; the existence of disorders typically linked to certain cultures; and the higher incidence of certain syndromes in one culture than in another.

The concept of psychological normality has deep cultural connotations. Behavioural traits that would be considered normal or even desirable in a certain society could be considered clearly pathological in others. Without having to recur to transcultural parameters, the relativity of the concept of normality in psychopathology becomes evident when we consider, for example, the different assessment that is made today, as compared with 30 or 40 years ago, in our society regarding the sexual activity of adolescents and young people, or homosexual behaviour.

Current Concepts of Mental Disorder and Mental Illness

Spitzer's definition (Spitzer and Endicott, 1978) differentiates the terms *mental illness* and *mental disorder*. The former refers to alterations with an observable pathophysiological process, such as organic brain syndromes or mental retardation. For the majority of categories, the different editions of the American Psychiatric Association's *Diagnostic and Statistical Manual* (known as *DSM-III, DSM-III-R*, and *DSM-IV*) refer to *mental disorder*, and define this quite adequately. However, the third condition in the

DSM's own definition, i.e., that a disorder be clearly different from other disorders, is not, obviously, always the case in psychiatry, which has led to the creation of marsinal diagnostic categories. Previously, Kendell (1975) had highlighted this concern over the lack of clear borders between one syndrome and another in modern classification systems.

Wing (1978) distinguished between two meanings of the term *mental illness*. The first is a wide-ranging concept including all of the deviations and abnormalities that lead a patient to seek professional help, and which result from the conjunction of two processes: statistical deviation and social attribution. The second is much more specific, and requires the existence of a clinical syndrome and underlying biological disorder. This dual definition stresses that, in such cases as personality disorder, there is no discernible syndrome or aetiology.

The *DSM-IV* classification (Frances, First and Pincus, 1997) notes that, for reasons of professional policy, terms such as *psychiatric disorder* or *psychological disorder* cannot be proposed, although they would be preferable to that of *mental disorder*. The biological model of mental health maintains that psychiatric disorders are true illnesses, and should be diagnosed as such. However, the definition of psychiatric illness has not been adequately formulated, either. Based on these conceptions, Guze includes, in one of his three consecutive definitions, the concept of suffering as necessary to define an illness, which was criticised by Kendell (1975). He affirms, in another definition, that illness is 'what doctors treat', and refers, in the third, to the concept of syndrome being comparable to that of *illness*. This follows the concepts of Sydenham, although that approach was surpassed in the 19th century by Virchow's conception, which stressed the need, when defining an illness, to discover, besides a definable course, a precise aetiology and pathophysiology.

DOCTRINAL TRENDS IN MENTAL HEALTH

If we make an inventory of the highly diverse activities of mental health professionals (especially of the most characteristic among them, the psychiatrist) in any given country, or even at a single work centre, we could catalogue them according to a typology of what we can call *extreme types* (Guimón, 1990).

We can consider as an extreme type on the scale that group of activities which supposes that mental health (above all psychiatry) focuses its research and interventions on the human brain, without any regard for the surrounding environment. At the other extreme, we find those conceptions which suppose that social phenomena should be studied globally, and modified. This bipolarity, is, naturally, artificial, and no professional from any psychiatric school would adhere to one or the other of these conceptions. If we establish a serial (or quasi-serial) relationship between them, we can see that, close to the extreme conception taking the human brain as its object of study, we would find the *biological* school in today's psychiatry. Going one step up the scale, we could refer to the reductionist behaviouralists, exemplified by Eysenck (1960). Further on up the scale, would be the position of the non-reductionist behaviouralists, such as Skinner (1953). Next we could find the partisans of introspective doctrines, such as phenomenology or psychoanalysis. Nearby on this scale would be those doctrines involving interpersonal relationships, such as those proposed by Sullivan (1967). Beyond that would cluster all of the approaches that relate psychiatric disorders to the interaction among people in the different groups to which they belong, and which propose group therapy techniques for their cure. Even further on the scale would be the schools assuming that the individual should not be treated as "mad"—that the person should not be considered ill, but rather the entire family system should be considered altered, a basic concept in family psychotherapy. At the other extreme of the scale would be the so-called antipsychiatric approaches, popularised by Laing (1967), Cooper (1967), and Szasz (1961), which consider that what needs to be treated is the alienating situation created by society, not the 'supposed mental patient'.

This typology not only throws light on the different positions regarding the acceptance of one or another object of mental health; it also serves to clarify somewhat the diversity of tasks that professionals carry out, and the diversity of theories to which they may be ascribed. According to Baselga (1975), theories may be considered as a set of systematically organised laws and rules that are the basis of a science, and which serve to relate and explain a certain order of phenomena. A set of theories may lead to the formation of what Tiryakian (1968, cited by Baselga, 1975) called a 'set of fundamental presuppositions, axioms, or premises that orient later investigation by pointing out those aspects that are immediately relevant to the phenomena under study'.

The spectacular progress of biological psychiatry, the advance of community psychiatry, and the growing participation of society as a whole in mental health programmes, have themselves originated different theoretical trends and different ways of operating within the health care system (Guimón, Fischer, Zbinden, and Goerg, 1997), which are usually grouped into three basic models: the *medical* model, the *psychological* model, and the *social* model. We believe that two others should be added: the *magical*

Table 1.1. Mental Health Concepts and Trends

Concept	Models	Doctrinal Tendencies	Theories
MAGICAL	SUPERNATURAL		
BIOLOGICAL	MEDICAL	Neuropsychiatry	1. Genetics
		Biological psychiatry	2. Metabolic
			3. Brain disorder
			4. Physical illness impairing adaptation
			5. Psychosomatic illness
		Behaviourism	6. Learning
		Cognitivism	7. Motivation
		Phenomenology	8. Excessive reaction to stress
			9. Cognitive disorders
RELATIONAL	PSYCHOLOGICAL	Psychoanalysis	
		Object relations	10. Characteristics of parents and children
			11. Fixation, regression
			12. Objects, container
			13. Family (double bind)
		General systems theory	14. Pathological communication
			15. Social isolation
			16. Social class and mobility
	SOCIAL		17. Cultural change
			18. Alienation
			19. Discrimination
POLITICAL		Sociology	
	ADMINISTRATIVE	Antipsychiatry	20. Human rights
		Humanitarian psychiatry	
		Ethics	21. Managed care
		Legal psychiatry	
		Management	

model, and the *politico-administrative* model. These major theoretical models, which determine psychiatry today, developed, as we shall see in the next chapter, progressively over the course of centuries.

REFERENCES

Baselga, E. (1975). Comentarios sobre teoría y modelo conceptual. Unpublished manuscript, Bilbao.

Cooper, D. (1967). *Psychiatry and antipsychiatry*. London: Penguin Books.

Devereux, G. (1961). Mohave ethnopsychiatry and suicide: The psychiatric knowledge and the psychic disturbances of an Indian tribe. *Bureau of American Ethnology Bulletin*. Washington, D.C.: United States Government Printing Office.
EU (1998). The recommendations on the situation of the mentally ill of the Council of Europe. *Recommendation Rec*. 98. Brussels: Council of Europe.
Eysenck, H. J. (1960). Handbook of abnormal psychology. London: Pitman.
Frances, A., First, M. B., and Pincus, H. A. (Eds.). (1997). *DSM-IV, Guía de uso*. Barcelona: Masson, Barcelona.
Guimón, J. (1981). Reflexiones sobre el carácter científico de la Psiquiatría. *Psiquis*, 2, 118–125.
Guimón, J. (1982). Definiciones de la psiquiatría. *Psiquis*, 3, 1–4.
Guimón, J. (1986). Ciencia y creencia en Psiquiatría. Paper presented at the European Congress on Science and Beliefs, Barcelona.
Guimón, J. (1990). *Psiquiatras: De brujos a burócratas*. Barcelona: Salvat Editores.
Guimón, J., Fischer, W., Zbinden, E., and Goerg, D. (1997). Consequences of recent changes in research and practice for the identity of psychiatrist. *European Psychiatry*, 12 (supp. 2), 92s–98s.
Guimón, J. (1998). La profession de psychiatre. *Evolution et devenir*. Paris: Masson.
Guimón, J. (2001). *Inequity and Madness. Psychosocial and Human Rihts Issues*. New York: Kluwer Academic.
Jaspers, K. (1946). *Psicopatología general*. Buenos Aires: Delta.
Kendell, R. E. (1975). The concept of disease and its implications for psychiatry. *British Journal of Psychiatry*, 127, 305–315.
Laing, R. D. (1967). *The politics of experience and the bird of paradise*. Middlesex: Penguin Books.
Skinner, B. F. (1953). *Science and Human Behavior*. New York: Macmillan.
Spitzer, R. L., and Endicott, J. (1978). Medical and mental disorder: Proposed definition and criteria. In R. L. Spitzer and D. F. Klein (Eds.), *Critical issues in psychiatric diagnosis*. New York: Raven Press.
Sullivan, H. S. (1967). *Clinical studies in psychiatry*. New York: W. W. Norton.
Sydenham, T. (1966). *Methodus Curandi Febres*. London: Crook.
Szasz, T. S. (1961). *The myth of mental illness: Foundations of a theory of personal conduct*. New York: Hoeber-Harper.
UN (1991). *The UN principles for the protection of persons with mental illness and the improvement of mental health care*. United Nations.
Wing, J. K. (1978). *Reasoning about madness*. London: Oxford University Press.
WPA. (1992). The General Assembly of the World Psychiatric Association. Hawaii: World Psychiatric Association.

2

Is Mental Health Founded on Truly Scientific Conceptions?

Mental health aims to be a movement, an endeavour that draws on various branches of the sciences. We shall briefly discuss here the scientific nature of the concepts on which these interventions are based.

SCIENCE AND PSYCHIATRY

Science has been defined in its widest sense as the 'body of objective knowledge regarding nature, society, man, and his thought' (Guimón, 1981, 1982). Using more restrictive criteria, science has been defined as the body of knowledge obtained through the so-called 'experimental method'. In any case, it would be excessive to claim that none of the knowledge attained by mankind before Galileo and Bacon (the founders of this method, in the early 16th century) can be considered scientific, although the form of acquisition and its very formulation may not meet this restrictive requirement demanded of the sciences by empiricist researchers.

Regarding this latter consideration, some recent authors have tried to establish wider criteria for distinguishing between science and other cognitive investigation, especially, eliminating the need for the requisite of causality as indispensable for considering something to be scientific. Psychiatry can, according to these criteria, be considered a science (Guimón, 1986). If we demand a more restrictive set of criteria, we see that a great deal of research has been carried out using the so-called 'scientific-natural method'—in the sense of Dilthey (1948) or Windelband's 'nomothetic' approach—not only in the field of the so-called psychoses with known bodily causes, but in other disorders. If we eliminate, using broader criteria, the need to refer to ideas of 'causality', then we can rely on a number of investigations inspired by psychological or sociological models and methods, based on what some authors called the 'historical-cultural method' (or Windelband's 'ideographic' approach). This method is based on understanding the connection between one event and another.

Be that as it may, it is evident that *human sciences* have made less progress than was initially hoped. In this sense, Ayer (1964) reflected on the limitations that arise when man is taken to be the subject of a science. He revised the optimism of the early 19th century positivists, who believed that what they called the *natural sciences* could be emulated by the *human sciences*. These hopes were not fulfilled by the social sciences, and according to Ayer, there are many reasons for this: the ruling factors behind human conduct are excessively complex; for moral and practical reasons, the number of experiments that can be carried out using human beings is limited; the methods used in the past have often been mistaken; the right questions have yet to be asked. However, many theorists have, in the end, accepted that the true reason for this difficulty lies in the fact that man is, in some way, beyond the order of nature, due to the *free will* that makes it virtually impossible to formulate any generalisations regarding his conduct.

These particular limitations of psychiatry as a human science, its diffuse boundaries, and the fact that it often has to recur, as noted above, to the methodology of the historic sciences, mean that its theoretical underpinnings suffer from a certain degree of vulnerability. Therefore, its domain can often be invaded by pseudoscientific conceptions (Guimón, 1998).

EXPLAINING *vs* UNDERSTANDING

The diversity of subjects studied in mental health matters (the central nervous system, behaviour, the unconscious, interpersonal relationships, family and social systems), as well as the professional's vast range of activities, have led to the emergence of different *doctrinal trends* (neuropsychiatry, biological psychiatry, behaviourism, cognitive science, psychoanalysis, social psychiatry) which can be grouped into two main models: the medical (or biological) model and the psychosocial model (Chapter 1 Table 1.1).

This is consistent with early 20th century German distinction, which in the field of psychology, led to an opposition between *comprehension* on the one hand, to 'understand intentions', belonging to the sciences of the mind (*historical* or *cultural sciences*), and causal *explanation* on the other, exclusive of the *natural* sciences.

But as Piaget pointed out, this opposition proved detrimental to the progress of the science of man and could even be criticised from an epistemological point of view. He contends that it is impossible, methodologically, to introduce an opposition between the science of man and the science of nature. Piaget (1967) also holds that the distinction between *explanation* (causal) and *comprehension* (the senses and intentions), however well founded, can in no way oppose the science of man and the science of nature. In reality, this dichotomy underlines two irreducible but indissociable aspects of knowledge, which all sciences attempt to reconcile in one way or another.

On the basis of these criteria, psychiatry can be seen as an empirical science focusing on the psychologically ill and employing one method or another, depending on the case.

As the various chapters of this book will show, there is no doubt that in the next two decades it is the medical model which will prevail and psychiatrists will thus increasingly become 'psychoneuroendocrinology' experts, delegating to other specialists (psychologists, educational specialists) some of the tasks linked to the psychosocial aspects of psychic illness specific to their profession.

THE NEED FOR EVIDENCE-BASED PSYCHIATRY

The language of medicine is simultaneously scientific, moral and political. These three languages make up a social body—which has come to be known as the 'body of medicine'. Medicine is a 'practical', 'operational science'. But as Gracia (1996) says, it is no longer quite as easy as it was a few decades ago to defend the scientific nature of medicine. Admittedly anatomy is a science, just like physiology, biochemistry or microbiology. But none of these sciences strictly identifies with medicine, even if the doctor has to be familiar with all of them to do his job:

> 'The doctor is in fact a social agent like any other, night watchman or street cleaner. The difference, it is true, is that the doctor needs complex scientific training to carry out his work effectively. But although he requires scientific knowledge, the doctor is not a scientist'.

Be that as it may, the assessment of efficacy and efficiency of treatment are presently taking on growing importance for medical practice (see chapter 7). An 'evidence-based' movement has appeared in medicine as a regulative idea, a method and a socio-political endeavour. Scientifically proven therapeutic measures or 'empirically supported treatments' are proposed through techniques such as randomised controlled trials, meta-analysis and 'consumer reports' studies. However, these procedures have advantages and disadvantages (Henningsen, 2000). They also have major ethical implications (Helmchen, 2001), since moral neutrality is a myth when referring to the incompatible ethical positions inherent in clinical and research practices (Miller, 2001).

Even if psychiatry has been one of the first medical specialties to use the tools of evidence-based medicine, this approach has, so far, been applied more often to pharmacological than to psychological treatments; however, Cochrane collaboration systematic reviews and other forms of review (e.g., the Patient Outcomes Research Team programme in Baltimore) have begun to appear (Thornicroft, 2001). This growing interest has led to the formation of task forces to define, identify, and disseminate information about empirically supported psychological interventions (Sanderson, 1998; Chambless, 1998; Barlow, 1999). The American Psychological Association Task Force on the Promotion and Dissemination of Psychological Procedures proposes some characteristics of empirically supported treatments (O'Donohue et al., 2000): they involve skill building, have a specific problem focus, incorporate continuous assessment of client progress, and involve brief treatment contact, requiring 20 or fewer sessions. To be 'well-established', treatments for specific disorders must be shown efficacious in at least two independent randomised clinical trials. However, the task force recognises that these findings are in part an artifact of sociological factors present in contemporary psychotherapy.

LIMITS OF THE EMPIRICAL APPROACH IN MENTAL HEALTH

Traditional clinical methods of assessing the effectiveness of psychological treatments (such as intelligence testing and objective personality tests such as the MMPI), are rarely used in empirically supported treatments, and have come under attack (O'Donohue et al., 2000).

On the other hand, many psychiatrists have reservations about the evidence-based medicine approach because of perceived limitations in its methodology, such as gaps in interpreting the available evidence and neglect of individual patient uniqueness in quantitative research through manualised treatment procedures (Beutler, 2000).

Furthermore, Cochrane studies also sheds light on psychological and practical obstacles which must be overcome before public health care systems can utilise new scientific results. The settings of psychotherapeutic randomised controlled trials to date have been highly artificial naturalistic psychotherapy, and studies should be complemented by efficiency studies and evaluation of whole health care systems if they pretend to be relevant to practice (Mundt and Backenstrass, 2001). Finally, empirically supported psychological treatments have not been effectively disseminated to the mental health professionals who deliver them, and thus are not readily available to the public that requires them (Barlow, Levitt, and Bufka, 1999; Goldfried et al., 1999).

Therapists complain that therapy research has only a remote resemblance to what goes on in actual clinical practice. There is a need for staff training to implement new psychological treatments, addressing professional barriers that may limit uptake, and investigations of the 'minimum effective dose' or the key active ingredients of the intervention (Lehmen and Steinwachs, 1998; National Institute for Mental Health, 1998).

To overcome these difficulties, some authors have proposed the need for more naturalistic studies; others urge adding criteria derived from mental health policy and economics (Buchkremer, 2001). In this sense, Barlow (1999) offers a way to overcome the problems of rigid manuals, as well as those associated with forcing clinicians to adhere to theories and practices that are outside of their interest, experience, and expertise.

New models of research have also been proposed. Margison (Margison et al., 2000) supports a model of professional self-management, 'practice-based evidence', as a complementary paradigm to improve clinical effectiveness in routine practice via the infrastructure of 'practice research networks'. For the prediction of courses of treatment response Lutz et al. (2001) combine a dose-response model with growth curve modelling to determine dose-response relations for well-being, symptoms, and functioning. Barkham (2001) argues for a core outcome measure (the 'Clinical Outcomes in Routine Evaluation-Outcome Measure') to provide practice-based evidence for the psychological therapies to complement the evidence-based practice paradigm. Kendall et al. (1999) propose 'normative comparisons', a procedure for evaluating the clinical significance of therapeutic interventions, consisting of comparing data on treated individuals with that of normative individuals. Mundt and Backenstrass (2001) emphasise the importance of more detailed psychopathology (through data that can be expected from neurosciences), which can then be matched to specific psychotherapy tools (Mundt, 2001).

REFERENCES

Ayer, A. J. (1964). *Man as a subject of science*. Londres: Athlone Press.

Barkham, M., Margison, F., Leach, C., Lucock, M., Mellor-Clark , J., Evans, C., Benson, L., Connell, J., Audin, K., & McGrath, G. (2001). Service profiling and outcomes benchmarking using the CORE-OM: toward practice-based evidence in the psychological

therapies. Clinical Outcomes in Routine Evaluation-Outcome Measures. *J Consult Clin Psychol*, 69(2), 184–196.
Barlow, D., Levitt, J., & Bufka, L. (1999). The dissemination of empirically supported treatments: a view to the future. *Behav Res Ther*, 37(Suppl 1), 147–162.
Beutler, L. (2000). David and Goliath. When empirical and clinical standards of practice meet. *Am Psychol*, 55(9), 997–1007.
Buchkremer, G., & Klingberg, S. (2001). What is science-based psychotherapy? On the discussion of guidelines for psychotherapy research. *Nervenarzt*, 72(1), 20–30
Chambless, D., & Ollendick, T. (2001). Empirically supported psychological interventions: controversies and evidence. *Annu Rev Psychol*, 52, 685–716.
Dilthey, W. (1948). *Introducción a las ciencias del espíritu*. Madrid-Buenos Aires: Espasa Calpe.
Goldfried, M., TD, B., Clarkin, J., Johnson, L., & Parry, G. (1999). Toward the development of a clinically useful approach to psychotherapy research. *J Clin Psychol*, 55(11), 1385–1405.
Gracia, D. (1996). El poder medico. In P. Ridruejo & A. Medina & J. L. Rubio (Eds.), *Psicologia Medica* (pp. 601–616). Madrid: McGraw Hill Interamericana.
Guimón, J. (1981). Reflexiones sobre el caracter cientifico de la psiquiatria. *Psiquis, 2*, 118–125.
Guimón, J. (1982). Definiciones de la Psiquiatría. *Psiquis, 3*, 1–4.
Guimón, J. (1986). *Ciencia y creencia en psiquiatria*. Paper presented at the Congreso Europeo de Ciencia y Creencia, Barcelona.
Guimón, J. (1998). *La profession de psychiatre. Evolution et devenir*. Paris: Masson.
Helmchen, H. (2001). Therapeutic effectiveness. Effects, effectiveness and value of therapeutic interventions. *Nervenarzt, 72*(1), 56–60.
Henningsen, P., & Rudolf, G. (2000). The use of evidence-based medicine in psychotherapeutic medicine (article in German). *Psychother Psychosom Med Psychol*, 50(9–10), 366–375.
Jacobson, N., Roberts, L., Berns, S., & McGlinchey, J. (1999). Methods for defining and determining the clinical significance of treatment effects: description, application, and alternatives. *J Consult Clin Psychol*, 67(3), 300–307
Kendall, P., Marrs-Garcia, A., Nath, S., & Sheldrick, R. (1999). Normative comparisons for the evaluation of clinical significance. *J Consult Clin Psychol*, 67(3), 285–299.
Lehman, A. F., & Steinwachs, D. M. (1998). Patterns of usual care for schizophrenia: initial results from the Schizophrenia Patient Outcomes Research Team (PORT) Client Survey. *Schizophr Bull*, 24(1), p11–20; discussion 20–32.
Lutz, W., Lowry, J., Kopta, S., Einstein, D., & Howard, K. (2001). Prediction of dose-response relations based on patient characteristics. *J Clin Psychol*, 57(7), 889–900.
Margison, F., Barkham, M., Evans, C., McGrath, G., Clark, J., Audin, K., & Connell, J. (2000). Measurement and psychotherapy. Evidence-based practice and practice-based evidence. *Br J Psychiatry* Aug, 177, 123–130.
Miller, R. (2001). Scientific vs. clinical-based knowledge in psychology: a concealed moral conflict. *Am J Psychother*, 55(3), 344–356.
Mundt, C., & Backenstrass, M. (2001). Prospects in psychotherapy research (article in German). *Nervenarzt*, 72(1), 11–19.
Myerson, A. (1994). The attitude of neurologists, psychiatrists and psychologists towards psychoanalysis (1939). *Am J Psychiatry*, 151(6), 48–54.
O'Donohue, W., Buchanan, J., & JE, F. (2000). Characteristics of empirically supported treatments. *J Psychother Pract Res*, 9(2), 69–74.
Piaget, J. (1967). Classification des sciences et principaux courants épistémologiques contemporains. In J. Piaget (Ed.), *Logique et connaissance scientifique* (pp. 1149–1224). Paris: Gallimard-Encyclopédie Pléiade.
Sanderson, W. (1998). The case for evidence-based psychotherapy treatment guidelines. *Am J Psychother*, 52(3), 382–387

Thornicroft , G., & Susser, E. (2001). Evidence-based psychotherapeutic interventions in the community care of schizophrenia. *Br J Psychiatry, 178*(1), 2–4.

Wolf, F., Miller, J., Gruppen, L., & Ensminger, W. (1997). Teaching skills for accessing and interpreting information from systematic reviews/meta-analyses, practice guidelines, and the Internet. Paper presented at the Proc AMIA Annu Fall Symp.

3

Aetiology

Vulnerability and Homeostasis

The differentiation between *endogenous* and *exogenous* has been in use since the late 19th century (Möbius, 1892) to distinguish between alterations stemming from biological predisposition—of a hereditary, degenerative nature—and those alterations induced by aggressions to the brain coming from the outside.

As we have already mentioned, Jaspers (1946) used the term *process* to describe a lasting alteration in the psyche, a permanent personality modification arising from known or suspected brain damage. He used the term *development* to refer to a personality modification occurring in the course of an individual's lifetime that depends on the environment or life experiences. The concept of a *reaction*, according to Jaspers, is the 'reaction of the psyche to an experience' that depends on 'the importance that certain processes have for the soul, to the point of provoking a reaction that is, in part, understandable: the reactive pathological state does not often appear in response to a particular experience, but rather to a sum of effects'. We can see in this concept a similarity to the psychoanalytical idea of *trauma*.

In the United States, Meyer (1957) developed a concept integrating biological and psychosocial knowledge, which he called *psychobiology*. It represents an attempt to understand the different types of psychopathological disorganisation in the face of stress, which he called *reactions*. Recognised as a pioneer in the study of life events, Meyer highlighted the importance of a patient's clinical history and personal biography, above all in those aspects related to stressful episodes and ways of reacting to them. According to this author, symptoms represent attempts at homeostatic reorganisation, and psychiatric pathology corresponds to a regression to primitive levels of organisation, so that nearly all psychopathology is reactive in origin.

Finally, some systems theorists, using a comprehensive approach to mental health, have examined all different levels of living systems, including cells and organs (structures involved in an individual's behaviour), as well as organisations, societies, and supranational systems (which are objects of interest to community psychiatry). Miller (1975), for example, proposed grouping disorders in accordance with these different levels.

VULNERABILITY

Although Meyer's concept of *reaction* no longer forms a fundamental part of the new classifications of mental illnesses, it is still generally accepted that there can be no single aetiological factor, whether external or internal, in mental disorders; rather, that their appearance depends on factors involving both the genotype and the phenotype. The consensus is that there can be a genetic or environmental predisposition (e.g., perinatal complications) towards certain alterations in the structure or functioning of the neuroendocrine system that condition vulnerability to stress. This biological vulnerability in itself does not justify (Miller, 1996) the appearance, or *expression*, of the disorder.

By the same token, most clinicians agree that defense mechanisms, which children acquire from their early infancy in relation to the significant others in their environment, enable them to modulate, more or less adequately, the external stimuli that contribute to onset and relapse, such as traumas or family and social conditions (Sullivan, 1962; Fromm-Reichmann, 1948; Arieti, 1974; Perris, 1989). These mechanisms and coping strategies have been called *resiliencies*, which sometimes enable the child to develop adequately, in spite of suffering from severe external aggressions or deprivations. Stressful life events can be counteracted by community support mechanisms (whether formal or informal). It is only when the latter are overwhelmed that it become necessary for defence mechanisms to intervene; if these are insufficient, then the biological adaptation systems are forced into action. When a hereditary weakness in these biological systems renders them incapable of counteracting stressful stimuli, the result can be a mental disorder.

This model of biological vulnerability is now widely accepted, under various names, such as Engel's *biopsychosocial model* (1980), or the idea of *integrative pluralism* expounded by Margison and Mace (1997). These are 'interactive' conceptions, because they suggest, as we have just discussed, that mental problems arise when a constitutional vulnerability is combined with a 'suboptimal' environment. More or less artificially, this predisposition can be divided into the following aspects.

Biological Vulnerability

Genetic studies have arrived at the conclusion that the hereditary factor is undoubtedly the dominant element of risk for the appearance of some psychiatric disorders, such as Alzheimer's disease, schizophrenia, depression, or autism. However, one's genetic inheritance is not a "cause", but rather a kind of vulnerability whose impact is, today, still largely unknown.

The Plasticity of the Dopaminergic System

The classic dopaminergic hypothesis has not received much support from recent biochemical research; even in a best-case scenario, the results of such investigation are often contradictory.

Friedhoff's research team, during the 1970s and early 80s, carried out major studies exploring the adaptation of neurons to the presence or absence of dopamine in the synapses. They showed that dopamine receptors can be regulated, adjusting the quantity of neurotransmitters. These and other findings paved the way for a new, more comprehensive vision of how the dopaminergic system functions. They proposed (Friedhoff et al., 1986) that schizophrenia is an alteration in the balance between the dopaminergic and cholinergic systems, and that this illness may involve an imbalance between the D1 and D2 receptors. Furthermore, they theorised that the high plasticity of the central nervous system reflects, among other things, the existence of a restitutive cerebral dopamine system. According to Friedhoff's theory, psychosis becomes manifest when this restitutive system is unable to act efficiently enough to compensate for the aetiological factors that tend to produce mental destabilisation, when there is a lack of plasticity in the dopaminergic system. This can occur if aetiological factors, whatever they may be, are so powerful that there is no way to counteract them, or because the restitutive system is inefficient and fails to respond adequately. In addition, Friedhoff et. al. described the effects of foetal exposure to psychotropic drugs, after administering neuroleptics to pregnant rats, which altered the post-natal cholinergic activity of the striatum, with a marked drop in dopaminergic activity. They suggested that this could have implications for an increase in vulnerability to extrapyramidal disorders during postnatal development, with possible clinical consequences.

However, in both schizophrenia and mental activity generally, it does not seem logical to believe that the dopaminergic system's sole function is to mediate in the action of neuroleptics. Given that, by reducing dopaminergic activity with the appropriate medication, psychotic symptoms can be ameliorated or eliminated; and given that the dopaminergic system is capable of adjusting its activity in the absence of medication, regulating the liberation of neurotransmitters and the number of receptors, then the system's physiological role could be that of homeostasis: avoiding the destabilisation of mental function in the face of noxious exogenous or endogenous agents. And it could do so by reducing its own activity, through an adaptation process—down-regulation—similar to that of the process evoked or provoked by neuroleptics (Dávila et al., 1989).

It did not seem reasonable, in Friedhoff's view, to think that the capacity to adjust pre- and post-synaptic function is present in the brain simply to compensate for the effects of medications. Carlsson proposed that the dopaminergic system could act as a filter to regulate sleep-wake activity and emotional tone. The dopaminergic system is surely able to adapt to psychological and physiological changes, as well. Friedhoff et al. found that a repeated and unavoidable stress produces an effect, similar to that of neuroleptics, in the conditioned avoidance response. Indeed, they showed that, under some circumstances, the dopaminergic system modulates a restitutive response, diminishing its activity. In humans, this response can serve as a protection against psychotic decompensation in the face of endogenous or exogenous aggressions. Later, Friedhoff studied in more detail how these adaptive systems interact with psychosocial factors and with learned coping mechanisms in psychiatric patients.

Monoamines and Depression

In affective disorders, it has been shown that there is an alteration in the urinary excretion of adrenaline and noradrenaline. It has also been confirmed that depressed patients excrete less tryptamine into their urine, and that these levels of excretion become normalised after electroshock treatment, which is in accordance with the observation regarding the antidepressant effect of tryptophan. However, recent studies have highlighted, above all, these patients' imbalance of noradrenaline and/or serotonine, showing that two compounds able to diminish cerebral noradrenaline (reserpine and alphametyldopa) induce depressive psychoses, and that dopamine has an antidepressant effect on some patients.

Studies in the last few decades have proved conclusively that in patients suffering from major depression, and in the brains of depressed patients who committed suicide, there are alterations in the regulation of noradrenaline and serotonine turnover in the synapses, particularly in the alpha2-adrenoreceptors that regulate this turnover in a delicate biofeedbck (García Sevilla et al., 1986, 1990, 1996, and 1998). It is a matter of increasing the presynaptic inhibitory activity of the brain's alpha2-autoreceptors and alpha2-heteroreceptors. This increase has been related to a deficit in noradrenergic and/or serotoninergic functions, more specifically with the drop in neurotransmitter turnover that has been postulated in depression.

GABA System and Panic Disorder

Studies using neuro-imaging techniques have shown structural anomalies in patients with different kinds of panic disorder, as well as differences in the circulation and glucose consumption in certain areas of the central nervous system when these subjects experienced certain symptoms. Studies examining the biological bases of anxiety have made it possible to discover a benzodiacepine-GABA receptor. More recently, investigators' efforts have begun to focus on proving the existence of certain agonists, partial agonists, and also antagonists of this receptor. In addition, they have postulated the existence of endogenous ligands. Their results have suggested that other neurotransmission systems (serotoninergic, dopaminergic, noradrenergic) could be implicated in anxiety. More recently, a hyposensitivity to alpha2-adrenergic autoreceptors, and alpha-adrenergic hypersensitivity in the locus coeruleus and other regions, have been found in panic disorder patients. Some authors have suggested different tests (e.g., pharmacological challenges, with yohimbine, sodium lactate, fenfluramine, or cholecystokinine) to provoke symptoms of panic and obsessive-compulsive disorder.

In the past few years it has been found a duplication in an extensive zone of chromosome 15, responsible for enhancing cerebral mechanisms that regulate alarm processes. This genetic predisposition would produce conditions including a higher number of neuronal connections in alarm mechanisms, or more sensitive ones (up-regulation). Under such conditions, certain environmental factors, as well as personality characteristics, can throw the delicate homeostasis out of balance, causing panic disorder.

Alzheimer's Disease

Although only 2% of these cases depends directly on heredity (Giannakopoulos et al., 1996), a high percentage of the remaining patients presents a genetically-based vulnerability towards protein deposits that damage cells, which, together with other external factors, can cause this disease. A vaccine is currently being developed, and studies with rats have shown that it is able to avoid these protein deposits. In humans, a study has been launched featuring 300 patients in some European countries and the United States.

Cognitive Vulnerability

Patients belonging to groups with higher risk of a severe outcome present many information-processing disorders, both during acute periods and during remissions or the period before onset of the illness. Sometimes this cognitive vulnerability appears early in life, as in certain schizophrenic patients, and hinders them from acquiring adaptive social skills or even learning how to efficiently use available social support structures. In addition, these deficiencies reduce or block their ability to react appropriately to changes caused by their illness or in the face of an inappropriate environment or one that fails to provide them with sufficient support.

Psychosocial Vulnerability

Vulnerability, according to the sociologist Brown (Brown, 1978), is related to the environment and to feelings of hopelessness or desperation. In the onset of mental illness, the inevitable losses that occur over the course of a lifetime could have a major influence if they overwhelm a person's protective resources for confronting them. Regarding depression, for example, Brown postulates that in an urban setting, the fact of belonging to a disfavoured social class raises the risk of major losses and setbacks, severe chronic difficulties, and feelings of low self-esteem. The assumption is that these feelings are powerfully influenced by the degree of 'impression of success' that we have in our social roles. Indeed, our feelings of self-worth and self-esteem come from the vision that we have of ourselves, and of our degree of satisfaction with the social roles that we play.

A sense of failure and low self-esteem can also stem from unresolved problems produced by previous life crises. For example, it has been postulated that indifference in the face of an early loss of the mother can lead to cognitive deformations able to produce depressive tendencies in adult life. How we see and feel about the world, based on our infancy, childhood, and adolescence, is constantly being modified by experience, which can serve to increase or diminish expectations for the future.

STRESS AND LIFE EVENTS

The "Stimuli Barrier" and Traumas

Psychophysiological research on stressful situations has, for its part, contributed data to help us understand how exterior events act upon our brains. It has been suggested that the brain has a 'stimuli barrier' that protects it against sudden or excessive external excitations, which could upset the balance or integration of essential functions. When external excitation overcomes the stimuli barrier, the result is psychic trauma, with the consequent disorganisation of mental functioning. With time, the barrier can be reorganised, in which case the trauma would have only a transitory effect.

Prominent psychoanalysts have gone deeper into defining psychic trauma, and determining its pathogenic potential. The assumption goes that the first, formative experiences in infancy, together with constitutional factors, condition this stimuli barrier's level of resistance (Titchener and Ross, 1974). Why some subjects are able to resist certain traumatic aggressions and not others can be explained by the fact that a traumatic experience can act as a screen on which previous conflicts and defences are projected. There is also a consensus that reactions to stress are conditioned by the degree of desperation, and that in the early mother-child relationship an acquisition of basic trust diminishes desperation in the face of traumatic situations. This confidence contributes to a certain sense of invulnerability or *resilience* (Werner and Smith, 1993).

Types of Stress Factors

Some investigators began to try to quantitatively assess—using scales—the life events that can provoke stress. The proposed scales were useful, but also widely criticised for oversimplification.

According to González de Rivera (2001), stress factors can be non-specific, semi-specific (i.e., external stress factors combine with other, independent pathogenic elements), and specific (when external stress factors play a determinant role in setting off a morbid process). This author defines stress syndromes as those psychiatric syndromes in which the defence or adaptation to extreme demands plays a determinant, specific aetio-pathogenic role. He establishes the classification of stress syndromes as acute (self-stress, acute reaction to stress, psychosocial crisis, post-traumatic syndrome, and adaptive disorders) and chronic (disorder stemming from extreme and persistent stress, Ochberg's victimisation syndrome, and professional burnout syndrome).

Change as a Pathogenic Factor

Although, as we have mentioned previously, cultural factors are 'sufficient' causes to set off a mental illness, but not 'necessary' in the aetiological sense (for example, on the contrary, the presence of a bacillus is a necessary but insufficient condition to produce certain infectious diseases), it should be kept in mind that in the most genuine psychiatric illnesses, i.e., endogenous psychoses, clinicians have usually been unable to find a convincing chronological relationship between social stress and the illness. The most probable explanation is that, since many psychiatric disorders are not easily diagnosed in their first, insidious stages, social stress, by intensifying their symptoms, makes it easier to identify them.

Among the most commonly cited cultural factors causing dissatisfaction and anxiety are oppression, poverty, malnutrition, urbanisation and industrialisation. There have been attempts to invoke psychological mechanisms common to these situations, such as object loss, separation anxiety, disorientation, and the stress of change. None of these general theories seems to be sufficiently satisfactory; therefore, we prefer to discuss below some of the stress-inducing circumstances that have been invoked as responsible for the differences in prevalence of some psychiatric illnesses.

Acculturation

A particularly stressful situation is the loss of one's culture in a short period of time, due to the invasion of another dominant culture. This leads to a loss in traditional values, a relaxation of traditional authority, and, overall, a 'disorientation' in the value system that produces an increase in behavioural disorders (e.g., drug addiction, sexual deviance, crime). The loss of more or less ritual group activities (such as religious practices) diminishes the population's psychological adaptation capacity.

Devereux (1961), following Durkheim (1951), stresses, in the genesis of emotional disorders, the transition from a so-called community of organic solidarity (*Gemelnschaft*) to a society of mechanical solidarity (*Gesellschaft*).

Urbanisation

The urbanisation process produces a conflict between old and new sets of rules, with the consequent increase in levels of anxiety, especially among older people, adolescents, and women—apparently the groups with the highest propensity to suffer breakdown from this kind of change. Schizophrenic patients seem to have difficulty functioning in situations that overemphasise competition and success, which is why they are particularly susceptible to breakdown in situations of cultural transition towards more competitive societies.

The Stress of Change in Itself

Situations of change can produce stress even when the change involves a more advantageous situation for the subject. Rising on the social scale, whether through economic enrichment or heightened prestige, can produce stress able to set off a psychological breakdown. By the same token, an improvement in the quality of life of an entire community (through automatisation, improvement in communications and transportation, and so on) can have deleterious effects on some of its members.

The effort to adapt one's values and behaviour to new and changing circumstances, as in the aforesaid case of an entire society undergoing an acculturation process, or of immigrants, can have severe psychiatric consequences. Paranoid, depressive, and psychosomatic symptoms among immigrants are a well-known phenomenon. However, when assessing the importance of immigration in the genesis of psychiatric disorders, it should also be borne in mind that there is a theory according to which immigrants are not more susceptible to illness; rather, that more psychologically weak individuals are the most likely to immigrate in the first place. Contrariwise, a recent study on Mexican immigrants in California showed that their mental health was actually better than that of native Californians, or those with immigrant parents.

Cultural Responses to Social Change

Societies as a whole try to create anxiety-reducing systems to facilitate the adaptation of those experiencing change. Both religious and lay organisations use their resources to help such people to adapt. In Spain, for example, cities with a large number of migrants from other parts of the country often have *casas regionales* (literally, 'regional houses'), where, say, Andalusians or Galicians can meet, socialise, and enjoy their local dishes and pastimes.

SOCIAL SUPPORT

Psychiatric illnesses can often become chronic, and produce a deterioration in the subject's previous level of social functioning. Such a deterioration is more marked when the care given to the patient involves admission to a psychiatric hospital. An alternative to inpatient treatment is the development of health care support resources within the community, which aim to assist patients in adapting to their environment. Sociologists tend to distinguish between formal and informal support systems. Formal elements are those that are considered, both by the providers and the users, as organised efforts towards the client's rehabilitation or improved functioning. These include all medical interventions, rehabilitation centres, protected housing, and so on. The different pre-existing social networks are considered informal elements because, although they can be very highly organised, they are not seen by their participants as specifically aimed at the treatment or rehabilitation of psychiatric patients.

Family

The most decisive informal support element is the family, although it is not always able to carry out this function. Family therapists have stressed the protective effect of the extended family, and the consistency of its relationship with a wider-ranging social network (Speck and Rueveni, 1969). These ideas have been confirmed by such research as the World Health Organization's *International Pilot Study on Schizophrenia* (WHO, 1973).

Social Networks

Their Impact on Mental Health

The results of sociological research have confirmed that certain characteristics of the social network in which an individual is immersed have a major impact on the appearance, course, treatment, and prognosis of different psychiatric disorders. There is almost universal agreement in the literature that, when compared with healthy individuals in the community, psychologically disturbed individuals have a smaller social network which provides them with less emotional support, information, and instrumental assistance. Many studies have shown that social support provides protection against the appearance of both physical and mental disorders (Guimón et al., 1985, 1986; Salcedo et al., 1987).

Social support networks have been considered protectors against such psychopathologies as neurosis and depression, but schizophrenia has been the illness of choice to demonstrate the deleterious effect that some networks can have on patients (Tolsdorf, 1976; Pattison and Loy, 1981; Garrison, 1978).

The social network also has an impact on the prognosis of mental disorders. Studies on the consequence of the loss of social support (e.g., from death, divorce, separation, or immigration), have shown that, when a person has no active social links or loses them, it is much more probable that he or she will become mentally ill (Bowlby, 1979).

Just as many transversal studies have related the so-called *life events* with mental pathology, the field of social networks research has transversally shown the correlation between low levels of social support and psychiatric morbidity. However, the lack of longitudinal studies, as well as the difficulty in measuring social support—due to frequent contamination from other variables—should make us cautious when trying to establish causal correlations.

Interventions aimed at modifying the characteristics of these networks can improve the prognosis for schizophrenia, according to some studies (Garrison, 1978; Hammer, 1981).

Self-Help Groups

In the context of actions that intend to modify the undesirable characteristics of social networks, pride of place should be given to the so-called *mutual-support groups*. We know that only 5–10% of those suffering from mental illness seek help from mental health professionals, while the rest seek it elsewhere. Among the latter segment of patients, *self-help groups* like Alcoholics Anonymous have proven to be powerful therapeutic resources. Similar groups have arisen to assist those presenting other problems.

HOMEOSTASIS

The galenic concept according to which illness is the result of change or imbalance in the four humours—sanguine, phlegmatic, choleric, and melancholic—predominated the entire Middle Ages.

The concept of *homeostasis* was later used by the French physician Claude Bernard to designate an organism's tendency to maintain, throughout its 'internal environment', an equilibrium, whose imbalance could produce different illnesses. Menninger (1963) expressed the same idea with his concept of *vital balance*, involving an appropriate distribution of the matter-energy and information processes between the organism and the environment, and which could undergo different alterations. Sullivan (1953) also postulated that psychological balance required an adaptation of the individual's internal psychological mechanisms to sociological conditions. This is the same concept, proposed by Meyer (1957), who believed that the different mental illnesses are psychopathological disorganisations in the face of stress.

For his part, Miller (1975) used general systems theory and mental pathology to define a system of balance between information and exchange of matter and energy, whose disequilibrium could provoke mental illness.

In our opinion, mental health, as we have tried to show in this chapter, is the result of an adequate functioning of the complicated homeostasis mechanisms described herein.

REFERENCES

Arieti, S. (1974). *Interpretation of schizophrenia*. New York: Basic Books, New York.

Bowlby, J. (1979). *La separación afectiva*. Buenos Aires: Paidós.

Brown, G. W., and Harris, T. D. (1978). *Social origins of depression*. London: Tavistock.

Dávila, R., Zumarraga, M., Andía, I., Manero, E., Retuerto, F., Bárcena, B., and Guimón, J. (1989). Dopaminergic balance and subtypes of schizophrenia. *British Journal of Psychiatry*, 154, 33–38.

Devereux, G. (1961). Mohave ethnopsychiatry and suicide: The psychiatric knowledge and the psychic disturbances of an Indian tribe. *Bureau of American Ethnology Bulletin*. Washington, D.C.: United States Government Printing Office.

Durkheim, E. (1951). *Suicide: A study of sociology*. New York: The Free Press.

Engel, G. L. (1980). The clinical application of the biopsychosocial model. *American Journal of Psychiatry*, 137, 535–544.

Escobar, J. I., Randolph, E. T., Puente, G., Spiwak, F., Asamen, J. K., Hill, M., and Hough, R. L. (1983). Post-traumatic stress disorder in Hispanic Vietnam veterans. Clinical phenomenology and sociocultural characteristics. *Journal of Nervous Mental Disorders*, 171(10), 585–596.

Friedhoff, A. J. (1986). A dopamine-dependent restitutive system for the maintenance of mental normality. *Annals of the N.Y. Academy of Science*, 463, 47–52.

Fromm-Reichmann, F. (1948). Notes on the development of treatment of schizophrenia by psychoanalytic psychotherapy. *Psychiatry*, 11, 263–273.

García Sevilla, J., Escribá, P. V., Ozaita, A., Walzer, C., and Guimón, J. (1998). Density of imidazoline receptors in platelets of euthymic patients with bipolar affective disorder and in brains of lithium-treated rats. *Biological Psychiatry*, 43, 616–618.

García Sevilla, J., Guimón, J., Vallejo, P., and Fuster, M. J. (1986). Biochemical and functional evidence of supersensitive platelet adrenoceptors in major affective disorder. *Archives of General Psychiatry*, 43, 51–57.

García Sevilla, J., Padro, D., Giralt, T., Guimón, J., and Areso, P. (1990). Adrenoceptor-mediated inhibition of platelet adenylate cyclase and induction of aggregation in major depression. *Archives of General Psychiatry*, 47, 125–132.

García-Sevilla, J. A., Escribá, P. V., Sastre, M., Walzer, C., Busquets, X., Jaquet, G., Reis, D. J., and Guimón, J. (1996). Immunodetection and quantification of imidazoline, receptor proteins in platelets of patients with major depression and in brains of suicide victims. *Archives of General Psychiatry*, 53, 801–810.

Garrison, V. (1978). Support systems of schizophrenic and nonschizophrenic Puerto Rican migrant women in New York City. *Schizophrenia Bulletin*, 4, 561–597.

Giannakopoulos, P., Hof, P. R., A. S., Guimón, J., Antonarakis, S. E., and Bouras, C. (1996). Early-onset dementias: clinical, neuropathological and genetic characteristics. Acta *Neuropathol.*, 91, 451–465.

González de Rivera, J. L. (2001). Clasificación de los síndromes de estrés. *Psiquis*, 22(1), 1–7.

Guimón, J., Dendaluce, I., Pascual, E., Ruiz, A., and Escobar, J. (1986). Red social en pacientes psiquiátricos del País Vasco. *Actas Luso-Españolas de Neurología, Psiquiatría y Ciencias Afines*, 14(2), 128–138.

Guimón, J., Ruiz, A., Apodaca, P., de Ros, P., and Sota, E. (1985). Red social en la población de Guecho. *Psiquis*, VI (126), 9–22.

Hammer, M. (1981). Social supports, social networks and schizophrenia. *Schizophrenia Bulletin*, 7(1), 45–58.

Jaspers, K. (1946). *Psicopatología general*. Buenos Aires: Delta.

Margison, F., and Mace, C. (1997). *Psychotherapy of psychosis*. London: Gaskell, London.
Menninger, K. (1963). *The vital balance*. New York: Viking Press.
Meyer, A. (1957). *Psychobiology: A science of man*. Springfield, Illinois: C. C. Thomas.
Miller, J. G. (1975). *General systems theory*.
Miller, T. W. (1996). *Theory and assessment of stressful life events*. Madison: International Universities Press.
Pattison, E. M., and Loy, M. (1981). Analysis of a schizophrenic psychosocial network. *Schizophrenia Bulletin*, 7, 135–144.
Perris, C. (1989). *Cognitive therapy with schizophrenic patients*. London: Guildford Press.
Salcedo, M., Pinilla, B., and Guimón, J. (1987). La red social en personas psicológicamente afectadas. *Psiquis*, 53–60.
Sullivan, H. S. (1953). *The interpersonal theory of psychiatry*. New York: W. W. Norton.
Sullivan, H. S. (1962). *Schizophrenia as a human process*. New York: Norton, New York.
Titchener, J. L., and Ross, W. A. (1974). In S. A. and. E. B. Brody (Ed.), *American handbook of psychiatry* (Vol. III). New York: Basic Books.
Tolsdorf, C. C. (1976). Social networks, support, and coping: an exploratory study. *Fam. Process*, 15(4), 407–417.
Werner, E. E. and Smith, S. S. (1993). *Overcoming the odds: high-risk children from birth to adulthood*. New York: Cornell University Press.
WHO (1973). *Report of the International Pilot Study on Schizophrenia*: World Health Organization.

4

Theories and Ideologies in Mental Health

Anyone who keeps abreast of the current psychiatric literature often has two contradictory attitudes about it. On the one hand, there is the admiration, even to the point of a sense of overload, inspired by the accumulation of discoveries that, using techniques from the basic medical sciences (genetics, neurobiochemistry, psychopharmacology, neurophysiology), have enriched, from the medical model's standpoint, our knowledge of psychiatric disorders. On the other, there is a certain degree of mistrust due to the impression that these data may lead to a decline in the importance of other factors, mainly psychological and socio-cultural, in considering the origins, manifestations, and evolution of mental illnesses.

Indeed, professionals in the mental health field seem to be divided into rival camps: those who preferably or exclusively apply biological treatments to their patients, and those who use psychosocial approaches. Without aiming to provide an exhaustive description, nor a critical evaluation of these models, the following is a summary of their underlying concepts (Guimón, Fischer, Zbinden, and Goerg, 1997).

THE MAGICAL MODEL AND SOCIAL CONTROL

Background

The magical conception of mental health prevailed in the times of so-called 'paleomedicine'. People believed that supernatural phenomena, in particular the influence of the spirits of tribal ancestors, were of vital importance in conditioning their behaviour. Breaking taboos, failure to fulfil traditional rights, and daemonic possession were considered the causes of madness. For centuries, mental illness was considered to be a form of daemonic possession, and was treated with exorcistic practices (Guimón, 1998).

The Current Situation

The Public's Point of View

Belief in magical or moral causes of mental illness are, today, less frequent in Western society (Guimón and Sartorius, 1999). In a German study (Angermeyer, Klusmann, and Walpuski, 1988; Angermeyer and Matschinger, 1996), only a small minority believed that schizophrenic disorders were influenced by supernatural powers (the will of God, witchcraft, possession by evil spirits, signs of the zodiac or one's horoscope). Contrary to researchers' expectations, this is also the case in less developed countries, and a recent study (Eker and Oner, 1999) failed to confirm the frequently cited finding that African peoples tend to give a predominantly supernatural or mystical explanation for mental illness. Another, somewhat earlier study (Eskin, 1989) in rural Turkey also failed to show the existence of a prevailing belief in a supernatural/mystical aetiology of mental illness. The study concluded that these Turkish peasants' opinions on the causes and treatment of mental illness were similar to the conceptualisations of modern psychiatry.

However, our own research in Geneva (Fischer, Goerg, Zbinden, and Guimón, 1999) showed that an important percentage of those surveyed believed that natural remedies were preferable to psychotropic medication. Only one-quarter of our subjects considered psychotropics to be more efficient than natural remedies.

Criticism

However, although they do not openly invoke supernatural or magical thinking, a number of scientifically doubtful—or frankly spurious—practices are extraordinarily frequent in the West (Guimón and Sartorius, 1999). The resurrection of homeopathy began in the 1980s, and it now widely disseminated throughout Europe. Acupuncture is practised all over the world, used beyond any reasonable indications. Folk healers and quacks of all stripes are making a killing (not literally, we can only hope) in cities large and small.

But if individual practitioners of these techniques can be dangerous for mental health, much more to be feared are the growing number of sects that aim to establish domains of social control with their activities.

Although these cults vary from those proposing new psychological theories to those preaching religious or political beliefs or strange health and eating practices, they tend to share certain social and psychological traits: they all offer new 'knowledge', more or less esoteric, transmitted by an indisputable and arbitrary authority; the majority of their leaders reject modern medicine, because they do not want to grant physicians any part of the control that they exercise over their followers; and they use 'brain-washing' techniques, i.e., systematic manipulation of their social and psychological influence over these individuals.

Many cults recruit people, who are frequently mentally ill, in order to indoctrinate them and then exploit them economically and control their lives. A trait common to all of them is the denial of the existence of mental illness, and attacks on psychiatry itself.

The so-called Church of Scientology is one of the most widespread cults in the world today. Its theoretical basis is 'Dianetics', which claims to be a 'modern science of mental health'. Scientology is fiercely critical of psychiatry and psychopharmacological medication (especially products like Prozac and Ritalin). Its methods include the use of psychological pressure to remain within the group, and brainwashing techniques, which lead its adepts to have serious difficulties when trying to make objective decisions or keep an open mind. It inculcates them with bizarre beliefs (e.g., about galactic emperors who bombard volcanoes with nuclear weapons) and rejects any criticism of this dogma, alluding to 'professional secrets' (Guimón, 2001).

THE MEDICAL MODEL: SCIENTISM

Background

The medical model (Maher, 1970) of illness assumes that the subject who presents certain alterations with regard to features considered normal within a population (behavioural alterations, when we refer to psychiatry) is ill, due to a demonstrable cause or aetiology (or one that it is assumed will be made manifest in the future), which produces certain symptoms, which in turn enables clinicians to determine a diagnostic label. Once the illness has been thus identified, it is possible to propose a symptomatic treatment, and ideally an aetiological one, and assume a certain course, so that the clinician can establish a prognosis. As a consequence of this process, carried out by the physician, the patient acquires the status of being a sick person, in the eyes of society, which situates him in the condition to demand from that society certain prerogatives: being excused from some responsibilities, special affective attention, economic protection, and so on. For its part, society demands that the patient fulfil the prerequisites of his role as a sick person: acceptance of his limitations, careful compliance with his doctor's advice, and so forth.

The Current Situation

The Public's Point of View

In spite of the medical model's amazing progress in mental health, its prestige is not so high with the general public. For example, in the previously cited German study (Angermeyer, 1997; Angermeyer and Matschinger, 1996), only one out of every two of those interviewed identified a brain disorder or constitutional weakness as the cause of a schizophrenic disorder, and genetic factors were invoked even less often. A study that we conducted in Geneva (Goerg, Fischer, Zbinden, and Guimón, 1999) found that the public viewed favourably some forms of treatment, such as relaxation techniques, meditation or yoga, and natural medicine, but only in very rare situations did our subjects take pharmacological therapy into consideration. The same seems to occur in other, less-developed countries (Erskin, 1989).

Criticism

Even within the health professions, the very concept of the medical model is subject to heated debate (Klerman, 1977). The most substantial criticisms of the indubitable progresses achieved by these medical conceptions focus on the fact that, today, we are still very far from being able to invoke biological causes for most disorders.

Indeed, biological psychiatry works on a wide variety of levels: molecular (neurotransmitters and receptors) and cellular, as well as at the level of neuronal groupings, whether isolated or in interaction. Therefore, we have yet to reach the point where we can relate structural or functional neurological alterations with a specific diagnosis.

The central nervous system is very complex. Biochemical data can only be classified locally, because there is no common unit of measurement able to characterise both the information produced on a local and molecular scale with that produced on a behavioural scale. The criteria offered for each organisational level differ from a taxonomic viewpoint (Bouguignon, 1989). It is possible to observe many differences among individuals on the psychological and behavioural levels, whereas on a biological level, the number of differences is still quite restricted. There is a high level of psychological specificity within each individual, but a weak consistency in the biochemical data.

Beyond space and time, the notion of causality loses all operativeness. The central nervous system functions according to the extraordinary heterochronicity of the different speeds of information transmission, and the latencies of response to messages. A nervous impulse, for example, runs through a cerebral neuron in a few milliseconds; a neurotransmitter (through an axon) can take a few hours; the response to a hormonal message has a latency of several minutes or hours; the immune response to an affective shock (Bartrop, Lazarus, Luckhurst, and Kiloh, 1972) has a latency of various days or even weeks. This, according to Bourguignon (1989), together with the multiplicity of the determinants of psychological cerebral activity (genetic, epigenetic, random) that ensures the development and maintenance of the system, opposes a one-to-one idea of causality, so that, at this time, we have no choice but to replace this idea of causality with one of correlation.

Also noteworthy here is the relative objectivity of measurement methods in psychopathology. Lehman (1975) stresses that a psychopathological investigator, when studying nosological entities such as organic brain disorders (e.g., senile dementia), looks for physical criteria; when studying functional psychoses (e.g., schizophrenia), he must be content to look for 'indicators' rather than 'criteria' of these psychoses, which, as nosological entities, are only hypothetical constructions. Psychopathology, by its very nature, is never characterised by physical, structural abnormalities. Its deviations are always functional and cannot be completely expressed by instrumental means. All instrumental exploration of psychopathology is fragmentary. This does not mean that psychopathology can only be studied by subjective methods, but it does mean that all of its direct and objective measurements are related only to its physical expression (e.g., movements, noise) or physical underpinnings (e.g., serological findings, electroencephalograms, biochemical indicators).

Symptoms, syndromes and nosological entities of a functional nature cannot be measured objectively. What we *can* measure objectively are only indicators; i.e., variables related to psychopathological phenomena. The phenomena themselves cannot be measured objectively; inferential traces will always separate them from a true 'criteria-based' measurement. According to Lehman, this problem is akin to that of meteorologists, who cannot dominate all of the variables involved in predicting the weather. Weather does not mean barometric pressure or wind direction. People want to know if it will be sunny, and what the temperature and humidity will be, all of which, combined, will determine good or bad weather. Meteorologists, then, depend on indicators.

The first objective indicator known in the history of psychopathology was what Exner called 'reaction time', and Wundt's school tried to use this to develop new objective indicators. In spite of the initial enthusiasm aroused by this idea, even its proponents soon arrived at the conclusion that the realisation of simple sensorial or psychomotor functions has little direct value in assessing complex personality factors.

PSYCHODYNAMIC CONCEPTS: INTERSUBJECTIVITY

Background

For its part, the psychoanalytical model (Maher, 1970) is based on certain formal suppositions. The fact that human behaviour can be depicted as the result of an energy system constitutes the first of these. This energy springs mainly from sexual instincts, and is called the *libido*. It can vary in intensity, even within the same individual; it is always present, even in early infancy; it is not limited only to the sex organs, but rather is linked successively to a variety of bodily zones related to nutrition and excretion, as well as procreation. The ties to one of these zones will determine an individual's character, through a process called *fixation*.

From a complementary viewpoint, Edelson (1984) formulated a psychoanalytical theory involving the following affirmations: 1) all 'meaningless' mental content calls for an explanation; 2) mental processes have a purpose; 3) there can be no meaningless mental content, without an unconscious purpose; 4) the relationship of meaningless mental content with unconscious purposes is governed by the so-called *primary process*; 5) at least one of the unconscious purposes with which unconscious mental content is related has as its aim or result the expression or gratification of sexual and hostile impulses or desires; 6) these sexual or hostile impulses have their origin in infancy, during which they are represented in psychic life by phantasies, which from then on become relatively inaccessible to the conscious mind; 7) if the gratification of a sexual or hostile impulse is impeded by an obstacle, the sequence oriented towards an end leads to a gratification phantasy; 8) there can be no meaningless mental content in the absence of an unconscious intrapsychic conflict.

As we shall see later on, many current psychoanalysts, when applying the dynamic model to mental health, are interested less in the 'intrapsychic' aspect (derived from Freud's *economic theory*) and prefer to adhere to the approach associated with the so-called British school of psychoanalysis, which involves a greater emphasis on object relationships. Consequently, today the literature refers to *relational theory* (Greenberg, 1996; Greenberg and Mitchell, 1993; Mitchell, 1988; Coderch, 2001).

The Current Situation

The Public's Point of View

Currently, in Western countries, the general public believes that psychological problems play a decisive role in the genesis of mental disorders. In Germany, (Angermeyer, 1997) there is a tendency to attribute the cause of psychosis to intrapsychic conflicts, lack of will, or overambition, more than to biological factors. Americans tend to see psychological problems as being caused by difficulties in life, and being susceptible to improvement through therapeutic efforts (Hillert et al., 1999). In Switzerland, a large percentage of the population stresses the importance of personal psychological factors, such as lack of willpower or being too demanding on oneself (Goerg et al., 1999). This also appears to be the case in less developed countries. For example, the aforementioned study in rural Turkey demonstrated the prevailing belief in the importance of psychological causes, followed by social and medical factors.

Regarding treatment, the general public has shown a marked preference for psychotherapy (Goerg, 1999). In fact, there is an enthusiastic sector of the public (Goerg, Zbinden, Fischer, and Guimón, 1997) that Kadushin has called 'the champions of psychotherapy'.

Criticism

However, in certain circles, the utility of psychoanalytical treatment of mental disorders has been called into question. Responsibility for the decline in psychoanalysis's prestige as a therapeutic technique can be attributed, in part, to psychoanalysts ourselves, who (due to our *furor curandis*) have tried for decades to use it systematically on certain disorders for which it is inappropriate, while simultaneously putting up energetic opposition to attempts to subject our practice to close scientific examination.

In reality, for psychiatric patients, psychoanalysis is long and painful, with results that are difficult to assess. Even though, for some diagnoses, analysis still represents one of the best possible approaches, patients are asking for quick relief from their suffering, and for most disorders, medication and certain non-analytical therapies offer more clear-cut symptomatic results. But it is no less true that an informed attitude from a dynamic standpoint is beneficial for the majority of psychiatric patients.

Like all other fields of study, science is in any case subject to the influence of fashion and economic factors. In this sense, individual long-term psychotherapy is, today, not held in very high esteem (Rutan, 1993), whether due to the new psychiatric classification systems that stress symptoms over the patient's underlying personality traits, or to economic factors (Tuttman, 1997). Nor is psychoanalysis any longer, as it was some years ago, the model used for training the greater part of mental health professionals. Now, the idea is to offer 'cost-effective' therapies (behavioural, cognitive) with the help of non-specialist personnel, supported by occasional specialist supervision. On the other hand, from a theoretical standpoint, the psychoanalytical model has been going through a crisis over the last few decades. A review of the Social Science Citation Index (Fonagy, 1996) revealed that the two most important psychoanalytical journals (*International Journal of Psychoanalysis* and *The Journal of the American Psychoanalytic Association*) were cited in other journals far less than the major psychiatry or psychology journals, which was an indication that the scientific impact of psychoanalysis on other disciplines could be in decline. This was not because the non-analysts (i.e., those publishing in journals featuring psychiatric or literary studies) were less interested in the subject than in previous years; rather, it was precisely the psychoanalysts themselves who did not often cite their own colleagues in psychoanalytical journals. One could argue that the major psychoanalytical schools that arose over the course of the 20th century are becoming fragmented: (Fonagy, 2000). Fonagy also points out that psychoanalysts, when discussing the data obtained in their research, fail to seriously consider alternative explanations proceeding from theoretical frameworks different from our own.

Kandel (1998), however, believes that, far from being a threat to psychoanalysis with the potential to destroy it, a closer integration with biological psychiatry could actually reinforce psychoanalysis's rich insights. He bases this argument on certain general principles (Fonagy, 2000). On the one hand, all functions of the mind reflect functions of the brain, but Kandel demonstrates convincingly that the ability of a particular gene to control the production of specific proteins in a cell is subject to environmental factors, and the fact that only 10–20% of our genes are transcribed or expressed in each cell gives a great deal of leeway to social factors.

In spite of its critics, psychodynamic theory continues to prosper (Rutan, 1993). The contributions of modern schools of dynamic theory are important, and abundant. There are many elaborations, modifications, and improvements on Freud's original theories about personality, and some of them, as we have seen, have obtained excellent results in their clinical application.

Dynamic Psychiatry

Psychoanalysis, as a science and as an exceptional instrument for self-knowledge, will continue to grow through its institutes and associations.

However, psychoanalysis is long and expensive, and its results are difficult to evaluate. Patients demand quick relief for their suffering so that modifications (short time, group) of the classic psychoanalytic technique are the only ones being applied to the general public. Probably, the only way for psychoanalysis to play a relevant role in the future of mental health will be through this kind of 'decaffeinated' dynamic psychiatry. In order for a form of psychiatry to be considered 'dynamic', it should at least acknowledge the importance of the unconscious and of transference. Moreover, dynamic psychiatry has traditionally been linked with the concept of 'conflict' arising between wishes and defences, between different parts of the personality and between impulses and external reality. It also takes into account concepts such as psychic determinism, deficits in intrapsychic structures, or internal object relationships. Dynamic psychiatry focuses on phantasies, dreams, fears, hopes, impulses, wishes, and self-image, rather than on the careful description of observable behaviour.

Most mental illnesses are not relieved by psychodynamic treatment, but, for some diagnoses, it is still one of the treatments of choice: personality disorders, paraphilias, anxiety disorders, eating disorders, certain conditions resistant to biological treatments, dual diagnoses, and so on. Additionally, a dynamically informed attitude is beneficial for the majority of psychiatric patients. Indeed, apart from the fact that as many as 71% of hospitalised patients have an Axis II diagnosis, character-based resistance to drugs and negative placebo effects also require a dynamic approach.

Moreover, as shown by recent epidemiological data (e.g., the ECA project), only a small percentage of the population with mental disturbances seek specialised psychiatric help. Between 25% and 40% of the patients visiting a general practitioner have an undiagnosed psychiatric disorder. General practitioners have to 'contain' the overwhelming mental suffering of these individuals, and they generally do so without having any specialised training. This function of 'containment' (in Bion's sense) is best understood within a psychoanalytic framework. Balint's groups represent one of the only ways of adequately facing this enormous challenge in mental health, which has been neglected to date.

THE SOCIAL MODEL: UTOPIA

Background

The social model of mental illness, fed by epidemiological data that suggests the influence of certain social factors in the development or genesis of certain disorders, proposes, in its most extreme version, that society itself is ill, not the patient, and that the diagnostic process is nothing other than an attempt to label people who try to free themselves from society's generalised alienation. Derivatives of this model would be the so-called *conspiracy* and *psychedelic* models. The radicalisation of the social model in the 1960s led to a movement that came to be called *antipsychiatry*.

For its part, the contributions of general systems theory to modern conceptions of family therapy have made it possible to develop new forms of theory and practice. From a theoretical standpoint, the idea that systems have a certain kind of isomorphism and specific laws of action (input, output, permeability, exchange of material and energy) was already included, although formulated in different terms, in Freudian psychoanalysis or Sullivan's interpersonal psychiatry (Sullivan, 1953).

However, there are elements from general systems theory that can indeed be considered original contributions. One is the principle of *equifinality*, which affirms that open systems can reach a certain state conditioned only by the parameters of the systems themselves, regardless of environmental and genetic factors. This concept, proposed by Miller (1975), would make it possible to minimise what he called the 'genetic fallacy of psychoanalysis' and avoid the dichotomy between biology and culture, which has, for so long, confronted individual and group therapies. Another of these original contributions is Von Bertalanffy's *stable state* concept (Von Bertalanffy, 1968), which refers to the capacity of structures or systems to remain constant over the course of their continual transformations. According to Durkin (1975), the term 'stable state' is preferable to that of *homeostasis*, to which, in Miller's opinion, psychoanalysis has been too closely linked. A third element from general systems theory is the concept of *negative entropy*, which is related to the second law of thermodynamics (i.e., that energy in the form of work can be applied to systems to maintain organisation and avoid entropy). This term has been used by theoreticians of systematic psychotherapy in order, they say, to offer a more appropriate energetic theory than that proposed by Freud, who was unaware of the second law of thermodynamics.

The Current Situation

Criticism

Antipsychiatry's radical criticism of the very existence of mental illness, the excessive power of psychiatrists in society, and the justification of psychiatric hospitals, has had a decisive impact on some aspects of the current status of psychiatric patients and psychiatry as a profession.

On the one hand, psychiatric nurses, psychologists, and other workers in the mental health field now share a good part of the responsibilities formerly held exclusively by psychiatrists—which, as we have pointed out, diffuses the confines of our speciality. On the other hand, the traditional psychiatric hospital has undergone major modifications in most Western countries, progressing from a more or less alienating holding area for patients to an active therapeutic environment. However, according to Berrios (1989), the most important consequence has been renewed interest on the part of psychiatrists in improving symptoms description to make it more rigorous, in an attempt to create a common language that would make psychiatric diagnoses more reliable. This effort was largely behind the extraordinary progress made over the last decade in the neurosciences, which has enabled investigators to provide us with better knowledge of psychiatric disorders, and better treatments for them. All of this contradicted the criticism of those who denied the very existence of mental illness, or who proposed to treat it exclusively with non-medical methods. Over the years, although antipsychiatry has seen itself forced to accept the existence of mental disorders, the movement has responded by going beyond the discussion of the heuristic value of different models of madness (biological, psychological, social, or even religious and literary). Psychologists and social workers have already been given their share of 'psychiatric power', and are now themselves the targets of updated criticism that no longer doubts the existence of mental illness or whether it can be treated (descriptive level of the problem), but rather whether a patient 'should be' categorised as a patient, or whether he 'should be' treated (prescriptive level).

Having reached this point, says Berrios, there is little that science, through new investigation, can do. The problems that are coming to the fore at this point include such issues as the 'right to be crazy', the 'power of the patient', the 'democratisation of management', and questioning society's right to force a madman to be treated rather than to 'leave him alone', even when it can be shown that he is indeed ill. Such iconoclastic stances cannot be countered with more intensive and rigorous medical research, but rather require a conceptual approach, using tools from the history and philosophy of psychiatry. Thus, the 'scientific' effort should be complemented by a philosophical and ethical one. The psychiatrist, concludes Berrios, will not only have to convince the citizenry that there are mental illnesses, but also that these illnesses should be treated, both for the good of the patient and that of society as a whole.

The Public's Point of View

Psychiatric deinstitutionalisation, which began in the 1950s, not only opened a door to the outside world and to society, but also multiplied the contacts between mental patients and people considered to be normal (Guimón, Fischer, and Sartorius, 1999). The stigma that, at first, was centred on an entity, a concept—madness—and its almost exclusive field of action—the psychiatric hospital—changed, influencing the public's behaviour towards mental patients in the community, and its relationship with and attitudes towards them. This step towards a more open society led to other transformations, for example the creation of negative, differentiated stereotypes regarding a specific behaviour, a specific psychopathology. Mental patients, in the early 19th century, were classified into categories susceptible to psychiatric treatment. The 'medicalisation' of this particular form of deviance has not resulted in mitigation, or even a neutralisation, of the negative response that it inspires. Entirely on the contrary, this stigma has spread to psychiatry itself, which had been put in charge of controlling and correcting manifestations of mental illness. Such continues to be the case today, since the term 'psychiatrisation', despite some semantic modifications, is unanimously defined as a depreciative description of patients' behaviour, attitudes, and thoughts.

The general public today expresses different concerns regarding mental health than the antipsychiatry camp. A recent study by Angermeyer and Matschinger (1999) revealed the widespread belief that in our postindustrial society, we are exposed to increasing levels of stress, which is considered the explanation for why psychiatric disorders have risen recently in areas where the process of social change has been particularly striking. On the other hand, the general public considers less important such decisive influences on the socialisation of children as broken homes, absentee fathers, or hyperprotectiveness, or the impact on adults of social change (e.g., destruction of natural lifestyles, decadence of traditional values, exploitation of persons in industrial society). The influence of socialisation, in this study, was ranked in fourth place; coming from a broken home was considered aetiologically the most significant, followed by the absence of parental affect and overly protective parents. In our own study in Geneva (Goerg et al., 1999), these childhood socialisation factors were considered very important by a segment of the population that excluded other factors, whether biological (brain disorders, constitutional weakness, heredity), psychological (life events, workplace difficulties, family or marital problems), social (social inequality, disappearance of traditional values, lifestyles not in harmony with nature), or supernatural (the will of God, astrology, witchcraft).

POLITICAL-ADMINISTRATIVE APPROACHES

Background

1. Politics can be defined as the set of operations aimed at guaranteeing social cohesion, and it is obvious that mental health has major political connotations.

2. Mental patients, due to the very nature of their problems, are not good at defending their own rights.
3. Political power, defined as the capacity to modify the will of others, should use the resources at its disposal—information, money, and legislation—to benefit mental patients.
4. Legislation should include specific measures for people with these kinds of difficulties, and apply different strategies to dignify their care.

Even though mental patients are not in a good position to defend themselves, professionals, certain religious orders, and more recently, associations of patients' relatives have collectively voiced their demands to the organs of power, around the world.

Western governments have been slowly waking up to the alarming dimensions of mental health problems. Unfortunately, however, politicians have generally shown more concern for cutting the growth of costs than for ensuring the quality of services and patients' rights.

The Current Situation

Managed Psychiatry

Over the last few decades, the major concern of all governments has been the containment of spiralling health costs, especially those related to mental health. The consequent reform of medical care initiated in the United States led to the current situation in that country, where 75% of psychiatrists treat patients within the framework of managed care organisations, especially the so-called *health maintenance organisations* (HMOs) which, altogether, involve some 125 million Americans. The large American health insurance carriers sold off part of their mental health portfolios, because they were problematical, to specialised companies that had been specifically developed for mental patients. Such firms have become an extremely powerful force within the insurance industry, and are currently dictating the course of psychiatric treatment in the United States. They have made major efforts to directly offer treatments, renting beds in local hospitals and creating their own outpatient clinics, in order to compete directly with the practices of established psychiatrists.

Although these rigid cost management approaches have yet to catch on in most of Europe, there is the fear that they could rapidly become generalised around the world. Indeed, new forms of reimbursement are already being introduced in many countries.

The application of reimbursements involving *diagnosis related groupings* (DRGs) came later in mental health than in other health care areas, because it was found that the reimbursement models that depended on psychiatric diagnoses lacked predictive value (Siegler, Axelband, and Isikoff, 1993). This favoured, at first, the treatment of psychiatric patients, but new, more-or-less fruitful attempts were soon made.

When *resource-based relative value scales* (RBRVS) were introduced into the medical system, it was a proposal that offered a certain amount of hope to psychiatric patients that they would receive privileged treatment, but, at the last moment, such a decision was overturned. The managed mental health care organisations have, in the end, established their own parameters for revising psychiatric services utilisation and needs. The majority of psychiatrists and mental health professionals have had no choice but to accept the rules laid down by psychiatric HMOs (Fink 1996).

The term *capitation* designates a relatively new formula according to which a service provider negotiates an overall budget for a certain population, based on the number of persons involved. Thus, in many managed psychiatry programmes, risk is shifted to the providers. When providers accept a capitation system, the *third-party payers* (i.e., insurance companies) introduce what is called a *utilisation review* (UR). This technique, first used in purely epidemiological studies, has become the basis for determining reimbursement mechanisms, treatment intensity, and patient needs. However, as various authors have suggested (e.g., Glazer and Gray, 1996), in managing psychiatric care, the UR should not be carried out by an outside unit, but rather be fully integrated into the health care process itself.

Criticism

This form of insuring psychiatric care, often called *managed mental health care*, has aroused passionate controversy among both radical critics and enthusiastic defenders, not only within our profession, but also among the general public (England and Goff, 1993).

Perhaps it is possible that, through transformations of this kind, quality can improve due to the elimination of useless or overly restrictive treatments; it is also possible for the consumer to have more complete information, leading to a better choice of available services. However, these treatment models are being continually modified for economic reasons, since providers' behaviour inevitably responds to the laws of supply and demand; the result is that psychiatrists are being forced to adjust to marketing decisions, with constant violations of their clinical autonomy.

The majority of professionals have shown resistance to managed mental health care, and so have their patients, in many different ways (Lazarus et al., 1996): verbal aggression towards psychiatrists who work for HMOs; the involvement of patients and their families in insurance disputes;

sending patients who are unstable, from a psychiatric point of view, to other professionals; refusal to co-operate with managed care procedures; and the appearance of lawsuits. Critics of the HMO system have focused on various shortcomings, such as the probability of insufficient or inadequate treatment; the risk of dehumanising mental health care; and the loss of autonomy on the part of professionals.

Favourable Opinions

Certain authors have suggested (Panzetta, 1996) that managed care can improve the quality of services while also cutting costs, through innovative agreements between managed mental health care providers and government organisations.

These defenders stress that the *practice guidelines* developed in the 1990s under the auspices of professional groups, such as the American Psychiatric Association, are generally accepted by insurance providers, and make it possible to clarify treatment methods. Given that these guidelines are presented in tandem with the managed health care companies' regulations, psychiatrists' resistance to them is higher than if they had arisen independently. However, the synergy created by these developments can empower physicians because, without direct medical participation in every step of the development of these guidelines, they would be neither efficient nor even usable. Other authors have said that managed mental health care can improve the overall mental health of children and adolescents (Geraty and Fox, 1996), and others maintain that emergency psychiatry, liaison psychiatry, and crisis intervention will become more important (Fink, 1993), and therefore, in the future psychiatrists should become more familiar with these fields.

Human Rights Legislation

The legal consideration of mental patients has changed over the course of history, but especially in the last few decades. In the 1960s, for example, the antipsychiatry movement, inspired by the counterculture, vindicated the rights of minorities suffering from discrimination (e.g., due to their race, gender, or sexual orientation), and criticised psychiatrists. Today, however, ex-mental patients and their families, with only some exceptions, understand the problems involved with mental illness, and the difficulties that professionals have in combating them. When we are able to establish a good relationship with associations that bring together patients and their families, these groups become our best allies in making the necessary efforts to change the laws that maintain, or even reinforce, the stigma and exclusion that burdens them.

Recommendations on equity and non-discrimination, diagnoses, treatment, research, and other relevant issues have been adopted by national legislatures. Despite these advances, rights violations continue to be reported in many countries. Therefore, it is advisable to establish these recommendations in an operative format that would make it possible to create instruments for assessing the quality of mental health care.

Anti-stigma programmes have gathered in force, not only in medicine and psychiatry, but also in the socio-political sphere, and in community-based support movements. The existing prejudice stems not only from cognitive factors, but also from deeply rooted feelings, so that merely intellectual interventions are inefficient, and can even be counterproductive.

CURRENT PERSPECTIVES ON INTEGRATION

The Danger of Reductionism

As Quintanilla (1986) points out, the term *reductionism* is generally brandished when discussing the reduction of theories, and refers to extrapolating this concept to the point of making it an indispensable prerequisite for a theory to deserve being considered 'scientific'. Quintanilla maintains that one of the implicit rational motives in *biologism* resides in the acceptable ideal that the organic level of a human individual's organisation is more basic than the psychosocial level. But the error of biological reductionism lies in the belief that this basic characteristic can only be guaranteed if it is considered exclusive.

According to Tizón et al. (1985) *biologism* is the abusive extension or generalisation of biological explanations and models into other fields of science and technology (particularly into the psychosocial sciences) with the aim of hiding the conscious or unconscious meaning of certain practices. These authors consider the roots of biologism to be an attempt to deny the limits of our knowledge of the world, based on providing falsely explicative 'pseudo-knowledge'.

Regarding this issue, as Castillo del Pino (1986) put it: 'given a specific behavioural act, it is perfectly legitimate for the investigator to propose, in a given case, the study of modifications that occur at a molecular level, since every act is of a material nature. However, it is also legitimate for the investigator to rule out exploring the changes occurring at the level of the biological structures that make this act possible. Finally, the act in question, insofar as it represents significant behaviour, is susceptible to codification and is, therefore, a social act which can be treated as such, regardless of its psychological or biological level'. Therefore, as Castillo del Pino observes, no line of research should aim to take in the totality of knowledge proceeding from the major theoretical fields of psychiatry, but rather should specify at which epistemological level it intends to operate.

A professional's decision to adopt one or another of these frameworks of reference is influenced, besides cognitive aspects, by other sociological aspects, such as religious beliefs, metaphysical and socio-economic conceptions, and certain aspects of the internal policies of the scientific field involved. Generally, these aspects have been ignored, but the new *sociology of science* suggests that there are certain principles that have a major impact on the transformations of scientific thought and practice: the scientific literature is growing exponentially; due to the so-called 'Mateo effect', 50% of all articles cited are by only 10% of the authors in a given field; there are 'invisible colleges' which, through their behind-the-scenes political power, also promote changes in the sciences.

Eclecticism or Syncretism?

Adopting a pragmatic conception of mental health, the majority of professionals around the world tends to adhere to a vision of the field focusing on therapeutic practice. Indeed, it has been possible to confirm that common factors are able to explain the majority of the benefits deriving from therapeutic interventions complementary to purely medication-based approaches. Clinicians' theoretical orientation only partially explains what they do in their work, since efficient therapists often use a mixture of common therapeutic ingredients, which they justify after the fact with the jargon of their preferred theoretical models.

Empirical studies have shown, for example, that different models of psychotherapy lead, from a symptomatic standpoint, to more or less the same result (Smith, Glass, and Miller, 1980). Therefore, a 'generic' model has been proposed (Orlinsky and Howard, 1986) based on universal data from all kinds of psychotherapy, regardless of their theoretical orientation (Bergin and Garfield, 1994). An integrative psychotherapy is thus born (Holmes and Bateman, 2002).

In any case, the dynamic orientation makes it possible to adopt an appropriate generic focus, a coherent conceptual model for all other treatments (be they pharmacological, cognitive-behavioural, systemic, or whatever) that could be prescribed (Gabbard, 1995), because the concepts of the unconscious, of transference, of defence mechanisms, and so on, are central to any therapy, whether hospital-based or at an outpatient centre.

A study involving 4000 mental health professionals (Davidovitz and Levenson, 1995) showed that half of psychiatrists, as well as a quarter of psychologists and social workers, identified themselves as having a purely psychodynamic orientation. The remainder reported an eclectic or integrating attitude. Indeed, at many community care centres, professionals of very different orientations (including pharmacological, psychodynamic, behaviouralist, and cognitive) have become aware of the fact that a single focus cannot be used adequately for every problem, and that the results stemming from the use of different techniques are actually comparable. This has led them to seek out the common components of these different techniques, and made manifest the importance of the patient's own characteristics, and of the therapeutic relationship.

This closing of the theoretical gap has been particularly important where dynamic psychotherapists and cognitive-behaviouralists are concerned. Indeed, in a survey conducted by Dies (1994), 30% of cognitive-behaviourist therapists said that they were interested in transference and countertransference (compared with 88% of psychodynamically oriented clinicians), and 20% took into account latent mental processes (compared with 82% of the psychodynamic group). According to Ellis (1992), this convergence should be intensified. Indeed, these therapies, in their early development, had no interest whatsoever in the 'black box', whereas today, cognitive-behavioural therapists are interested in dynamic processes.

If we review the literature on this topic (Guimón, 1998), we can see that, during the 1960s, the behaviourists treating anxiety based on a 'stimulus-response' model soon found that neither the hypothesis of extinction through exposure, nor cognitive formulations, were able to explain such phenomena as the improvement through abreaction of certain neurotic conditions, the appearance of truly acute panic attacks in certain patients over the course of their autogenic training, or the tendency of certain patients suffering from phobia to seek out so-called *phobic companions*. To explain these phenomena, they had to refer to the unconscious. Panic is related to internal terrors that fade with the remission of the symptom, but which persist if they are not approached in a more global manner. To ignore this internal, or psychic, vision of panic and reduce it to observable phenomena or to 'internal events' is excessive simplification.

Cognitive behaviourists have, therefore, found themselves with no choice but to accept the role played by what they have come to call, somewhat shyly, 'private events' in the genesis of symptoms and the development of treatments. It has become obvious that, in practice, behaviour therapy was indeed very close to certain psychoanalytically oriented psychotherapies. It has been shown that factors such as the therapeutic relationship, suggestion, and manipulation of patients' expectations regarding the improvement of their problems, all play an important role.

Progressively, behaviour therapy has begun to take into account patients' beliefs, thoughts, and feelings.

Family therapy was initiated by analytically-oriented practitioners, but it is also true that, as observed above, certain elements proceeding from general systems theory can be considered original contributions (Durkin, 1975): the principle of 'equifinality' (Miller, 1975), Von Bertalanffy's stable state concept (Von Bertalanffy, 1968), the concept of negative entropy, and others. Certain theoretical and technical aspects of the systems approach come out of psychoanalysis: there is a parallelism between the idea of 'family secrets' and the Freudian unconscious; the technique of 'reformulation' (underlying the positive connotations of negative messages) that had already been used in psychotherapy in order to ease the acceptance of an interpretation that was difficult to accept, showing its more 'digestible' side; the 'symptom prescription' was already frequently used in analytical psychotherapy to combat 'masochistic defences'; the re-creation of more appropriate behaviours than the ones actually manifested in a certain situation ('sculpting') comes from psychodrama, and so on.

Looking at the long-term picture, therapeutic programmes have frequently been adopted that featured activities following a variety of orientations, sometimes carried out by different therapists, which often brings up the problem of limits. In spite of this, a plural focus, in the sense used by Coderch (2001), is possible, and desirable.

Referring to psychoanalysis, Fonagy (2000) underlines the need to increase our sophistication concerning social influences. The classical psychoanalytical focus would be intrapsychic, the individualised self. Relational explanations were often, at first, limited to blaming the mother for her child's difficulties, although later it was admitted that the influences between the child and the environment are reciprocal.

With notable exceptions that we shall discuss in another chapter (Erikson, 1960; Fromm, 1947; Horney, 1937; Sullivan, 1953), the wider cultural and social context in which object relations develop is unknown to psychoanalytical theorists. According to Fonagy, the absence of psychoanalytic sophistication regarding the social environment represents a major challenge in psychoanalysis's evolution, beyond the question of its scientific status. In any case, given the intensive nature of psychoanalytical treatment, its influence will always be reduced to a relatively small group of individuals able to benefit from this form of psychotherapy.

The Dynamic, the Relational, and the Communicational

It is important to bear in mind that at this time, all of the doctrinal tendencies agree when it comes to highlighting the importance of relationships in the formation of the personality, the aetiology of psychopathology, and the treatment of psychiatric symptoms. Although they stress different aspects of the interpersonal world, and use different concepts to explain it, all of them put it at the forefront. Regarding this, we should not forget that Foulkes (1964) already used the term *social hunger* to describe the true drive behind inter-relating.

In the present text, we use the concept of *relational psychiatry* to refer to the approaches that are especially interested in psychodynamic and social theories in mental health. In the early 1980s, Tizón entitled one of his books *Relation-based Psychology* (1982), an alternative concept to *dynamic psychology*, and Coderch (2001) has provided a wide-ranging description of its implications in psychoanalysis.

Besides psychoanalytically oriented psychology, Gestalt psychology and the psychology derived from bioenergetics could also be considered 'dynamic'. The term *dynamic psychology* is very directly based on a Freudian point of view, and the energetic hypothesis. This analogical hypothesis of psychic energy should, according to Tizón, be replaced, at least in part, by postulates such as those that Rapaport (1960) called 'psychosocial' and 'adaptive' with a 'communicational' intent.

For its part, relational mental health is mostly based on the paradigm of object relations, although it maintains such basic postulates as psychic, genetic, structural dynamic, and interactionist determinism, and of 'overdetermination by the unconscious'.

Relational mental health studies behavioural disturbances—but with a different level of inter-relational meticulousness—later drawing up hypotheses regarding intrapersonal (representational) and interpersonal reality. It is based, above on, on interiorised environmental relationship experiences (internal reality), unlike dynamic psychology, more focused on representation. Klein's work has been decisive in indicating the importance of the first year of life in the structuring of psychobiological identity, both of 'fundamental psychobiological reaction characteristics' (constitution) and of 'basic anxieties and defences' (personality) (Klein, 1971). There are even those who use the term *imprinting* to refer to the importance and persistence of the infant's social acquisitions, metabolised and organised through a mediator, a barrier of contact with the environment (Lorenz, 1970; and Bowlby, 1979). Other forerunners of relational theory include Ferenczi (1967) and Fairbairn (1962), and among the contemporary theorists are Greenberg (1966, 1983, 2001) and Mitchell (1988, 1993).

The fields where relational mental health concepts can be applied are not limited to the relationship with patients and their families, but should also include relationships among professionals, and those involving professionals, their patients, and the community.

General Systems Theory

As is well known, general systems theory (Von Bertalanffy, 1968) affirms that the universe comprises a hierarchy of concrete systems, defined as accumulations of material and energy organised in inter-related components or subsystems acting together, which exist in a space-time continuum. General systems theory makes it possible to integrate the biological and social sciences with the physical sciences, which, as far as psychiatry is concerned, means an opportunity to throw light on mind-body problems, try to achieve a biological and social integration of human nature, and seek new approaches towards psychopathology, diagnoses, and the treatment of mental illness. Here, a 'system' is a set of units related among them. The state of each unit is conditioned by the state of the other units. Cells, organs, organisms, groups, organisations, societies, and nations can be considered 'concrete living systems' that can be classified into 'types', (such as different kinds of cells and organisms, or societies) with different kinds of social organisation (primitive, agricultural, or industrial). A suprasystem of any living system is the system immediately above its subsystem. For example, the suprasystem of a cell is the organ in which it is situated.

Matter and energy (terms used in the same sense as in the physical sciences) are organised through 'information'. Systems exchange matter, energy and information across their borders. All systems are subject to the second law of thermodynamics: their entropy increases over time as their available energy or internal order diminishes. Therefore, in systems, generally, randomness is a more probable state than orderliness.

General systems theory provides a new vision of the mind-body dilemma, by formulating this dichotomy in computer-science terms, as an 'information process' and a 'matter-energy process'. It also provides insight into the process of language codification. A step beyond was proposed by Menninger (1963), in the sense of describing normal and psychopathological personalities in terms of systems theory. But here, we are more interested in highlighting the application of general systems theory to diagnosis, treatment, and especially, pathology.

According to Miller (1975), general systems theory can contribute to improving diagnoses in mental health. A basic principle is that each process should be identified, if possible, with the structure that carries it out. A second principle is to include, as part of the diagnosis, all of the routing patterns for matter-energy and information that are transmitted through systems and subsystems. The third principle refers to the existence of 19 critical subsystems in all living systems, enabling the diagnostician to know which are the system's basic parts and processes. After taking these steps, says Miller, the clinician can indicate the specific types of treatment to be applied. If the basic alteration involves the matter-energy process, perhaps it can be corrected through diet, medication acting on the metabolism, or surgical interventions that modify the matter-energy currents. If the basic defect resides in information processes, the specialist can use psychotherapy techniques that alter neurotic habits, or medication that blocks pathological signals, such as tranquillisers able to diminish some types of anxiety. By determining the exact subsystem affected, the precise variables that are outside of normality, or the feedback or adjustment processes that do not operate correctly, it is possible to improve the precision with which the appropriate type of treatment can be applied.

Although these conceptions have yet to be fully fleshed out in the field of mental health, they are highly noteworthy when approaching new holistic concepts, with a comprehensive vision of clinical and therapeutic aspects of treatment. These options dovetail nicely with postmodern philosophical attitudes, as set forth by Coderch (2001).

REFERENCES

Angermeyer, M. C., Klusmann, D., and Walpuski, O. (1988). The causes of functional psychoses as seen by patients and their relatives II. The relatives' point of view. European *Archives of Psychiatry and Neurological Sciences, 238,* 55–61.

Angermeyer, M. C., and Matschinger, H. (1996). Public attitude towards psychiatric treatment. *Acta Psychiatrica Scandinavia, 94* (5), p326–336.

Angermeyer, M. C., and Matschinger, H. (1996). Relatives' beliefs about the causes of schizophrenia. *Acta Psychiatrica Scandinavia, 93,* 199–204.

Angermeyer, M. C. (1997). Social Representations of mental illness among the public. *European Psychiatry, 12* (suppl. 2), 114s.

Angermeyer, M. C., and Matschinger, H. (1999). Lay beliefs about mental disorders: a comparison between the western and the eastern parts of Germany. *Social Psychiatry and Psychiatric Epidemiology, 34,* 275–281.

Bateman, A. (2002). Integrative therapy from an analytic perspective. In J. Holmes and A. Bateman (Eds.). *Integration in psychotherapy. Models and methods.* (pp. 11–27). New York: Oxford University Press.

Bartrop, R. W., Lazarus, L., Luckhurst, E., and Kiloh, L. G. (1977). Depressed lymphocyte function after bereavement. *Lancet, 8016,* 834–836.

Bergin, A. E., and Garfield, S. L. (1994). *Handbook of psychotherapy and behavior change.* New York: Wiley.

Berrios, G. (1992). *Personal communication.*

Bouguignon, A. (1989). Biologie et classification en psychiatrie. *Confront Psychiat, 24,* 157–181.

Bowlby, J. (1979). *La separación afectiva.* Buenos Aires: Paidós.

Castillo del Pino, C. (1986). El biologismo en psicopatología y en psiquiatría. *Informaciones Psiquiatricas, 104,* 148–159.

Coderch, J. (2001). *La relación paciente-terapeuta. El campo del psicoanálisis y la psicoterapia psicoanalítica.* Barcelona: Paidos.

Davidovitz, D., and Levenson, H. (1995). *National survey on practice and training in brief*

therapy: comparison of psychologists, psychiatrists and social workers. In A. P. Association (Ed.). New York.
Durkin, H. E. (1975). The development of systems theory and its implications for the theory and practice. In L. R. Wolberg and M. L. Aronson (Eds.), *Group therapy* (pp. 8–20). New York: Stratton International.
Durkin, H. E. (1982). Change in group psychotherapy: Therapy and practice: A systems perspective. *International Journal of Group Psychotherapy, 32*(4), 431–439.
Edelson, M. (1984). Hypothesis and evidence in psychoanalysis. Chicago: University of Chicago Press.
Eker, D., and Oner, B. (1999). Attitudes toward mental illness among the general public and professionals, social representations and change. In J. Guimon, W. Fischer and N. Sartorius (Eds.), *The image of madness* (pp. 1–13). Basel: Karger.
Ellis, A. (1992). Group rational-emotive and cognitive-behavioral therapy. *International Journal Of Group Psychotherapy, 42*(1), 63–80.
England, M. J., and Goff, V. V. (1993). Health reform and organized systems of care. In W. Goldman and S. Feldman (Eds.), *Managed mental health care.* San Francisco: Jossey-Bass.
Erikson, E. H. (1960). The problem of ego identity. In M. Stein, A. H. Vidich and D. M. White (Eds.), *Identity and anxiety.* New York: The Free Press.
Eskin, M. (1989). Rural population's opinions about the causes of mental illness, modern psychiatric help-sources and traditional healers in Turkey. *Int. J. Soc. Psychiatry, 35,* 324–328.
Fairbairn, W. R. (1962). *Estudio psicoanalitico de la personalidad.* Buenos Aires:Ed. Hormé.
Ferenczi, S. (1967). Teoría y técnica del psicoanálisis. Buenos Aires: Paidós.
Fink, P. J. (1993). Psychiatrist's roles in managed care programs. *Hospital and Community Psychiatry, 44*(723–724).
Fink, P. J. (1996). Are psychiatrists replaceable? In A. Lazarus (Ed.), *Controversies in Managed Mental Health Care* (pp. 3–16). Washington: American Psychiatric Press.
Fischer, W., Goerg, D., Zbinden, E., and Guimón, J. (1999). Determining factors and the effects of attitudes towards psychotropic medication. In J. Guimón, W. Fischer and N. Sartorius (Eds.), *The image of madness* (pp. 162–186). Basel: Karger Medical and Scientific Publishers.
Fonagy, P. (1996). The future of an empirical psychoanalysis. *British Journal of Psychotherapy, 13,* 106–118.
Fonagy, P. (2000). *An Open Door Review of Outcome Studies in Psychoanalysis* (www.ipa.org.uk/research/complete.htm). London: IPA.
Foulkes, S. H. (1964). *Therapeutic group analysis.* London: Wheaton and Co.
Fromm, E. (1947). *Man for himself.* New York: Penguin.
Gabbard, G. O. (1995). Psychodynamic psychotherapies. In G. O. Gabbard (Ed.), *Treatments of psychiatric disorders* (Vol. 2). Washington: American Psychiatric Press, Inc.
Geraty, R. D., & Fox, R. J. (1996). Can managed care improve mental health outcomes for children and adolescents? In A. Lazarus (Ed.), *Controversies in Managed Mental Health Care* (pp. 57–68). Washington: American Psychiatric Press.
Glazer, W. M., and Gray, G. V. (1996). How effective is utilization review? In A. Lazarus (Ed.), *Controversies in managed mental health care* (Vol. ch. 13, pp. 179–194). Washington: American Psychiatric Press.
Goerg, D., Fischer, W., Zbinden, E., and Guimón, J. (1999). Public attitudes towards deviant situation in daily life: Interventions proposed. In J. Guimón and W. Fischer and N. Sartorius (Eds.), *The image of madness* (pp. 38–55). Basel: Karger Medical and Scientific Publishers.
Goerg, D., Zbinden, E., Fischer, W., and Guimón, J. (1997). Stereotypes of the public concerning psychotropic drugs and compliance with medication. *European Psychiatry, 12* (suppl. 2), 115s.
Greenberg, J. (1996). Psychoanalytic interaction. *Psychoanal. Inquiry, 16,* 25–38.

Greenberg, J., and Mitchell, S. (1983). *Object relations in psychoanalytic theory*. Cambridge: Harvard University Press.
Greenberg, J. R. (2001). The analyst participation: A new look. *Journal of the American Psychoanalytical Association, 49* (2), 359–398.
Guimón, J. (1998). *La profession de psychiatre. Evolution et devenir*. Paris: Masson.
Guimón, J., Fischer, W., and Sartorius, N. (1999). *The image of madness*. Basel: Karger.
Guimón, J., Fischer, W., Zbinden, E., and Goerg, D. (1997). Consequences of recent changes in research and practice for the identity of psychiatrist. *European Psychiatry, 12* (supp. 2), 92s–98s.
Guimón, J., and Sartorius, N. (Eds.). (1999). *Manage or perish? The challenges of managed mental health care in Europe*. New York: Kluwer Academic/Plenum Publishers.
Guimón, J. (2001). Inequity and Madness. Psychosocial and Human Rihts Issues. New York: Kluwer Academic.
Hillert, A., Sandmann, J., Ehmig, S., Wisbecker, H., Kepplinger, H. M., and Benkert, O. (1999). The general public's cognitive and emotional perception of mental illnesses: an alternative to attitudes research. In J. Guimón and W. Fischer and N. Sartorius (Eds.), *The image of madness*. Basel: Karger.
Holmes, J., and Bateman, A. (Eds.). (2002). *Integration in psychotherapy. Models and methods*. New York: Oxford University Press.
Horney, K. (1937). *The neurotic personality of our time*. New York.
Kiloh, L. G., Andrews, G., Nelson, M., & Bianchi, G. N. (1972). The relationships of the syndromes called endogenous and neurotic depressions. *Br. J. Psychiatry, 121*, 183–196.
Klein, M. (1971). Algunas conclusiones teóricas sobre la vida emocional del bebé. In M. Klein (Ed.), *Desarrollos en psicoanálisis*. Buenos Aires: Hormé.
Klerman, G. L. (1977). Mental illness, the medical model and psychiatry. *Journal of Medicine and Philosophy* (2), 220–243.
Lazarus, A., et al. (1996). Controversies in managed mental health care. Washington DC: American Psychiatric Press Inc. Lorenz, K. (1970). The establishment of the instinct concept. In K. Lorenz (Ed.), *Studies in animal and human behaviour*. London: Methuen.
Lorenz, K. (1970). The Stablishment of the Instinct Concept. In K. Lorenz (Ed.), *Studies in Animal and Human Behaviour*. Londres: Methuen.
Maher, B. (1970). *Introduction to research in psychopathology*. New York: McGraw-Hill Books.
Menninger, K. (1963). *The vital balance*. New York: Viking Press.
Miller, J. G. (1975a). General systems theory. In A. M. Freedman, H. I. Kaplan and B. J. Saddock (Eds.), *Comprehensive textbook of psychiatry*. Baltimore: Eds. The Williams and Wilkins Co.
Miller, J. G. (1975b). *General systems theory*.
Mitchell, S. (1988). *Relational concepts in psychoanalysis*. Cambridge: Harvard University Press.
Mitchell, S. (1993). *Hope and dread in psychoanalysis*. New York: Basic Books.
Orlinsky, D. E., and Howard, K. I. (1986). Process and outcome in psychotherapy. In S. L. G. A. E. Bergin (Ed.), *Handbook of psychotherapy and behavior change* (pp. 311–381). New York: Wiley.
Panzetta, A. F. (1996). Is public behavioral health care manageable? In A. Lazarus (Ed.), *Controversies in Managed Mental Health Care* (pp. 69–80). Washington: American Psychiatric Press.
Quitanilla, I. (1986). El biologismo en psicopatología y en psiquiatría. *Informaciones Psiquiátricas, 104*, 148–159.
Rapaport, D. (1960). The structure of psychoanalysis. *Psychological Issues*, II (2).
Rutan, J. S., & Stone, W. N. (1993). *Psychodynamic Group Psychotherapy*. New York: Guilford.
Siegler, J. E., Axelband, M., and Isikoff, J. (1993). Psychiatry: taking a leadership role in managed health care. *Psychiatric Times* (July), 32.

Smith, M. L., Glass, G. V., and Miller, T. I. (1980). *The benefits of psychotherapy*. Baltimore: Johns Hopkins University Press.
Sullivan, H. S. (1953). *The interpersonal theory of psychiatry*. New York: W. W. Norton.
Tizón, J. (1982). *Psicología basada en la relación*. Barcelona: Hora.
Tizón, J., Salamero, M., de la Alama, E., and Diez Munguira, J. M. (1985). Introducción al biologismo; implicaciones teóricas, repercusiones en la asistencia. *Informaciones Psiquiátricas, 103*, 1–18.
Tuttman, S. (1997). Protecting the therapeutic alliance in this time of changing health-care delivery systems. *International Journal of Group Psychotherapy, 47*(1), 3–16.
Von Bertalanffy, L. (1968). *General systems theory*. New York: Braziller.

5

Relational Aspects of Mental Health

Part 1: Psychological Factors

PHENOMENOLOGY: A RELIC OF THE PAST?

Within the field of relational psychiatry, a number of psychological schools have tried to integrate themselves into a 'comprehensive' vision of the human. They do not aim to directly explain reality with laws, which they consider more within the realm of the natural sciences, but rather to understand the life of an individual, and describe its uniqueness.

Phenomenology as a philosophical system was created by Husserl (1940) as an orientation that tried to get back to 'the things themselves', with a 'naked and naïve' soul. In order to achieve this goal, he said, any observational elements lacking in interest for the research at hand must be eliminated, using so-called 'phenomenological reduction' techniques.

Jaspers applied this system to psychopathology and psychiatry. For him, the psychopathologist's mission is to 'apprehend experience' in order to intuitively capture the psychic states that patients go through. To do this, he must approach the patient's experiences not merely as an observer, but trying to experience them himself, which means stimulating the patient's 'self-unfolding' while avoiding applying any influence on his own part, and creating an ideal atmosphere for this. The result is an interviewing method with unmistakable relational overtones.

Following Dilthey (1948), Jaspers (1946) calls *understanding* the vision of the psychic state obtained from within; on the contrary, *explanation* stems from knowledge of objective, causal relationships. For Jaspers, 'the psyche arises from the psyche in a way understandable to us: one who is attacked becomes angry, and we understand when he carries out defensive acts; one who has been tricked becomes mistrustful'. Both the ideas of the 'understandability' or 'non-understandability' of a patient's life experiences, as well as their 'explicability' or 'inexplicability', are very important contributions to psychopathology, especially the study of psychosis.

Jaspers used the term *process* to describe a lasting alteration in the patient's psyche, stemming from a known or suspected organic brain lesion. On the contrary, he used the term *development* for a modification of the personality in the course of a patient's lifetime that depended on the environment, or specific experiences. His existential psychology is derived from existential philosophy, represented, principally, by such figures as Heidegger, Hegel, Kierkegard, and Sartre, who had a major influence on Husserl's phenomenological thought. The existential movement opted for 'life experience', for man faced with himself, vertiginous with freedom and singularity, as opposed to the man of 'social organisation'.

PSYCHOANALYSIS

It was Freud who first explored in depth the affective and relational aspects of personality, elaborating an original doctrine that transformed psychology.

Freudian Psychoanalysis

By analysing traumatic experiences, called up under hypnosis, Freud observed that they were usually of a sexual nature, and were not consciously remembered by the subject. In Vienna, he worked with Breuer in this field, soon arriving at the conclusion that to explore this subconscious area (an idea that already existed prior to Freud), dialogue with the patient was more useful, as proposed by Bernheim, with whom he had worked in France. This was the true beginning of relational psychology.

Instinctive Vicissitudes: from Narcissism to Relationships

According to Freud, each individual's outer reality and inner world combine to determine each and every one of our actions. The first infantile experiences are fundamental to understanding adult behaviour. Part of his theory of the instincts is clearly biological: the child comes into the world loaded with libidinal drives for which he tries to find release in order to obtain pleasure. This tendency, which he called the *pleasure principle,* represents the drive to maintain the amount of excitement felt at as low and as constant a level as possible. A stimulus provokes displeasure, and the tendency to diminish tension leads to the search for immediate satisfaction through a reduction in tension. In a small child, the search for satisfaction can even be carried out via inadequate means (e.g., crying to discharge the tension produced by a feeling of hunger) or through phantasy. This means of satisfaction characterises the so-called *primary process*, a mode of psychological functioning belonging to the realm of our dream life, and which is also present in the mental life of psychotics and during certain moments of artistic creativity.

The other part of the theory acquires a clearly relational tinge. The obstacles that reality imposes on the immediate satisfaction of desires forces the psychic apparatus to adapt its mode of action to these demands, submitting itself to the reality principle. Action, here, is characterised by the norms of efficiency, judgement, choice, and decision belonging to the so-called *secondary process* prevailing during waking activity. The sublimation of repressed instincts is thus the basis of the genesis of culture.

Freud, between 1900 and 1910, developed his theory that the libido is deposited either in the self (*narcissistic libido*) or other 'objects', i.e., persons, things, values (*object libido*). In this concept of the *object*, he more clearly introduces the idea of relationships with others. Freud also described the vicissitudes in the affective relationship between children and their parents, including the so-called *Oedipus complex* (erotic desires directed towards the parent of the opposite sex, and hostility towards the one of the same sex, and contrary desires in the so-called *inverted Oedipus*), and the *castration complex* (fear of being punished as a result of these desires).

During the last phase of his life, Freud spoke of a *death instinct* reflecting a basic (biological) human need to seek a drop in the level of tension. He progressively attributed more and more importance to this instinct in such phenomena as children's games, recurring dreams after a traumatic event, and *transference*.

The Psychic Apparatus: Relational Aspects of the Second Topic

After his first model of personality (*first topic*), consisting of a *conscious* zone and an *unconscious* one, Freud proposed a new definition of the psychic apparatus (*second topic*), this one tripartite. The first of its three levels, the *id*, is the primitive, original form of the psychic apparatus, containing first libidinal (sexual and aggressive) energy, and then products of denial. Governing by the pleasure principle through the primary process, the id is, in its totality, unconscious.

Up to this point, these Freudian models have a biological basis, but the environment comes in at the point where Freud postulates how the other two levels become differentiated from the id in the course of development. Indeed, the psychic apparatus, in contact with reality, elaborates the *ego*, which is like a differentiation from the more superficial layers of the *id*. The ego acts by adapting itself to the reality principle through the secondary process.

The *superego* arises as a later differentiation from the ego. It contains, first, repressive forces that are opposed to the unconditional gratification of desires. The superego represents the interiorisation of the norm. Freud dates its appearance in the boys to the post-Oedipal period, during which, after his incestuous desires have been rejected, the child identifies himself with his father. What the child incorporates is not his father's persona, but *his* father's superego, which he, in turn, incorporated from his father's superego. Melanie Klein, among others, believed that rudiments of the superego can be seen in pre-Oedipal periods.

Whereas renouncing the satisfaction of a desire due to outside demands produces only displeasure, renouncing it for superego-related, internal reasons, besides this natural displeasure, can, itself, produce satisfaction: the ego feels exalted, and considers its renunciation of the instinctive drive to be a meritorious act. However, besides its repressive norms, the superego contains a differentiation from the ego, the *ego ideal*, based on self-observation and consciousness. It is generally accepted that, in spite of being almost totally unconscious, the superego is conscious, or at least pre-conscious, in these functions of the ego ideal.

Relational Aspects of Defence Mechanisms

The ego can defend itself against the dangers that it experiences in its relationship with the outside by means of flight mechanisms or by trying to change the outside world. But these reactions are not useful in defending itself against the dangers of the id's contents (i.e., drives). To do this, it needs psychological defence mechanisms. These unconscious mechanisms are found to a greater or lesser degree in all personalities, and influence human activities. They only acquire a pathological nature when they are repeated compulsively, or when they persist at ages in which they are no longer necessary. In psychological pathologies, defence mechanisms are distributed characteristically in different disorders.

Among the mechanisms described by Freud (e.g., *fixation, regression, denial, isolation, undoing, reaction formation, somatisation*), fixation, regression, and somatisation have more to do with narcissistic libidinal development than with object relations.

However, other defence mechanisms involve a relational context. *Projection* consists of exteriorisation, onto the surrounding world, of our own feelings and thoughts, which then come back to us as if they were foreign. *Introjection*, on the contrary, enables us, through fantasy, to pass certain objects, or qualities inherent to these objects, from 'outside' to 'inside'. It is very similar to *identification*, whereby we assimilate an aspect, property, or attribute of the other, and then transform ourselves, completely or partially, based on this model. Without projection or introjection, there would be no valid identification, which is so necessary to the child's development. On the other hand, *Sublimation* is the channelling of instinctive tendencies towards altruistic and spiritual ends.

Psychopathology According to Freud

Freud considered anxiety to be either a response to external dangers (*realistic*, or *objective anxiety*) or internal ones (*neurotic anxiety*). According to his first explanation, such dangers, if they overcome the individual's elaboration capacity, produce a discharge in the form of automatic (or *primary*) anxiety. According to his second interpretation, these dangers, upon being perceived, cause the ego to produce an anxiety signal, putting the psyche on alert, and setting off defence mechanisms.

Regarding his first, clearly biologist hypothesis (1894), Freud, when maintaining his so-called *economic model* of the psyche, believed that anxiety neurosis was caused by a dissatisfaction of the libido, which if not naturally channelled through the sex act (due to abstinence or *coitus interruptus*), would be channelled into anxiety creation. Thus, this description of anxiety is aetiological, incorporating, to a certain extent, the concepts of Freud's former 'spinal theory of neurosis', which assumed the existence of functional disorders in the spinal medula. According to this theory, the process is biological, but the consequences are psychological. In this sense, Freud was a precursor of the modern conception of anxiety's biochemical bases.

However, when later defending his second model of the psychic apparatus, Freud accepted that this blocking of libidinal discharge could occur not only due to physical causes, but to relational ones, stemming from the repression of unacceptable libidinal drives and infantile traumas.

On the other hand, in his *Project*, Freud accepted that besides an inadeequate discharge of sexuality, both hunger and breathing difficulties (present at the moment of birth) could be stimuli able to overcome the child's elaboration capacity, producing anxiety.

But he added in his *Three Essays* (1905) that, since the child is dependent on the mother, anxiety could also be produced by separation from her; this would explain, for example, children's fear of the dark. He later discovered other causes for anxiety besides separation from, or loss of, the mother:

loss of the penis, loss of the object's love, and loss of the superego's love. These could all be termed *traumas*, dangers threatening the integrity of the ego.

Some of Freud's followers developed conceptions based partly on relational ideas, such as Wilhelm Reich (1942) with his *character armour*, which are of interest in the psychotherapeutic relationship. Ferenczi, for his part, was the precursor of what would later come to be called *active techniques*, which produced major modifications in the analyst-patient relationship.

Psychoanalysis and Object Relations

Melanie Klein: Early Relationships

Object relations form the basis of an approach to psychoanalysis often called the British School, which are of great interest to relational studies generally. Remember that the *object* is any person, thing, or animate, inanimate or abstract entity—or any part of these—towards which we direct our drives, our desires. These objects may be external to the subject, but he processes them inside himself, creating an *internal object*, which represents the external one.

Human beings experience, with regard to their internal objects, a series of sensations to which they add feelings, and which have bodily and behavioural effects, although they are not usually expressed in words. These are *unconscious phantasies*, primary content of the unconscious mental processes of attachment (Bowlby, 1973) and aggression.

For authors from the British School, followers of Melanie Klein, the infant faces a variety of dangers: some proceed from differentiation/indifferentiation anxieties; others from persecutions, internal or external; and yet others are produced by experiences of loss and guilt. Each one of these situations can give rise to different anxieties, unconscious phantasies, and defence mechanisms. Differentiation anxieties—sometimes called *primitive confusions*—have to do with the first weeks of life, during which the infant's 'inside' and 'outside' are not well defined. Outside, exist *objects* (persons, things) that satisfy its needs with more or less regularity. When the infant feels some displeasure, 'something comes' to calm this unpleasant sensation, and the anxiety that it sets off. Therefore, all infants should have during these first stages as stable and affectionate a psychological environment as possible. The 'outside' is sometimes 'caring', but at others frustrating (persecutory), so that anxieties arise in the infant based on the psychological experience of the threat of disintegration by this 'bad mother' who does not care for it, but also by the 'badness' that it feels within itself. All 'no care' is, for the child, an attack, a persecution, but also a projection of his own aggressiveness (excrete the bad, the faeces; drive away the persecutor) (Klein 1937; 1957).

The child tries to control these anxieties, whether through actual flight or through defence mechanisms or by accepting his own innate aggressiveness (and the resultant guilt), until then only projected. This last step gives rise to a third kind of anxieties, those related to loss, error, or guilt, what Klein called *depressive anxieties* (Klein 1940).

The child winds up perceiving clearly that the source of his satisfactions, of his pleasure, is outside himself, in his mother—who can disappear. This realisation leads the child to fear that his attacks on her could make him lose her, which leads to attitudes of mourning for her loss. If he is able to have confidence in his own reparative capacities, he establishes a good relationship with reality, with total objects (simultaneously good and bad). The defensive manoeuvres of this 'depressive' position enable him to see an external reality less deformed by his own needs.

Narcissism

Freud used the concept of narcissism, with different connotations, throughout his oeuvre. In the paper 'Leonardo da Vinci and a Memory of his Childhood" (Freud, S., 1910), he linked narcissism to the homosexual object choice of a man who, after repressing his love towards his mother, identifies with her by loving men as his mother loved him. In 1914, in one of his major works, *Introduction to Narcissism*, Freud distinguished between a primary narcissism (which develops with the ego after autoeroticism) and a secondary narcissism, which is a reinvestment in the ego of that which was previously invested in the object. He compared the first with the body of an amoeba, and the second with the pseudopods that it emits. In this work, Freud explained that human beings sometimes make a 'narcissistic' amorous choice, when they take themselves (narcissistic choice) or similar persons (homosexual choice) as an object. On the contrary, they make a 'cathectic' object choice when they seek objects based on the model of the woman who raised them. Freud here also links narcissism to the aggression that springs from the primordial rejection that the narcissistic ego opposes, in early life, to the exterior world that is the source of stimuli. In hypochondria, Freud saw a stasis, a storage of the libido in the organ, which produces displeasure.

In this same work, Freud developed the concept of *self-esteem*, which implies an ego function able to positively or negatively judge the self. When self-esteem is threatened, this sets off narcissistic activities to protect it.

The concept of narcissism has undergone interesting developments in post-Freudian authors. Klein denied the existence of instinctive drives that do not involve external or internal objects, so she considered that both autoeroticism and narcissism include a relationship with interiorised objects. Among her followers, Rosenfeld believed that it is necessary to differentiate between the libidinal and destructive aspects that co-exist in narcissism, and stressed the self-idealisation and the devaluation of objects that narcissistic individuals present. These ideas were very influential in the work of Kohut and Kernberg.

Kohut pointed out that primary narcissism is threatened in infancy due to the inevitable defects in maternal caregiving, so that the child seeks the former state of perfection. He therefore creates a grandiose and exhibitionistic self-image, called the *grandiose self*, idealising an object of the self, called the *idealised parental imago*. These two images are adequately integrated in the healthy adult personality; but if the child has suffered major frustrations, when he becomes an adult, he will present a narcissistic personality.

Kernberg stressed that the development of normal and pathological narcissism always involves the self's relationship with representations of internal and external objects. Narcissistic personalities do not develop a true relationship between the self and the object, but rather between the primitive, grandiose self and its projection onto objects, i.e., 'a narcissistic relationship of the self with the self'. According to Kernberg, there are external regulators of narcissism: libidinal gratifications coming from external objects, gratifications obtained by egotistical means, and gratifications of cultural aspirations, whose balance is essential in the economy of self-esteem.

Mourning

Melanie Klein (1946) noted that the early onset of guilt seems to be one of the consequences of excessive envy. If this premature guilt is experienced by the ego when it is not yet in a position to deal with it, it is then experienced as a persecution, and the object that arouses it becomes a persecutor. Several months later, when the depressive position arises, the ego has a greater capacity to stand the pain of guilt and develop the corresponding defences, above all the tendency to repair.

Persecutory guilt co-exists with persecutory anxiety. The essence of guilt, according to Klein, resides in the feeling that the damage done to the loved object was caused by the subject's aggressive impulses. The need to cancel or repair this damage comes from the sense of guilt.

The main emotions involved in persecutory guilt are resentment, pain, desperation, fear, and self-reproach. In depressive guilt, the most important feelings are worry about the object and about the ego, pain, nostalgia, and responsibility. It is manifested, especially in normal mourning, by sublimatory and reparation activities, and is dominated by the life instinct.

The proportion of guilt intervention after a loss, and the persecutory or depressive quality of this loss, will determine the quality and intensity of the reaction that is experienced due to this loss. In some clinical situations, mainly melancholia, patients carry to extremes their self-punishing tendencies determined by persecutory guilt, to the point that they actually mutilate or even kill themselves. Depressive and persecutory guilt can coexist throughout a patient's lifetime, with one or the other predominating according to whether the love instinct or the destructive instinct is predominating. An especially characteristic trait of depressive guilt is the desire to repair the object that the patient imagines he has damaged through his own destructive drives.

The feeling of pain contained in depressive mourning, together with its reparatory drives, form the basis for creativity and sublimation, which arise when the patient overcomes the psychotic mechanisms that become neurotic ones: inhibition, repression, and displacement. Manic reparation, unlike the depressive variety, is a defence, since, although it also aims to repair the object, feelings of guilt or loss do not appear, and it is oriented not towards original objects but towards distant ones, as is the case for some among those who work with charitable organisations.

Bowlby and Attachment

Bowlby (1973, 1979) described the so-called *attachment behaviours* as being based on four possible hypotheses (Tizón, 1982). The *secondary relational tendency* hypothesis states that the basis for attachment is the satisfaction of needs for food, clothing, cleanliness, and movement, through the relationship with the mother or her substitutes. The *first object suction* maintains that it is the innate tendency to suckle at the breast which establishes the first relationship. The *primary desire of return to the maternal womb* (Rank) has fallen out of favour today. The *primary attachment to the object* hypothesis is based on Harlow's observations concerning higher mammals and human beings, showing with teddy bears that, although the need to suckle is very strong, once it was satisfied something remained, and which made the monkeys seek contact with their own kind. This 'something' is called *attachment behaviour* or *affective link*, the search for a relationship for itself, unrelated even to food.

Epigenetic Development: Erickson

Erickson (Erickson, 1960) described a *diagram of epigenetic development* parallel to Freud's phases of libidinal development. The first phase of development is the oral or sensory-oral phase, during which the infant's dominant tendency is 'incorporation' (suckling)–incorporating not only food but also odours and cutaneous and auditory experiences. In the phase that Erickson called *muscular-anal* (*anal sadism* in Freud), the small child develops feelings of autonomy (respect, shame, and doubt); the mode of social relations is to grab and let go of the object, and the basic feelings are the desire to 'do things well', which gives him a feeling of autonomy. In the *locomotor genital* phase, the child becomes more demanding and dependent. During the *generative genital* phase, which begins after weaning, the conflicts of early infancy are revived.

Based on these phases, Erickson developed a model of the principal psychosocial phases that human beings go through during their development.

Psychoanalysis and Society

Certain psychoanalysts have come to be called *culturalists* because of the importance that they laid on culture in the genesis of behaviour and symptoms. Although one could include a number of authors in this group, we shall limit ourselves to Erich Fromm, Harry S. Sullivan, and Karen Horney, who constitute a homogeneous group that served as the nucleus and catalyst for an entire school of American psychoanalysis, laying the groundwork for a better understanding of interpersonal relations.

All of them received orthodox psychoanalytical training at the beginning of their careers. It is noteworthy that their therapeutic technique never varied substantially from Freud's over the course of their development. It is in the theoretical conception of personality, in the consideration of the genesis of psychic levels, in their description of the ego's defence mechanisms, and, especially, in the role they attributed to society, where they dissented fundamentally from the tenets of Freudian orthodoxy. In their works, they criticised many of the premises considered basic until that time: Freud's biological orientation in his explanation of instincts and the psychological differentiation between the two sexes; the universality and inevitability of the phases of libidinal development; and, in particular, the Oedipus complex.

Karen Horney

Horney's most notable theoretical dissensions centred on Freud's instinct theory: she believed that it is mistaken to think that libidinal energy is the prime mover behind any behaviour, and rejected the biological genesis of complexes, proposing that their origin was actually social. She also rejected the Freudian interpretation of the origin of society, based on the repression of primarily aggressive instincts. Rather, she believed that, since natural selection tends to eliminate traits that are harmful for survival, it would be odd for aggressiveness to persist over the course of human evolution. With this argumentation, however, she forgot that aggressive drives are not always harmful to the development of personality and society. She criticised the Freudian affirmation that these instincts are innate, pointing to findings in cultural anthropology, principally those of Mead (1939), who described 'non-aggressive' social groups in New Guinea.

She formulated categorically—and here she was a forerunner of antipsychiatry—that there was no such thing as a normal psychology and another, abnormal psychology. Norms can only be established with relation to the culture in which an individual is immersed, and in which he has developed.

For Horney (1942), our culture offers four escape routes for the anxiety produced by conflict: to rationalise it, deny it, narcotise it (as addicts do), and to avoid it (which produces inhibitions for feeling or doing certain things).

She proposed the existence of traits common to all neurotic personalities: rigidity in reactions, and discrepancy between possibilities and realisations. The basis for all neurosis, according to Horney, is found in the *basic anxiety* of infancy and early childhood. The later conformation of a neurotic disorder would be in accordance with the conflicts inherent in the individual's culture.

Thus, she described ten neurotic traits of modern industrialised man, which involve three basic attitudes: moving towards people, against people, or fleeing from people. These mechanisms can only be considered pathological if they are not forms of acceptable behaviour in a particular society. In the American society in which Horney developed her theories, these conflicts could be caused by: the ambivalence between the competitive attitudes that lead to the search for success, and those of fraternal love demanded as premises by the culture; the continual, instinctive temptations of consumer society in the face of an inability to satisfy them; and the contradiction between the proclamation of individual freedom and the growing, real limitations placed on that freedom. These situations of ambivalence, in reality, are similar to those that Laing discussed regarding the relationship between schizophrenics and their families, in the form of what Bateson called a 'double bind'.

Horney, whose work reached a wide audience in America through mass-market publications, also influenced the theoretical evolution of psychoanalytical specialists. The antipsychiatric theorists owe some of their ideas to this author. A certain tendency to oversimplification of concepts, and the absence of a solid theoretical explanation for some of her most important ideas, are perhaps the reasons why Horney's work has not had an even greater impact on the theoretical development of psychoanalysis worldwide.

Erich Fromm

Fromm was interested, above all, in the relationship between the individual and society. He severely criticised Freud's biological orientation, especially his doctrine of instincts. Although Fromm agreed that there are impulses—hunger, sex, and thirst—that are common to all human beings, he stressed that the factors which truly differentiate individuals (love, hate, desire for power, sexuality, and so on) have their origin in the social process. Society does not only repress; it also creates, and so human energies can become productive forces that mould the social process: 'Not only is man made by history. History is made by man'. What conditions our behaviour, according to Fromm, is not the satisfaction or frustration of any instinct, but the individual's relationship with his world, a world that is constantly changing and is not, as Freud assumed, static. The Freudian explanation for behaviour, based on the repression of sexual instincts was excessively simplistic, in Fromm's view. Man has the same biological drives as other animals, but the manner in which they are satisfied is determined culturally. What differentiates human beings from other animals is our capacity to store knowledge from the past in the form of symbolic memory, and our ability to foresee future possibilities, which enables us to reach imaginary conclusions that go beyond the limits of our senses.

Therefore, we are able to be conscious of the limitation of our existence; of the fact of having been born without any choice in the matter; of the inexorable law of death; and that our personal development cannot go beyond the limits marked by the level of culture achieved in our time. These fundamental facts of existence were described by Fromm under the name of *existential dichotomies;* these are opposed to what he called the *historical dichotomies* (e.g., social injustice, war, hunger), which are susceptible to resolution.

The existence of historical dichotomies provokes contradictions, in the face of which man cannot remain passive. Oppressive social classes try to convince the oppressed that these historical dichotomies are an inevitable part of human life; in other words, that they are really existential dichotomies. During the Middle Ages, the theory of a social order ordained by God, with fixed classes, served, according to Fromm, to rationalise the exploitation of the oppressed by the ruling classes, just as in our capitalist society, the rationalisation is that the free market enables anyone to reach his maximum level of achievement, and therefore 'the poor are necessarily lazy'.

The existence of these contradictions forces man to try to seek a balance between himself and society, which inclines him to create ties like religions, or political theories, such as Marxism. Based on this affirmation, Fromm turns Freud's opinion that religion 'is the obsessive neurosis of humanity' on its head, saying that 'neurosis is a personal form of religion'. In the face of these existential contradictions, man could take three stances: the most frequent, is that of voluntarily conforming to the modules imposed by society; the neurotic stance involves an intimate disagreement, but a conformist attitude; and the creative stance involves the desire to realise oneself as an individual.

In this process of self-realisation, this search for individuality, the individual is conscious of the fact that he must confront, with only his own efforts, the pathological conditions of social life, and try to escape from the feelings of despair and loneliness that they produce, with certain psychic mechanisms (moral masochism, sadism, destructiveness, and automatic conformity). Out of the individual's struggle with society, certain *social characters* arise in individuals (perceptive, exploiter, avaricious, manager, productive).

Although society continually frustrates such desires of individualisation, human beings can progress, thanks to in-depth knowledge of these problems, in love and in work.

Harry Stack Sullivan

Sullivan, born and educated in the United States, devoted himself for some time to psychotherapy with schizophrenics (Sullivan, 1927), with notable success. He shared the orientations of Horney and Fromm, with whom he soon formed an ideological group known by commentators as that of *cultural psychoanalysis*. His theories, often difficult to understand, are set forth in a number of essential texts (Sullivan, 1953, 1954, 1962, 1967). Sullivan accepted, for the most part, Freud's doctrine of the instincts, but added to the innate physical needs (sex, sleep, hunger, thirst) the human species's desire to develop socially. Anxiety, according to Sullivan, is the opposite of euphoria, and stems from the impossibility of achieving security, and the fear of disapproval. One of his fundamental contributions to psychoanalysis was to stress the importance of relationships in the genesis of neurosis, and its treatment (*interpersonal theory*). In this sense, he is considered, together with Ferenczi, the precursor of *relational psychoanalysis*.

Relational Psychoanalysis

The relational perspective (Greenberg, 2001) was developed explicitly as a reaction to previous excesses. In the first place, there was the excess consisting of conceptualising relationships with others as the transformation of our instictual phantasies.

In this sense, Greenberg points out that during nearly a century, psychoanalysts have shown a more or less phobic avoidance of accepting their participation in the analysis process, but today, it is necessary to recognise that the analyst influences the analysand's experience in many different ways, and to a much greater extent than the first authors thought; this impact of the analyst's behaviour can never be understood while it is happening; an effective analysis can only be carried out in fits and starts, as the result of negotiations within each individual dyad; the objective of these negotiations is to find a way to work, unique to a particular dyad, which is fitting for both participants (Pizer, 1992, 1998; Greenberg, 1995); analytical objectivity is very relative, because one cannot be objective about anything, and because the analyst's memory and desire can never be avoided or prohibited; our countertransference is, then, 'the air that our patients breathe'. It is true, says Greenberg, that, working with these premises, the classical analytical framework is broken, and the analyst runs a risk and puts himself on the line in a very personal way. But experience shows that the analyst can then, in a movement which has not been sufficiently taken into consideration in the classical descriptions, offer himself, as a person, to contain the tensions and anxieties that the patient is experiencing as a consequence of being in treatment. It is, therefore, futile to try to develop a fixed psychoanalytical methodology applicable to all analysts, all analysands, and all dyads.

In Greenberg's view, however, there has been an abuse of relational approaches, because the majority of publications that discuss this perspective centre on periods of analysis during which the tensions about what is going on become unbearable for both participants. They present a series of examples about the way in which we should all work, which pressure the reader/analyst to be open enough, flexible enough, and concerned enough to respond in an appropriate manner.

Greenberg reminds us that Freud already pointed out that patients also have to experience a 'positive, non-censurable transference' able to motivate their participation in the analysis (Freud, 1912). The ideas contained in the patient's 'non-censurable' transference include belief in the value of the treatment, based on favourable views of analysis as a discipline and the analyst as a professional. The patient is a member of a social group that shares these beliefs, and comes to the analysis with the expectation of being helped, and that the analyst whom he has chosen is interested in providing him with this help, and competent to do so. It is believed that positive, non-censurable transference acts in two ways: first, it involves, for patients, the conviction that analysis, although difficult, will help them to improve their lives; second, it lends authority to the figure of the analyst, which involves realistic desires to please, to be a 'good' patient. Positive, non-censurable transference facilitates the analytical work at hand, and is based on socially validated beliefs, and therefore presumably 'realistic' ones, regarding what analysis and the analyst can provide.

In fact, it would be fair to say that the relational critique tends to cast doubt on many of the beliefs that lie at the heart of unconditional positive transference.

The roots of a relational response, like those of so many foundational principles of relational psychoanalysis, have their origins in the writings of Sandor Ferenczi. The analyst, maintained Ferenczi, gives the patient more than a simple insight into the mechanisms of his unconscious mind. Whether he is conscious of it or not, he inevitably also provides the patient with a new and crucial kind of relational experience (Ferenczi and Rank, 1924).

It is possible, says Greenberg, that psychoanalysis has lost much of the cultural prestige that it used to have, and that its philosophical origins make it, today, somewhat suspicious. However, in each analytical dyad a much more important reality is created, in which a series of needs and desires are satisfied. Because of this, the motivation for treatment evolves within the relational matrix created by the analyst and the analysand.

REFERENCES

Alonso Fernández, F. (1982). *Compendio de psiquiatría*. Madrid: Oteo.

Binswanger, L. (1955). *Daseinsanalyse und Psychiatrie*. Berne.

Bowlby, J. (1973). *Attachment and loss. Separation anxiety and anger*. London: Hogarth Press.

Bowlby, J. (1979). *La separación afectiva*. Buenos Aires: Paidós.

Coderch, J. (2001). *La relación paciente-terapeuta.El campo del psicoanálisis y la psicoterapia psicoanalítica*. Barcelona: Paidos.

Dilthey, W. (1948). *Introducción a las ciencias del espíritu*. Madrid-Buenos Aires: Espasa Calpe.

Erickson, E. H. (1960). The problem of ego identity. In M. Stein, A. H. Vidich and D. M. White (Eds.), *Identity and anxiety*. New York: The Free Press.

Fonagy, P. (2000). An open door review of outcome studies in psychoanalysis (www.ipa.org.uk/research/complete.htm). London: IPA.

Fonagy, P. (1996). The future of an empirical psychoanalysis. *British Journal of Psychotherapy*, 13, 106–118.

Freud, A. (1960). *El yo y los mecanismos de defensa*. Buenos Aires: Paidos, Biblioteca del hombre contemporáneo.

Freud, S. (1929a). *Introductory lessons on psychoanalysis*. London: Hogarth Press.
Freud, S. (1929b). *Introductory lessons on psychoanalysis* (complete works). London: Hogarth Press.
Freud, S. (1962). On the grounds for detaching a particular syndrome from neurasthenia under the description 'anxiety neurosis'. *Standard Edition of the complete psychological works of Sigmund Freud* (Vol. 3, pp. 90). London: Hogarth Press.
Freud, S. Fragment of analysis of a case of hysteria. *Standard Edition of the complete psychological works of Sigmund Freud* (Vol. 7, pp. 7–122). London: Hogarth Press.
Freud, S. (150). Repression. *Standard Edition of the complete psychological works of Sigmund Freud* (Vol. 14, pp. 1915). London: Hogarth Press.
Freud, S. (1900). The interpretation of dreams. *Standard Edition of the complete psychological works of Sigmund Freud* (Vol. 4, pp. 163–277). London: Hogarth Press.
Freud, S. (1905). Three essays on the theory of sexuality. *Standard Edition of the complete psychological works of Sigmund Freud* (Vol. 7, pp. 123–231). London: Hogarth Press.
Freud, S. (1910). Leonardo da Vinci and a Memory of his Childhood, *S.E.* (pp. 63–137).
Fromm, E. (1947). *Man for himself.* New York: Penguin.
Fromm, E. (1949). Psychoanalytic characterology and its application to the understanding of culture. In S. S. Sargent and M. W. Smith (Eds.), *Culture and personality*. New York: Jenner-Gren Foundation for Anthropological Resarch.
Heidegger, M. (1951). *El ser y el tiempo*. Mexico City: Fondo Cult. Econ.
Greenberg, J. (1996). Psychoanalytic interaction. *Psychoanal. Inquiry*, 16, 25–38.
Greenberg, J., and Mitchell, S. (1983). *Object relations in psychoanalytic theory*. Cambridge: Harvard University Press.
Greenberg, J., (2001). The analyst participation. A new look. *Journal of the American Psychoanalytical Association*, 49 (2), 359–398.
Grinberg, L. (1962). On a specific aspect of countertransference due to the patient's projective identification. *International Journal of Psychoanalysis*, 43, 436–440.
Horney, K. (1937). *The neurotic personality of our time*. New York.
Horney, K. (1955). *La neurosis y el desarrollo humano*. Buenos Aires: Psique.
Husserl, E. (1940). *Ideas relativas a una fenomenología pura y una filosofía fenomenológica*. Mexico City: Fondo Cult. Econ.
Jaspers, K. (1946). *Psicopatología general*. Buenos Aires: Delta.
Kernberg, O. (1980). *Internal world and external reality*. New York: Jason Aronson.
Kernberg, O. F. (1980). Neurosis, psychosis and the borderline states. In H. I. Kaplan and A. M. Freedman and B. J. Sadock (Eds.), *Textbook of psychiatry* (Vol. Vol 1). Baltimore: Williams and Wilkins.
Kernberg, O. F. (1982). The theory of psychoanalytic psychotherapy. In S. Slipp (Ed.), *Curative factors in dynamic psychotherapy* (pp. 21–43). New York: McGraw-Hill.
Kernberg, O. (1986). *Internal world and external reality. Object relations theory applied.* New York: Jason Aronson.
Kernberg, O. F. (1993). The current status of psychoanalysis. *Journal of the American Psychoanalytic Association*, 41 (1), 45–62.
Kierkegard, S. (1961). *Obras y papeles*. Madrid: Guadarrama.
Klein, M. (1946). Notes on some schizoid mechanisms. In *The Writings of Melanie Klein* (Vol. 1). London: Hogarth Press.
Klein, M. (1969). *La psychanalyse des enfants*. Paris: P.U.F.
Mead, M. (1939). *From South Seas: Coming of age in Samoa. Growing up in New Guinea, sex and temperament*. New York: Morrow.
Mitchell, S. (1988). *Relational concepts in psychoanalysis*. Cambridge: Harvard University Press.
Mitchell, S. (1993). *Hope and dread in psychoanalysis*. New York: Basic Books.

Sartre, J. P. (1961). *El ser y la nada*. Buenos Aires: Ibero América.
Sullivan, H. S. (1927). The onset of schizophrenia. *American Journal of Psychiatry*, 105, 135–139.
Sullivan, H. S. (1953). *The interpersonal theory of psychiatry*. New York: W.W. Norton.
Sullivan, H. S. (1954). *The psychiatric interview*. New York: W.W. Norton.
Sullivan, H. S. (1962). *Schizophrenia as a human process*. New York: Norton, New York.
Sullivan, H. S. (1967). *Clinical studies in psychiatry*. New York: W.W. Norton.
Tizón, J. (1982). *Psicología basada en la relación*. Barcelona: Hora.

6

Relational Aspects of Mental Health

Part 2: Social Factors

UNCLEAR EPIDEMIOLOGICAL FINDINGS

Psychiatric epidemiology has clearly shown the existence of disorders that are typically linked to certain cultures, as well as the higher incidence of certain syndromes in one culture than in another, and different forms of presentation of the same syndromes in different cultures or during different historical periods (Durkheim, 1951). It has also enabled investigators to formulate a number of hypotheses regarding the conditioning factors of symptomatic variation within a single culture.

Differences in the Incidence of Certain Syndromes in Different Cultures

There are certain behaviours which would be considered undoubtedly pathological in our Western society, and which are part of the cultural landscape in others. Many authors cite such behaviours, including *amok* (Malayan race to the death, a word incorporated into English in the phrase 'to run amok'), *latah* (a behaviour involving the imitation of other people's gestures), the so-called 'mad-dog-who-wants-to-die' (headlong race into battle, highly aggressive and with complete disregard for one's own life, which was typical of certain Crow Indians in battle); *berserk* (warlike fierceness of Vikings before battle, also incorporated into English as the phrase 'to go berserk'); *'heart-bursting'* behaviour (Mohave mourning attitudes

(Devereux, 1961)—all attitudes well documented in various transcultural studies.

Moreover, some authors have tried to deny the very existence of some disorders (above all, schizophrenia) in primitive societies, whereas others have shown that they are indeed present in such settings. Lanbscher reported finding schizophrenics among the Tembu, in a paper criticised by Devereux (1961). A review of the literature by Alonso Fernández (1977) showed contradictory opinions in this regard.

Apart from the question of whether or not some disorders exist in certain cultures, what is indeed unquestionable is the difference in the incidence and the prevalence of certain disorders from one culture to another—a phenomenon, of course, also seen in non-psychiatric illnesses, depending on the differing geographical distribution of aetiological factors (e.g., malaria is unknown among the Eskimos, and there is no snow blindness among the Mongos). However, different transcultural epidemiological studies give conflicting incidence and prevalence statistics, which must be attributed more often to the lack of unanimity in their diagnostic criteria than to other factors. In any case, it is indisputable that, for example, the incidence and prevalence of alcoholism and drug addiction present a notable variance in different societies.

Pathoplasty in Mental Disorders

Cultural conditions undoubtedly modify the presentation of mental disorders. Society confers a role on the patient, conditioning the moment when the alteration appears, its shape, and outcome. Everything happens as if the subject's society had said, 'don't get sick, but if you do, do it this or that way'. Thus, the cultural forms of madness are imitated a *grosso modo* by simulators, or unconsciously symbolised in Ganser's syndrome or conversion hysteria. Many erstwhile investigators studying the behaviour of alcoholics in certain districts, such as New York'sonce infamous Bowery, where the prevalence of alcoholism was unusually high, arrived at the conclusion that their inhabitants' strange antics could not be ascribed solely to excessive alcohol consumption. Just as there is a 'culture of poverty', with far-reaching effects on the behaviour of many people, regardless of their actual economic income (as Oscar Lewis observed), other segments of the population present a 'culture of alcoholism', conditioning the behaviour of their members, and the symptoms of alcohol-related illnesses.

Cultural differences at different moments in history also have a deep influence on how symptoms present. Depressive delusions, which only a few decades ago tended to focus on condemnation, and less frequently referred to bankruptcy or illness, are currently much more likely to focus on economic problems than on religious ones or hypochondria. Schizophrenic hallucinations also vary in content from one society to another, or even within the same society over short periods of time, with reference to important local events, and so on.

Variations in Frequency within the Same Culture

Many epidemiological studies have called attention to the difference in the incidence and prevalence of certain illnesses in different social classes. However, different studies often have varying results, due to methodological difficulties. The conclusions that they draw from their data are also ambiguous. For example, regarding the higher frequency of schizophrenia among disfavoured social classes, some authors attribute its prevalence precisely to socio-economic limitations; others prefer to cite possible biological factors associated with belonging to a disfavoured social class; yet others suppose, on the contrary, that schizophrenia itself contributes to the patient's slide down the social scale, which would explain why such subjects are more frequently found in these strata than in others.

An American study, carried out in New Haven by Hollingshead and Redlich (1958), on the prevalence of mental illness with relation to social class is now considered a landmark in sociological research in the field of psychiatry. The study concluded that there was indeed a higher number of mental disorders among subjects belonging to disfavoured social classes, who had access to psychiatric care of a quality inferior to that of subjects from more economically advantaged classes.

RELATION AND COMMUNICATION

General Systems Theory and Mental Pathology

Regarding the genesis of mental disorders, general systems theory states that they derive fundamentally from an alteration in the relationship between members of the family system (synchronic communications alteration). Certain authors, however, attribute a major pathogenic role to certain diachronic characteristics of communication: those derived from the existence of family myths, secrets, and themes.

Sensory deprivation experiments show that the organism requires a minimal level of certain informative inputs to function normally, so that isolation and monotony can produce disassociative phenomena, hallucinatory experiences, and so on. On the contrary, information overload can produce behavioural alterations, as has been shown in rats, and human beings, as well (Miller, 1975).

In severe pathologies, it is known that, for example, difficulty in filtering information can be related to schizophrenic behaviour. A genetically determined metabolic defect could be responsible for diminishing the capabilities of as-yet undiscovered channels involved in processing cognitive information. Schizophrenics' tendency to isolate themselves has been interpreted as an attempt to escape an excess of information, which they are incapable of handling.

Communication in Psychiatry

It is not surprising (Ruesch, 1975) that mental health professionals have become interested in the matter-energy or information transactions in the systems they work with, which has familiarised them with the basic computer-science concept of feedback. This term means that the impact of a message is sent back to the information control centre, so that the observed effects can be taken into account on the next step.

Human communications operations are based on two different symbol systems:

—*Non-verbal communication* is based on an analogic principle. Man develops a small-scale inner model of the world, based on recognition of similarities and differences, and which enables him to prepare the quick reactions necessary for survival in the face of external events.

—*Verbal communication* is based on a digital principle. When someone has time to analyse a situation, he uses words or numbers, which are able to denote detailed aspects of events.

Distortions in communication among human beings can produce behavioural alterations (Ruesch, 1975) able to lead an individual to commit non-gratifying or unsuccessful actions that are intolerable to the group. The therapist, in psychoanalysis, tries to modify the patient's body of information, deliberately imparting new information, or he may try to mobilise information of which the patient is not conscious. In social therapies, he may try to modify the patient's forms of response by modifying his surrounding environment.

Therapeutic communication in individual psychotherapy is used to increase the patient's self-knowledge; to verbalise unnecessary presuppositions; to modify attitudes; to increase tolerance of others' conduct; to formulate objectives; and to qualify the patient's personal lifestyle. In group psychotherapy, more attention is paid to the impact of one person's communications and actions on others, so that the therapist may clarify rules, specify roles, and discuss the group's organisation.

Psychotherapy exercises its influence through some fundamental processes (Ruesch, 1975): *recognition* refers to the therapist's response to the patient's presence, and his intention to communicate; *understanding* refers to the establishment, in the therapist's mind, of an appropriate model of the patient's behaviour.

REFERENCES

Alonso Fernández, F. (1977). *Fundamentos de la Psiquiatría actual*. Madrid: Paz Montalvo.

Devereux, G. (1961). Mohave ethnopsychiatry and suicide: The psychiatric knowledge and the psychic disturbances of an Indian tribe. *Bureau of American Ethnology Bulletin*. Washington, D.C.: United States Government Printing Office.

Durkheim, E. (1951). *Suicide: A study of sociology*. New York: The Free Press.

Hollingshead, A. B., and Redlich, F. C. (1958). *Social class and mental illness*. New York: John Wiley and Sons.

Miller, J. G. (1975). General systems theory. In A. M. Freedman and H. I. Kaplan and B. J. Sadock (Eds.), *Comprehensive textbook of psychiatry*. Baltimore: Williams and Wilkins Co.

Ruesch, J. (1975). Communication and psychiatry. In A. M. Friedman, H. I. Kaplan and B. J. Sadock (Eds.), *Comprehensive textbook of psychiatry*. Baltimore: The Williams and Wilkins Co.

7

Clinical Assessment

Created in Europe during the first half of the 19th century, descriptive psychopathology (Berrios, 1984), the foundation of clinical assessment, comprises a vocabulary, a syntaxis, and certain propositions about the nature of the language and behaviour of mental patients. Since language and behaviour are charged with meanings which must be interpreted through theories, a truly atheoretical description, based on pure observation, is impossible (Berrios, 1997).

In our times, the progressive introduction of the scientific method has given rise to the development of experimental psychopathology.

DESCRIPTIVE PSYCHOPATHOLOGY

As discussed in Chapter 1, the classification of the sciences set forth by the so-called Freiburg School, which distinguishes between *natural sciences* and *human sciences*, led, in the terrain of psychopathology, to the opposition between *understanding* (of meanings and intentions) belonging to the human sciences, causal *explanation*, which could only be used, in psychiatry, in the realm of *exogenous* or *organic psychoses*. A current within this school (*comprehensive and biographical psychology*) tried to understand the individual's life and describe it 'in its uniqueness', but the school that had the most subsequent influence on psychiatry was developed by Karl Jaspers, with his *General Psychopathology*.

In psychopathology, Jaspers (1946), as we have already discussed, used phenomenology in order to try to understand the pathological experience, eliminating remaining elements by a process called *phenomenological reduction*, which forces the interviewer to situate himself vis-à-vis the patient's experiences not as a mere observer, but as someone trying to experience them, and act them out for him (Guimón, 2001). This leads to an *understanding*, or *vision of the psyche obtained from within*, as opposed to an *explanation* that aims to find objective, causal relationships. Piaget (1967) criticised this dichotomy, which manifests two uncompromising, but indivisible, aspects of knowledge, and said that the status that it enjoyed for decades was, to a large extent, responsible for the fact that the human sciences had progressed less than was originally hoped. In any case, the use of this procedure and these differentiations has fallen into disuse in today's clinical practice.

Something similar may be said of the concepts of *process, development*, and *reaction* discussed previously, and which in the current semiology are found only indirectly present in some chapters referring to reactions to stress, schizophrenia, and psychic syndromes due to cerebral disorders. Altogether, these types of morbid development, so dear to the classical psychopathologists, have fallen almost completely out of use, and have, for young psychiatrists, 'theological', if not an esoteric, connotations (Guimón, 2001).

For its part, so-called *existential psychology*, in its clinical and descriptive aspects, above all in everything regarding affect (*existential analysis*), is based on Scheler's classification of feelings by strata. Whereas, as we have pointed out, phenomenology aims to limit itself to observing, sensing, and reflecting, existential analysis not only observes, senses, and reflects, but also interprets. Existential analysis demands, in fact, that the therapist participate in the patient's existence, in a reciprocal 'you/me' relationship (Zutt, 1958). This tendency had a certain resonance in Central Europe, above all insofar as it referred to the doctor-patient relational dynamic, and even today it still has some followers. However, like other phenomenological concepts, the terms and techniques of existential analysis no longer interest most professionals.

The Phenomenological Method

The so-called experimental method can be used rigorously, as we have discussed, in mental health research, especially in biological research. But let us not think that this experimental method is the only way to further knowledge in our field. The ideographic or historico-cultural method, and the phenomenological method, even though they have not been submitted to experimentation in the strictest sense of the word, have made undoubted contributions to advances in the field of psychopathology (Guimón, 2001). Finally, in psychoanalysis, which functions with its own method, it has also provided important mental health findings.

According to Husserl (1940), psychophysiology and psychophysics can only explain the external structure of experiences, not their essence, which is the aspect that interests phenomenology, which must transcend empirical phenomena, with their concrete data, to capture through phenomenological analysis the universal essence, or *eidos*, of all phenomena. In the realm of perception, for example, it would extract from the perceptive phenomenon the *eidos* or essence of all possible perception.

From a phenomenologist standpoint, the aim of psychology is to describe our states of consciousness; however, according to Husserl, conscience is intentionality, directed towards anything exterior to the individual: 'all consciousness is consciousness of something.' Psychology thus describes, by means of 'participatory intuition' the intentionalities of consciousness.

It was Jaspers who applied Husserl's system to psychopathology. In his view, we must 'act out intuitively those psychic states that patients really experience, consider them according to their relationships of affinity, delimit them and differentiate them as strictly as possible, and apply precise terminology'. We must situate ourselves vis-à-vis the patient's morbid life experiences 'not as mere observers, but trying to experience them and act them out for ourselves'.

Throughout most of his later career, Jaspers devoted himself more to philosophy than to clinical practice, and the phenomenological psychologists and psychiatrists who came after him tended to follow this criterion of phenomenological reductionism only very relatively. In our times, these interesting concepts have fallen out of favour, although they are included, to a certain extent, in the general guidelines for carrying out a clinical interview (Guimón, 2001) and in some 'humanist' psychotherapies.

Binswanger's existential analytical method (Binswanger, 1955), applied to mental health, continues to be of some interest today in the assessment of reactions to life events, and in psychoses; however, as early as Zutt (1958) it was argued that they could not be linked to nosography.

Is Descriptive Psychopathology Useful Today?

Given the acceptance enjoyed today by experimental approaches to descriptive psychopathology, it is worth asking to what extent the proud, new science of psychiatry demands that those who practise it be familiar with the now-forgotten tenets of descriptive psychopathology.

The prevailing ignorance among mental health professionals (admittedly somewhat less so in psychiatrists) regarding psychiatric semiology, their manifest inability to define basic terms such as hallucination, illusion, pseudoperception, delusion, overvalued ideas, confusion, perplexity, stupor, catalepsy, and so on; the ease with which they accept data from assessment scales badly translated from English–all of this is seriously compromising the validity of their findings and psychopathological research (Guimón, 2001). The basic psychiatric syndromes will continue to exist for decades to come, and their reliable diagnosis will continue to be impossible unless we recur to descriptive psychopathology, which today has at its disposal more or less structured interviews to facilitate their assessment.

EXPERIMENTAL PSYCHOPATHOLOGY

During the 1950s, interest in diagnosis grew when new, efficient medication appeared; another fresh wave of interest came later, with the discovery of specific treatments for certain disorders, and of biological markers with the potential to provide concurrent validation of diagnoses, and enable clinicians to prescribe more appropriate treatment. A new generation of biological psychiatrists started to take over the Departments of Psychiatry in the United States, replacing the older, more psychoanalytically oriented generation. The third edition of the American Psychiatric Association's *Diagnostic and Statistical Manual* (1980), known as the *DSM-III*, even though it aimed to be atheoretical, was really based on a medical model, and aimed to facilitate the adoption of more or less 'aetiological' treatments. This is why, although the symptoms were originally taken from traditional descriptive psychopathology, 'experimental' psychopathology was introduced progressively, backed by major developments in what we have come to call the *cognitive neurosciences*. Soon, a series of 'dimensional' visions of personality (such as the 'five great factors' theory, Cloninger's seven factors, or Livesley's 18 dimensions) were found to be more useful when seeking correlations with neuropsychological or biochemical markers.

The Neo-Kraepelinians

World psychiatry, so globalised today, has been hugely influenced by the group of investigators in the United States which, since the 1970s, has tried to elaborate a scientific approach to diagnosis able to avoid aetiological references, focusing instead on detailed clinical case descriptions, as Kraepelin (1920) had done, in order to achieve the aim of reliable diagnoses. This movement, which Klerman (1978) dubbed 'neo-Kraepelinian', defends the importance of classification in psychiatry, opposes the psychoanalytical perspective, and is highly interested in research. These authors have carried out a persistent effort to come up with methods for the reliable detection of certain psychiatric syndromes by examining their symptoms and evolution. However, they have attempted to immediately raise these syndromes to the rank of illnesses, trying to attribute them, too hastily, to biological alterations in general, or cerebral alterations (Guimón, 1990).

And we say 'too hastily' because, in reality, we are forced to accept the limited objectivity of the measurement methods used in psychopathology. Indeed, when we study organic cerebral disorders, we are looking for 'physical' criteria, but when we study functional psychoses (e.g., schizophrenia), we have to content ourselves with looking, not for criteria, but for 'indicators' – variables related to the psychopathological phenomenon.

Phenomenologists used subjective methods ranging from empathy to the so-called *immediate impression*, as well as the traditional clinical history. Later, *focal* methods were described, interviews aimed at stimulating specific areas of the subject's mental processes, facilitating more structured responses in these areas. If interviews are conducted in a more structured manner (e.g., personality questionnaires and assessment scales), then more quantifiable clinical observations are obtained, but in reality, they are not any more objective (Guimón, 1981). When other kinds of tests are introduced, as well–such as cognitive tests, behavioural response tests, and psychophysiological measurements–we can refer to 'quasi-objective' methods, but only completely involuntary and unconscious physiological measures (e.g., cerebral neurophysiological measures, the new neuro-imaging techniques, or biochemical tests) can be considered 'objective'. Even in the case of these methods, as we have already observed, there are many intervening variables, such as motivation, affect, adaptation, introspective elaboration, personality type, and socio-economic level (Guimón, 1998).

Over the last ten years, all aspects of medicine have been under scrutiny. Both the financial backers of clinical services and their programme directors have become more and more convinced of the utility of *evidence-based medicine* (Sackett et al., 1996). Clinical judgement is no longer accepted as a sufficient reason for offering psychiatric treatment. Increasingly both national policy recommendations and local health care administration decisions are made based on proof of their efficiency.

Evidence-Based Mental Health

Evidence-based mental health tries, in clinical practice, to make decisions regarding the individual care of mental patients based on the best existing evidence (see Chapter 2). However, this evidence, widely disseminated in clinical guidelines, has limitations, because in many areas there is only a small body of research, or it has been conducted using populations very different from those in the clinician's own setting. In addition, the recommended interventions are not often available to any professional, such as certain expensive medications or highly sophisticated psychotherapies (Holloway, 2001).

As Fonagy (1996) put it, evidence-based medicine was founded on the ideal that decisions regarding the care of individual patients should involve the conscientious, explicit, and judicious use of the best current evidence. This focus has been strongly defended, particularly in North America and Western Europe. The arguments in its favour include: more efficient resource utilisation; better clinical knowledge; better communication with patients; its potential for identifying the best health care methods, and enabling patients and professionals to make better-informed decisions. These are good reasons, but all of them were as relevant to medicine in the past as they are today. So why the current insistence on this approach?.

Fonagy's answer is that the movement is based on economic considerations: on the hope that the organisation of health care will be able to cut its spiralling costs by finding the most profitable option within the range of available treatments. Both governments and insurance companies find the idea of allocating health resources on the basis of evidence to be quite attractive. In the United States, for example, it has been suggested that health care funds cover interventions only if sufficient evidence exists they will produce the desired effects. Many politicians and administrators affirm that only those interventions that, according to available evidence, can be shown to work, should be paid.

The Experimental Method

The scientific, or experimental method advocated by Galileo Galilei (1600–1680) and Francis Bacon (1561–1626), and later enhanced by Descartes's concept of 'methodical doubt' and 'the criteria of evidence' consists of observing significant facts, forming hypotheses to explain them, and then submitting them to experimental observation. Thus, a series of propositions can be established and ordered hierarchically in such a way that some serve as a basis for others, with the more general propositions being formulated as laws. The term *experimental design* refers to five interrelated activities that are required for any investigation using scientific or experimental hypotheses: 1) formulating a hypothesis, and planning data collection and analysis in order to prove it; 2) formulating the guidelines to follow in proving the hypothesis; 3) collecting data in accordance with the designed plan; 4) data analysis in accordance with the plan; 5) making a decision regarding the hypothesis, based on the guidelines, and inductive inferences concerning the probable truth or falsehood of the research hypothesis.

The term *experimental design* is also used in a stricter sense, referring to a type of planning used when assigning the experiment's subjects to experimental conditions, and sometimes to the statistical analysis associated with such a plan. The investigator should use this procedure because it enables the resulting data to be comparable with the results of other studies.

In any case, statistical tests are useless if the assessment of variables is not carried out with sensitive instruments that will provide reliable, valid measures.

REFERENCES

Berrios, G. E. (1984). Descriptive psychopathology: A conceptual history. *J. Psychol. Med.*, 14, 303–313.

Berrios, G. E. (1997). *The history of mental symptoms*. Cambridge: Cambridge University Press.

Binswanger, L. (1955). *Daseinsanalyse und Psychiatrie*. Berne.

Fonagy, P. (1996). The future of an empirical psychoanalysis. *British Journal of Psychotherapy, 13*, 106–118.

Guimón, J. (1981). Reflexiones sobre el carácter científico de la Psiquiatría. *Psiquis*, 2, 118–125.

Guimón, J. (1990). *Psiquiatras: De brujos a burócratas*. Barcelona: Salvat.

Guimón, J. (1998). *La profession de psychiatre. Evolution et devenir*. Paris: Masson.

Guimón, J. (2001). Prologue. In J. I. Eguiluz (Ed.), *Introducción a la Psicopatología* (pp. 19–24). Madrid: Wyeth.

Holloway, F. (2001). Balancing clinical value and finite resources. In G. Thornicroft and G. Szmukler (Eds.), *Textbook of community psychiatry* (pp. 167–179). New York: Oxford University Press.

Husserl, E. (1940). *Ideas relativas a una fenomenología pura y una filosofía fenomenológica*. Mexico City: Fondo Cult. Econ.

Jaspers, K. (1946). *Psicopatología general*. Buenos Aires: Delta.

Klerman, G. L. (1978). The evolution of a scientific nosology. In J. C. Shershow (Ed.), *Schizophrenia: Science and practice*. Cambridge: Harvard University Press

Kraeplin, E. (1920). *Psyhiatrie, ein Lehrbuch für Studierende und Aertze*. Leipzig: A. Label.

Piaget, J. (1967). Classification des sciences et principaux courants épistémologiques contemporains. In J. Piaget (Ed.), *Logique et connaissance scientifique* (pp. 1149–1224). Paris: Gallimard-Encyclopédie Pléiade.

8

Relational Assessment

Dynamic Aspects

Psychoanalysis is (not only, but fundamentally) a clinical intervention. Patients and society demand proof of its efficacy, and therefore we need to standardise our techniques and establish reliable, valid methods for assessing them. Fonagy (2000) expressed scepticism about the value of this 'evidence' in supporting the generalisation of psychoanalytical treatments, since he considers it improbable that, even in the face of overwhelming evidence in favour of this relatively expensive treatment, resources will ever be available to provide psychoanalysis to a significant proportion of those who need it.

In any case, it should be noted that psychoanalytical research is inevitably a compromise between the usual clinical procedures and the demands of experimental science.

SEMIOLOGICAL ELEMENTS

The psychoanalyst uses a semiology corresponding to the descriptions of mental functioning provided by the different psychoanalytical schools over the years.

Thought

During treatment, the psychoanalyst's interest centres on the patient's *thought resistances* and *associations* in reaction to his interpretations. In the patient's thoughts, there is a *manifest content* and a *latent content*, as well as *primary* and *secondary thought processes*.

Inner World

From an object-relations viewpoint, we can refer to an *inner world* and *object representations*, as well as a set of *subordinate functions*, such as *empathy*, the *quality of self-objects representation*, the affective *tone* of relations, the ability to maintain them and to invest in them emotionally, and so on.

Libidinal Evolution

The *libido* (mental representation of sexual instincts) is satisfied in different parts of the body during the child's first years of development, which marks the personality's different evolutionary phases or stages (oral, anal, phallic, latent, genital). Individuals' greater or lesser *fixation* on these phases will have a major influence on their adult personalities, and their proneness to different mental illnesses.

The *tanathos* (mental representation of the death drive, from which aggressiveness derives) follows a parallel evolution.

Types of Anxiety

Rycroft (1986) described the following forms of anxiety: *automatic* or *primary* anxiety (the ego's response to an accumulation of stimuli); *signal* anxiety (the ego's alert mechanism in the face of threat); *castration* anxiety (stemming from threats to sexual functioning, bodily harm, or loss of status); *separation* anxiety (fear of separation from objects that are essential to survival); *depressive* anxiety (fear of the individual's own hostility towards 'good objects); *paranoid* or *persecutory* anxiety (fear of being attacked by 'bad objects'); *real* or *objective* anxiety (in the face of external dangers); *neurotic* anxiety (in the face of internal dangers); *psychotic* anxiety (referring to primary, paranoid, and sometimes depressive anxiety which threatens the individual's very identity); *generalised* or *free-floating* anxiety; and *acute* anxiety or *panic attack* (which refers, in psychoanalysis, to the forms of presentation of *signal* anxiety).

Defence Mechanisms

Sigmund Freud and Anna Freud described a set of defence mechanisms against anxiety (see chapter 5).

Processes of Change

In the course of analytic work, *processes of change* and *resistance* to change occur. Terms such as *repetition compulsion, negative therapeutic reaction* and *guilt* are used.

Limitations of Psychoanalytical Semiology

Psychoanalytical semiology suffers from low inter-rater reliability. Although some authors have published attempts to define psychoanalytical concepts in dictionary form, different psychoanalytical schools and different authors assign different meanings to the same terms. Obviously, it would be in our interest to agree, if not on true operative definition criteria, at least on a glossary of psychoanalytical terms of reference.

CRITIQUES OF PSYCHOANALYTICAL ASSESSMENT

The scientific validity of the psychoanalytical method has been the target of much criticism. To verify its validity, there are four possible perspectives (Shakow, 1960): developmental, experimental (using animal or human subjects); transcultural, and that of the psychoanalytical interview (Fonagy, 1996, 2000).

Psychoanalytical research is usually carried out through studying the sessions of individual patients (the so-called *single-case methodology*). Fonagy (2000) observes that it would be more advantageous to study series of cases, as, for example, Clarkin et al. (1991) did with patients suffering from borderline personality disorders, grouped with a combined *DSM-IV* and *structural object-relations* theory approach. Psychoanalytical theories are rarely able to predict the specific disorders that an individual may develop given a certain type of early life experiences.

The psychoanalytical interview technique is, therefore, the basic instrument of psychoanalytical investigation. The psychoanalytical interview makes manifest some of the basic phenomena that constitute its theoretical foundations. These phenomena appear repeatedly and in various degrees of intensity, under relatively controlled conditions. On the other hand, given the very special conditions under which psychoanalysis occurs, the interviews provide psychologically significant material, which can rarely be attained with laboratory experiments. For example, procedures such as free association offer possibilities that other approaches do not. Finally, interviews provide us with an exceptional opportunity to make a relational connection among internal psychological states, and some specific aspects of external behaviour that are manifested by the patient or observed by the analyst.

Be that as it may, the psychoanalytical interview presents many drawbacks as a research method.

Data Collection Problems

There are serious data collection problems, due principally to the fact that the data are collected by a therapist who is simultaneously an observer and a participant; i.e., the data are limited by the human observer's limitations as an instrument. Moreover, it is difficult to combine research and therapy, because the demand for the analyst to give the patient *free-floating attention* (to offer a *third ear*) is the antithesis of objective observation.

It is possible to improve on transcriptions of sessions, by filming interviews or disassociating the functions of the psychoanalyst and the observer. The data thus obtained could be complemented by recording the analyst's own associations and feelings after the session. However, these techniques involve an invasion of patients' privacy, and place demands on the therapist that are difficult to ignore. Finally, the study of the enormous amount of material thus collected is very cumbersome.

Such psychoanalytical interviews offer merely descriptive facts to the investigator, which naturally have very subjective value. There have been many high-profile debates regarding whether, in reality, the psychoanalyst can be considered an investigator during the interview. There are those who believe that this is indeed the case, because at the end of the day, he is continually trying to prove hypotheses in the form of interpretations. Shakow (1960) differed on this point, arguing that, in a real-world situation, it is impossible to isolate individual variables and follow them systematically, and so he prefers to call this form of interview a *semi-naturalist approach*. The psychoanalyst, for his part, is an integral element of a treatment process, more than an experimental manipulator of the situation, which limits his objectivity. Finally, the prediction value of the results (such as the patient's degree of adaptation in his daily life, for example) is limited by the multiplicity of concurrent factors, except insofar as they refer to relationships that take place in the analytical setting, which can be examined quite rigorously.

Data Obtained from Psychoanalytical Interviews

Data obtained from psychoanalytical interviews are 'soft' (changing, diffuse), so that filming the interviews can improve the assessment of some variables (vocal tone, gestures). Unexpressed thoughts and feelings, and hidden physiological responses, cannot be filmed, but the analyst can reconstruct, in part, after the session, some of these non-verbalised expressions occurring during the session, but not without a certain degree of distortion. Investigators should not demand that the patient make the same reconstruction effort, because free association obtained after the session would interfere with the psychoanalytical process.

For now, it also remains impossible for us to collect the patient's hidden physiological reactions. These responses, presumably significant for understanding what has occurred, have no special intercommunicative value for the therapist who, as far as we know, is rarely aware of them;

however, they undoubtedly play a highly significant role in the patient's intercommunicative process, and therefore, indirectly, in what is communicated to the therapist. This is probably true for the therapist, as well.

Data Analysis

Regarding data analysis, we can distinguish three major problems: 1) Those related to the moment (the time) when the data were collected (e.g., what happens during the session itself, events reported several weeks after they occur, or data referring to early childhood). Rapaport (1960) has noted the fact that, even to understand the 'here and now' it is necessary to have some kind of material from childhood (regardless of whether these involve real events or early phantasies). 2) Data regarding the therapy itself obviously have a different degree of relevance. 3) Verbal or kinaesthetic data (fine and gross bodily movements) are easy to assess from films, but not hidden physiological responses.

In addition, the therapist should recuse himself as a data evaluator, and use the services of a professional data analyst. The type of data that we can collect are divided into various types which enable us to look at different relational problems: 1) the psychoanalytical process, e.g., transference, resistance, interventions, interpretations, and reconstructions; 2) aspects of the patient's relational adaptations, which include symptoms and defences, and certain conditions that modify them; 3) problems related to the discharge and inhibition of needs, the forms taken by attempts to fight against these needs, and the changes that occur in these forms, and so on.

In sum, it is clear that, even under optimal conditions, it is very difficult for a psychoanalytical interview to meet the demands of the so-called experimental method.

PSYCHODIAGNOSTIC ASSESSMENT

The so-called *dynamic psychodiagnostic* plays a less important role in mental health today than it did a few decades ago. Dynamic assessment, in any case, naturally runs into greater difficulties than measuring other characteristics of patients.

A diagnosis in dynamic psychiatry today should take into account such factors as ego strength or weakness, the nature of the unconscious (Luborsky et al., 1998), defence mechanisms, and superego structure. The influence of the British object-relations school has led to stressing the importance of assessing family relationships, transferential modules, and object relations in general.

There are a number of instruments for comprehensive psychodynamic assessment, such as Bellak's Ego Function Assessment (EFA) questionnaire (Bellak, 1973); another developed by Weinryb et al. (1991) for the Karolinska Institute (KAPP); and the Cierpka's *Operationalised Psychodynamic Diagnostics* (Cierpka et al., 1995).

Other questionnaires have been developed to measure specific dynamic aspects, such as ego strength, object relations, coping styles, or defence mechanisms. In addition, different psychodynamically oriented studies have used instruments to measure modification variables in psychotherapy (Frank, 1968; Rapaport, 1968; National Institute of Mental Health, 1975; Piper, 1984; Hamilton, 1993; Strup, 1984; Zanello, 2000), sometimes grouped together in the form of batteries. MacKenzie (1987) created a *Core Battery* which was adapted for use in Bilbao (Guimón, 1988); however, it turned out that it was not very sensitive when dealing with non-severe pathologies. Recently, we have created our own battery (Guimón et al, 2000).

When the American Psychiatric Association (APA) developed its revolutionary DSM-III classification, a group of prestigious psychoanalysts failed to convince the APA to include an additional, psychodynamic axis. However, Axis II included, within the personality disorders, categories that had clearly been influenced by psychoanalytical thought. The fact that the DSM-III recommended always filling in the diagnosis with a descriptive personality category left a certain margin for a dynamic understanding of the patient's diagnosis. The DSM-IV (Frances, First, and Pincus, 1997) proposed an additional scale of defence mechanisms as an optional addition to Axis II.

The World Health Organization's new classification, the ICD-10, arranges things differently by including personality disorders as just another section of the main axis. In addition, personality disorders are defined in a purely descriptive manner, without considering differentiations of a dynamic variety.

In reality, perhaps it is preferable for psychiatric classifications to remain based exclusively on descriptive criteria, and for investigators to try to define parallel psychodynamic classifications until the latter are sufficiently developed to be able to converge with the former.

Projective Tests

Over the last two decades, major progress has been made in dynamic psychiatry assessment, both in term of psychopathology assessment and in assessment of the psychotherapeutic process, which we shall not discuss here. Regarding psychodynamic diagnosis, projective tests have been less frequently used; these include Rorschach's psychodiagnostic test, or

Bellak's Thematic Apperception Test (TAT), as well as questionnaires, such as the Minnesota Multiphasic Personality Inventory (MMPI). All of these tests represent an attempt to reflect the subject's pathological reality, in measurable terms, but also going beyond mere symptomatic description. In sum, their creators were searching for a reliable measurement of intrapsychic functions. However, most research using these instruments has shown that they are not very reliable. In addition, the assessments using these instruments are based on drive theory or ego psychology, and the forms of mental action are defined in terms of *fixation points* and *ego functions*. In order for them to be useful, the instruments derived from these theories demand very experienced personnel in order to be used properly.

The Ego Function Assessment Test

A major step forward in psychodynamic assessment was made by Leopoldo Bellak, who, after starting out in the 1950s investigating the aetiopathogeny and evolution of schizophrenia, focused his research on developing a more effective assessment instrument. This culminated in the publication of a paper in 1968, under the auspices of the National Institute of Mental Health (NIMH), proposing an assessment scale for ego functions, with both a diagnostic and prognostic objective, and which summed up the work of the Menninger Foundation in its effort to link the dynamic functioning of schizophrenia with its clinical pathology, thus creating a reliable and valid predictor of long-term treatment prospects.

This scale, the EFA, is based on a psychoanalytical approach, and comprises twelve subscales corresponding to as many ego functions. The quantitative assessment is made with data provided by the patient using an intermediate instrument, a semistructured interview with 144 questions. After its definitive validation, the original version of the EFA has been widely used in English-speaking settings, applied as a predictor of different pathologies, from schizophrenia to personality disorders. In spite of this, critical examination of this instrument has aroused a considerable number of objections to its reliability. Therefore, although we were considering the possibility of validating a Spanish version of the EFA, we finally decided to abandon the idea, due to the lack of guarantee that we could later use it in our clinical practice.

DSM-IV Defence Mechanisms Scale

The DSM-IV, to meet the needs of psychodynamic professionals, has created a scale of 27 predominant defence mechanisms and coping styles, which can also be listed in Axis II, and is defined according to seven different levels.

Relational Capacity Assessment

Some interesting relational capacity assessment systems have been proposed, including Horney's *interpersonal nosology*, an idea also taken up by Fromm, and Leary's *circumplex model*; however, they have not been widely used.

Schutz described, in 1958, the *Fundamental Interpersonal Relations Orientation* (FIRO), for creating an interpersonal profile of the individual. It has been used in some research with the aim of studying the selection of roommates with a 'compatibility index', and seems useful for predicting interpersonal behaviour in a psychiatric ward.

Another method, closer to clinical reality, involves conducting an interpersonally oriented initial interview. Many of the interview techniques proposed by Sullivan (1954) are useful in such a situation. For example, the interviewer tries to determine whether the patient is able to make comments on the process of the interview in which he is involved, or to accept the interviewer's comments on it. The interviewer also observes whether the patient is tense, but denies it when asked, and whether he is able to detect the most unpleasant or pleasant parts of the interview. The patient is asked about his interpersonal and group relationships and his closest friends, and about his degree of intimacy with people of both sexes. He may also be asked for detailed information about the formal and informal groups (such as clubs) to which he belongs.

Along the same lines, Frank (1968) described an *interpersonal relations interview* which enabled him to establish hypotheses regarding interpersonal behaviour.

The Bel Air Battery

At the University of Geneva Medical School's Department of Psychiatry, we use a battery of tests developed by the author (Guimón, 2000).

REFERENCES

Bellak, L. (1968). Research on ego function patterns: A progress report. Rating scales for scoring ego functions from clinical interview material. In L. Bellak and L. Loeb (Eds.), *The schizophrenic syndrome*. New York: Grune and Stratton.

Cierpka, M., et al. (1995). Die erste Version einer Operationalisierten Psychodynamischen Diagnostik. *Psychoterapeut*, 40 (69–78).

Clarkin, J. F., Marziali, E., & Munroe-Blum, H. (1991). Group and family treatments for borderline personality disorder. *Hospital Community Psychiatry*, *42*, 1038–1043.

Fonagy, P. (2000). An open door review of outcome studies in psychoanalysis (www.ipa.org.uk/research/complete.htm). London: IPA.

Fonagy, P. (1996). The future of an empirical psychoanalysis. *British Journal of Psychotherapy*, 13, 106–118

Frances, A., First, M. B., and Pincus, H. A. (Eds.). (1997). DSM-IV, *Guía de uso*. Barcelona: Masson, Barcelona

Frank, K. (1968). Indications for psychoanalytic group therapy. *Psyche*, 22(778–785).

Guimón, J., Gonzalez-Pinto, A., Sanz, C., & Gonzalez-Ceinos, M. (1988). Efectos terapeuticos en un programa de sensibilizacion grupal. *Psiquis*, *1*, 11–28.

Guimón, J., Erehnsperger, S., Weber, B., Fredenrich, A., Vucetic, V., Zanello, A., Zinetti, A., & Maercker, A. (2000). Evaluación de la psicoterapia grupal en la asistencia psiquiátrica: la Batería " Bel-Air ". *Psiquis*, *21*(6), 277–287.

Guimón, J. (2001). *Intervenciones en psiquiatría comunitaria*. Madrid: Core

Guimón, J., Gonzalez-Pinto, A., Sanz, C., & Gonzalez-Ceinos, M. (1988). Efectos terapeuticos en un programa de sensibilizacion grupal. *Psiquis*, *1*, 11–28.

Guimón, J., Erehnsperger, S., Weber, B., Fredenrich, A., Vucetic, V., Zanello, A., Zinetti, A., & Maercker, A. (2000). Evaluación de la psicoterapia grupal en la asistencia psiquiátrica: la Batería " Bel-Air ". *Psiquis*, *21*(6), 277–287.

Hamilton, J. D., Courville, T. J., Richman, B., Hanson, P., Swanson, C., & Stafford, J. (1993). Quality assessment and improvement in group psychotherapy. *American Journal Of Psychiatry*, *150*(2), 316–320.

Luborsky, L., and Crits-Christoph, P. (1998). *Understanding transference: The core conflictual relationship theme method*. Washington, DC: American Psychological Association Press.

McKenzie, K., & Dies, R. (1982). *Core Battery clinical outcome results*. Calgary: University of Calgary.

Piper, W. E., Debbane, E. G., Bienvenu, J. P., & Garant, J. (1984). A comparative study of four forms of psychotherapy. *Journal of Consulting and Clinical Psychology*, *52*, 268–279.

Rapaport, D. (1960). The Structure of Psychoanalysis. *Psychological Issues*, *II*(2).

Rycroft, Y. (1986). *Psychoanalysis and beyond*. London: Hogarth Press.

Strup, H., & Binder, J. (1984). *Psychotherapy in a New Key*. New York: Basic Books.

Sullivan, H. S. (1954). *The Psychiatric Interview*. New York.: W.W. Norton.

Weinryb, R., Rössel, R., and Asberg, M. (1991). The Karolinska psychodynamic profile II. Interdisciplinal and cross-cultural reliability. *Acta Psychiatrica Scandinavica*, 83, 73–76.

Weinryb, R., Gustavsson, J. P., Asberg, M., and Rössel, R. J. (1992). Stability over time of character assessment using a psychodynamic instrument and personality inventories. *Acta Psychiatr. Scand*. 1992.

Weinryb, R. (1992). *Construction and evaluation of a rating instrument for psychodynamic assessment. The Karolinska Psychodynamic Profile (KAPP)*. Stockholm: Kongl Carolinska Medico Chirurgiska Institutet.

Zanello, A., Weber Rouget, B., Maier, K., & Gex-Fabry, M. (2000). Le questionnaire de fonctionnement social (QFS): premiers résultats de validation auprès d'une population controle: Paper presented at the thhird scientifical research meeting of the University Hospital Vaud-Genève.

9

Relational Assessment

Social Aspects

Although the importance of the patient's environment in psychological disorders' genesis and forms of presentation has been known for centuries, it is only during the period between the two World Wars that attempts were made to conceptualise these inter-relationships. Foulkes (1964), influenced by the work of Goldstein (1940) on the central nervous system, by Gestalt psychology's postulated relationship between *figure* and *background,* and by Lewin's field theory (1935), proposed what he called the *reticular theory of neurosis*. According to Foulkes, mental disorders are generated within the *plexus* of the family, develop in the context of the groups to which the patient later belongs, and can be treated ideally in therapeutic groups. Several decades later, the application of general systems theory to studying alterations in communication, especially in mental patients' families, marked another major step for research based on this approach. Finally, the application of findings on institutional organisation to the study of therapeutic settings has notably enriched our understanding of the environment in which mental illness develops.

Some research projects can be carried out by routine collection of social data, group interviews, observation during active participation in a task, description of routine tasks, and so on. However, surveys using a more complex design are often necessary.

EPIDEMIOLOGICAL METHODS

Epidemiology is a branch of medical ecology (Wing et al., 1974) that examines the relationship between human illness and the environment in which human beings live. As far as mental illness is concerned, epidemiologists are not only interested in the distribution of disorders across human populations and in estimating their rates of frequency, but also (Morris, 1970) in studying their course (and therefore, their treatment, management, and prognoses) and service organisation.

Estimating Mental Illnesses' Rates of Frequency

With the data obtained in epidemiological studies, it is indeed possible to find historical trends, describe the health of a community, determine individual risks, complement the clinical description of illnesses, identify syndromes, and discover causes. It is also possible to answer questions regarding a population's needs, and the number of persons who contact the existing services, which provides valuable orientation on the evolution of mental health and psychological disorders in a community.

Semiological Elements

The most frequently studied measures are the *incidence,* which is the number of new cases in a population during a period of time, and *prevalence,* i.e., the number of cases present in a given population.

Another important measure for a disorder is its *life prevalence,* which is the probability that an individual will develop it over the course of a lifetime.

The investigator should have precise operational definitions, in order to distinguish between subjects who are cases and normal subjects. Therefore, each study should establish a *case definition,* including the following elements: the definition should be appropriate for the study, the terms used in the definition should be sufficiently precise (features present), and there should be some artificial limit or *cut-off point* of severity.

Methods

Some of these variables may be studied using simple statistical description procedures, or more complex ones (such as *case registers*), and comparing these findings with data from other places. The case definition, using symptomatic or syndromic measurements from scales or questionnaires, is not very difficult as far as the major psychiatric illnesses – such as organic mental disorders and psychoses – are concerned. However, we still run into serious difficulties when dealing with milder syndromes, such as anxiety or depression, which do not have a clear-cut distribution across the population (in binary syndromic categories, i.e., 'yes or no'), but rather appear on a continuum, with a 'dimensional' presentation.

Systems Assessment

To provide mental health care, it is essential to have procedures for assessing the capacity of certain community systems (formal and informal) to provide support for those with psychological difficulties. It is also necessary to know to what extent these mental health services are prepared to meet the population's demands, in order to introduce modifications responding to unmet needs, and improve existing services.

The studies that have been carried out to date provide us with certain descriptions of patients' families and social networks, and the health care systems with which they are in contact. More or less objective methods have been set forth for assessing these contexts, and efforts have been made to provide them with the necessary validity and reliability. The following pages offer what must be a fragmentary, summarised vision of the attempts at diagnosis and assessment of families, social networks, institutions, and health care systems.

Semiological Elements

Families

It is difficult to define which are the families that function well, and which provide adequate support (Fleck, 1976; Howells, 1971). Stachowiak (1979) compared therapists' opinions regarding the normality of two sets of families. One comprised families of psychiatric outpatients from a public clinic. The others had been chosen by physicians, teachers, and other community counsellors as being very well adapted within their communities. The therapists, without exception, assessed the patients' families as being those that functioned best, and the others as being disturbed. Stachowiak believed that these errors came from such biases as mistakenly taking the so-called 'democratic model' as being equivalent to adequate functioning. He concluded that the truly well adapted families were able to make group decisions much more easily, and had a definite tendency to present a *matriarchal* or *patriarchal* structure, with flexible leadership. The poorly adapted families presented either too little or too much 'expressed emotion', and inadequate communication.

Social Networks

The concept of *social network* was coined by Barnes (1954) to characterise the social ties of 'persons who relate with each other, utilise their time together, like or dislike each other, and reciprocally give or ask for things' (Guimón, Ruiz, Apodaca, De Ros, and Sota, 1985). The concept of networks is inherent to the more general idea of *social* or *community support systems*, which have been shown to impact strongly on the prognoses of mental patients (Mosher and Keith, 1980).

Services

Some health care services show useful characteristics for certain patients, whereas others are aimed at patients with different disorders. Therefore, a real typology of therapeutic settings has been developed, with highly precise elements differentiating them (Liberman, 1983; Guimón, Sunyer, Sánchez de Vega, and Trojaola, 1992). These include, for example, 'hospitals that support or maintain the stereotype' (i.e., whose structure stigmatises patients), compared with those that 'confront the stereotype', and so on.

Assessment Methodology

Families

A family interview conducted with a systemic approach features some original techniques (such as avoiding the identification of a single member as the patient, seeking power alliances, and 'task prescription'). The *genogram* is a more complete way of exploring family antecedents; *role-playing* and *sculpting* have become an integral part of active group therapies based on the psychodrama, and are of interest as part of the assessment process.

Social Network Assessment Instruments

Axis IV of the DSM-III and the DSM-IV included guidelines on how to code absence of social support. More specifically, social network assessment instruments have been developed, among which one of the most complete is the one that we have used, in a Spanish adaptation (Guimón et al., 1985), developed by Escobar et al. in their studies at the University of California (Los Angeles). The instrument collects descriptive and interactional information, according to two criteria. 1) *Structural criteria.* These include the following variables: a) *size,* the number of persons belonging to the network; b) *density,* ratio between real and potential ties within the network; c) *degree,* average number of relationships that one member has with others within the same network; d) *interconnection,* concept related to elements of density and degree of a certain network's links. 2) *Interactional criteria.* These include: a) *social contact,* based on frequency of the contact; b) *direction,* defined as instrumental if the subject's usefulness to the network's members is higher than theirs to him, reciprocal if it is equal, and dependent if the network members are more helpful to the subject than vice-versa; c) *transactional content,* referring to the material or non-material elements exchanged in a relationship between two persons and/or the types of activity that unites the participants (this criterion separates emotional support from material support); d) *differences in ties*, i.e., single relationship if it has only one type of content, and multiple if it has more than one area of content; and e) capacity to *activate connections*, which determines the two major types of networks: f) *open*, characterised by having a relatively large number of members and connections, with weak ties (*low density*); and g) *closed*, presenting strong ties and small number of members, generally related to each other. Groups of the latter type tend to be culturally homogeneous, with face-to-face interaction, and its members are situated in the same geographical areas. We shall refer to these classifications again in Chapter 10.

Assessment of Health Care Units

Various instruments have been developed to measure different aspects of health care services, enabling us to draw up a 'taxonomy' of the units that can have a relationship with therapeutic response. For example, Kellam et al. (1966) developed a *Ward Information Form*, which quantifies certain visible aspects of psychiatric wards. Moos proposed a *Ward Atmosphere Scale*, which has been translated into Spanish and French, and which we have used in some studies (Moos, 1997). Another interesting instrument, the *Multiphasic Environmental Assessment Procedure*, evaluates the social and physical environment of treatment units.

ATTITUDES ASSESSMENT

Assessment Methodology

The methods most frequently used to study prejudices regarding mental illness are psychosocial research questionnaires and public opinion polls carried out using attitude scales, presentation of clinical scenarios, and text-content analyses.

Content Analyses

These techniques involve collecting, collating, and analysing material from the mass media (e.g., newspapers, radio, television, magazines), and then quantifying it for statistical analysis. It is also possible to study values and attitudes expressed in books aimed at the general public, or in different material involving mass dissemination. Castairs and Wing (1958) were pioneers in such research, studying the content of 1267 letters sent to the BBC in a television programme on mental illness.

ASSESSMENT OF STRESS AND LIFE EVENTS

Axis IV of DSM-III and DSM-III-R focused on the area of psychosocial stressors, but DSM-IV has replaced this with a method for enumerating psychosocial and environmental problems, which recognises the growing importance being attributed to relational problems, especially family ones, for approaching treatment. Examples of these include (Frances, 1997) the death of a relative, discrimination, workplace problems, scarcity of resources, and homelessness.

EXPERIMENTAL DESIGN IN SOCIOLOGICAL RESEARCH

Sometimes, in mental health research using social models, studies are conducted without a previous hypothesis, as when we study the prevalence of a given disorder in a community. However, the study design is generally based on an initial hypothesis, and the choice of method and instruments is made in consequence, after which a pilot study is often carried out to ensure that the method is indeed valid.

When questionnaires are used, a pilot study is essential in order to identify ambiguous or superfluous questions. Once the questionnaire has been corrected, and the investigator's behaviour has been modified if found to be inappropriate, then the principal study can be conducted. A special design case involves the analysis of trends through studying documents and clinical histories, which provide a great deal of information. However, clinical histories cannot usually be used to collect reliable data beyond such basic facts as sex and age, since anything else tends to be recorded imprecisely. Therefore, retrospective studies are frequently deceiving, and usually it is necessary to carry out prospective studies with the help of instruments aimed at the general population, which measure different social variables.

The so-called *deviant case* analysis shows the importance of precision in measuring variables. A deviant case is one that does not fit into the general theory that is accepted after a hypothesis is considered confirmed. *Content analysis* is an interesting research procedure, which transforms collected information without restructuring it into quantifiable data. For example, content analysis can be used to study press reports on mental health, the discrimination experienced by patients, or transcripts of clinical interviews. Patients' diaries can also be useful for epidemiological research.

An investigator can also make direct observations on activities carried out in a more or less closed setting, such as a ward in a psychiatric hospital.

Social interaction can be measured using simple sociometric procedures, such as graphing patients' movements or their interactions with treatment personnel. Such techniques have been used in assessing wards and groups.

Observation can also provide us with data for assessing institutions and intraprofessional interactions. Some things that happen to patients in a hospital can, for example, be related to the hierarchisation of personnel, the patients' age distribution, the presence of visitors, and so on. These factors can be compared from one ward to another, detecting the different presentations of a characteristic in patients according to these factors. This institutional analysis method is difficult to carry out due to the flexibility demands that it places on the investigator.

In the study of health care programmes and services, it is possible to have a *low degree of resolution* (e.g., the study of psychiatric wards in Spain by Sunyer et al., (1990) or a *high degree of resolution* (e.g., a study of a psycho-educational group at Basurto Hospital by Guimón et al. (1993). The methodologies used for these studies are, necessarily, different: the former are descriptive, and the latter are evaluative (including *ideographic* and *nomothetic* approaches); qualitative and quantitative; sociological and psychological.

Recently, there has been a trend towards conducting studies that combine various techniques of this sort, such as the mixed (or cross-institutional) design proposed by Moos for research on therapeutic communities.

Sometimes it can be interesting to take fieldwork outside the hospital walls, studying, for example, the behaviour of small, mental health-related groups, such as Alcoholics Anonymous meetings, paying attention to the groups' structural characteristics, communication systems, activities, and so on. Naturally, such studies require the authorisation of those involved. It may be necessary to forego publishing parts of the study, to avoid damage to the participants.

Thus, it is possible to study the behaviour of society in general regarding mental health. The *social ecology* method studies the distribution of certain behaviours, such as suicide, as they relate to social variables. The data thus obtained are always prone to the so-called *ecological fallacy:* it may be mistaken to believe, without further confirmation, that a person or small group of persons in a certain area necessarily shares the characteristics prevalent in that region. An example of this would be a city where schizophrenics are concentrated in a district with a high proportion of immigrants, although the schizophrenics themselves may be native-born.

REFERENCES

Fleck, S. (1976). A general systems approach to family pathology. *American Journal of Psychiatry*, 13, 669–673.

Foulkes, S. H. (1964). *Therapeutic group analysis*. London: Wheaton and Co.

Frances, A., First, M. B., & Pincus, H. A. (Eds.). (1997). *DSM-IV, Guia de uso*. Barcelona: Masson, Barcelona.

Goldstein, K. (1940). *Human Nature in the Light of Psychopathology*. Harvard: Harvard University Press.

Guimón, J., Ruiz, A., Apodaca, P., de Ros, P., and Sota, E. (1985). Red social en la población de Guecho. Psiquis, VI (126), 9–22.

Guimón, J., Sunyer, M., Sánchez de Vega, J., and Trojaola, B. (1992). Group analysis and ward atmosphere. In F. P. Ferrero, A. E. Haynal and N. Sartorius (Eds.), *Schizophrenia and affective psychoses. Nosology in contemporary psychiatry*. John Libbey CIC.

Guimón, J., Eguiluz I., and Bulbena, A. (1993): Group pharmacotherapy in schizophrenics. *European Journal of Psychiatry*, 7 (3), 147–154.

Howells, J. (1971). *Theory and practice of family psychiatry*. New York: Bunner-Mazel.

Kellam, S. G., Shmelzer, J. L., & Beman, A. (1966). Variation in the atmospheres of psychiatric wards. *Archives of General Psychiatry, 20*(1), 169–183.

Lewin, K. (1935). *A dynamic theory of personality*. New York: McGraw Hill.

Liberman, R. P. (1983). Research on the psychiatric milieu. In J. G. Gunderson (Ed.), *Principles and practice of milieu therapy*. New York: Jason Aronson.

MacKenzie, K. R. (Ed.). (1996). *Effective use of group therapy in managed care*. Washington. D.C.: American Psychiatric Press, Inc.

Moos, R. H. (1997). *Evaluating treatment environments. The quality of psychiatric and substance abuse programs*. New Brunswick: Transaction.

Morris, J. N. (1970). *Uses of epidemiology*. London: E. and Livington.

Mosher, L. R., and Keith, J. (1980). Psychosocial treatment, individual, group, family and community support approaches. *Schizophrenia Bulletin*, 6, 10–41.

Sunyer, J. M. (1990). *Evaluacion de la atmosfera en las Salas Psiquiatricas Espanolas*. Universidad Autonoma, Barcelona.

10

Relational Diagnosis

DIAGNOSTIC AMBIGUITIES IN THE DYNAMIC DIAGNOSIS

Patients asking for psychoanalysis still express their complaints (as do the referring professionals) in terms of traditional nosology. Analysts usually only make use of psychiatric classification systems to decide whether or not a particular patient should be analysed (e.g., a patient diagnosed as having dementia would be rejected) or to predict outcome (e.g., the prognosis of phobic symptoms is considered different according to whether the 'diagnosis' is of an anxiety disorder or schizophrenia). As a consequence, psychoanalysts tend to ignore recent research in psychiatric diagnosis and classification.

Freud's concept of diagnosis was closely related to his notion of 'analysability' (Widlocher, 1984). What he meant by this was, on the one hand, that there were 'psychoneuroses' which could be analysed and, on the other, that there were 'actual neuroses', 'traumatic neuroses', and 'narcissistic neuroses' which could not. Kart Abraham offered a classification of mental illnesses based on the states of libidinal development, and Melanie Klein used a similar principle. Although useful for clinical psychoanalytical work, these classificatory exercises were not based on empirical research.

Current psychiatric classifications (such as DSM-III and IV) have modified the realm of neuroses and character disorders, which have been replaced by headings for different disorders, e.g., anxiety, dissociative, somatoform, personality, psychosexual, factitious, impulse control, and adjustment disorders. This approach obscures the psychoanalytical understanding of these disorders. If empirically confirmed, Kernberg's (1980a) 'structural' approach to diagnosis could allow the reintroduction of psychodynamic factors into recent classifications. Kernberg (1980b) differentiates between neuroses, psychoses, and borderline states, on the basis of three main structural characteristics: degree of integration of identity, level of defensive operations, and capacity for reality testing.

On the other hand, as Widlocher (1984) has pointed out, psychoanalytic psychopathology includes categories such as *manifest* and *latent* content, *secondary* and *primary* processes of thought, *regression*, *transference*, and *mechanisms of defence*, and also makes use of categories such as *negative therapeutic reaction* to evaluate change and resistance to change. In addition, psychoanalysis has described new clinical entities that are now more or less widely used in psychiatry (*phobic neurosis*, *character neurosis*, *borderline states*, and so on). These and other concepts co-existed, and sometimes rivalled, those of descriptive psychopathology.

In any case, psychoanalysts generally have shown little interest in systematically organising these semiological findings into diagnostic constructions, although there have been some attempts at diagnostic classifications. Unfortunately, in the psychoanalytical community there has not been much enthusiasm about projects for systematising these constructs, and when this has been attempted, the resulting descriptions have generally been based on arcane observational systems and terminologies which place them beyond the use of the average psychiatric practitioner.

A diagnosis in dynamic psychiatry is particularly concerned with factors such as the *strengths* and *weaknesses of the ego*, the nature of unconscious conflicts, and defence mechanisms and the structure of the superego. Under the influence of the British school, the importance of the assessment of family relationships, transferential patterns, and the so-called *internal object relations* have been taken into account. These components have been appropriately approached through the development of increasingly sophisticated instruments, such as Bellak's EFA (Bellak et al., 1973)—which was, however, too complicated to be used widely. Recently, the KAPP has proved to be an instrument that is not only easier to use, but also offers a higher inter-rater and test-retest reliability. On the other hand, new propositions are been made by an IPA group working on the empirical formulation and evaluation of psychoanalysis including Kachele, Emde, and Fonagy (see Fonagy et al., 2000).

Although the theoretical orientation of psychiatrists has been modified throughout the last twenty years because of impressive advances in the biological model, most mental health professionals continue to be interested in eclectic or 'generic' approaches, which have frequently been called 'dynamic'.

As we said previously (see chapter 4), for psychiatry to be considered 'dynamic', it must take into account the importance of the unconscious and of transference. In addition, dynamic psychiatry stresses concepts such as 'conflict', 'psychological determinism', 'deficits in intrapsychic structures' or 'internal object relations'. Although Dynamic psychiatry focuses more on desires, fantasies, dreams or self-image, it nevertheless incorporates conceptions and procedures emanating from non-analytical psychotherapeutic models (behaviourism, cognitivism and general systems theory), which have shown their efficacy in the treatment of certain disorders.

RELATIONAL DIAGNOSIS: SOCIAL ASPECTS

Although it has been known for centuries that the patient's environment can have a major impact on the genesis and forms of presentation of psychological disorders, attempts were not made to conceptualise these inter-relations until the period between the two World Wars. Foulkes (Foulkes, 1965; Foulkes and Anthony, 1957) proposed, as discussed in Chapter 8, what he called a *reticular theory of neurosis*. The application, several decades later, of general systems theory to studying alterations in communication, especially in mental patients' families, was another landmark in research based on this approach. Finally, the application of findings on institutional organisation to the study of therapeutic settings has notably enriched our understanding of the environment in which mental illness develops.

These studies, collectively, have provided us with specific descriptions of patients' families and social networks, and the health care systems with which they are in contact. As we discussed in the previous chapter, more or less objective methods have been developed for assessing these contexts, and efforts have been made to endow them with the necessary validity and reliability.

The following pages offer a necessarily fragmentary, summarised vision of the attempts at diagnosis and assessment of families, social networks, institutions, and health care systems.

Family Diagnosis

Is It Possible to Diagnose Families?

Although, as we have seen, in psychiatry there has long been a lively discussion regarding the validity of, or need for, diagnoses, these doubts have been expressed even more vehemently among authors focusing on family therapy. Haley (1979) claimed that interest in diagnoses was typical of novices in family therapy; the more experienced family therapists tended to work with a minimum of information. They try to intervene as soon as they have an idea of what is going on, and they do not like to delay therapy due to some diagnostic or assessment overzealousness. Many of these therapists, according to Haley, believe that to carry out a careful diagnosis serves more to alleviate the therapist's own anxiety, rather than benefiting the family. Haley describes the family not as a set of problems independent from the therapist; rather, he includes the therapist in his descriptions, stressing how the family responds to the therapist's interventions. He believes that the attempt to propose a diagnosis is artificial.

On the contrary, other authors, such as Ackerman (1982), are of the opinion that, in any case, therapists inevitably make judgements about the families that they treat. They describe them, they compare them with others, and they establish significant differentiations among them. These authors believe that diagnosis and family therapy are parallel processes, and that the question is not so much whether or not therapists should make diagnoses, but rather how can they do it better.

To diagnose a family presupposes making a judgement regarding the normality or abnormality of its functioning. Howells (1971), Fleck (1976) and others have described family-system functions. The greatest difficulty arises when trying to establish criteria that make it possible to discern whether families are fulfilling these functions adequately.

Theories of Minuchin, Ackerman, and Bowen

Minuchin (1982) described families, in a well-known paper, in terms of structures, of development and adaptation states. According to this approach, the therapist, in order to make a diagnosis, must participate in the family's communication, making observations and asking questions. Thus, he can detect the transactional modules and boundaries, and propose hypotheses regarding which modules are functional, and which dysfunctional. In this way, he draws up a sort of family 'map'.

Ackerman (1982) set forth a different approach, assessing at what point the family has become stuck on a growth curve of different values, and to what point it achieves or falls short of achieving both its own expectations about itself and society's expectations, as well as the professional achievements that tend to define a 'healthy family'. The next step is to determine to what extent the alliances and divisions within the family group influence the individual members' expression of affect, emotional development, and health. Thus, the therapist's efforts focus on painting as clear a picture as possible of the balance of forces in the family, differentiating between those forces that predispose its members to illness, and those that protect health and growth.

For his part, Bowen (1961, 1976) stressed the importance of what he called greater or lesser 'differentiation of the self' in the origin and diagnosis of emotional disorders, both in individuals and the family. He proposed an assessment scale that places individuals on a continuum of 0–100, from the lowest level of human functioning to the highest. This author coined the concept of *undifferentiated family ego mass* for the set of fusions produced between the self and the family. This concept is particularly useful when it refers to the nuclear family, but Bowen also considered it applicable to the extended family and social networks. The higher the degree of 'undifferentation', the greater the possibility of potential problems. In Bowen's framework, undifferentiation resolves itself through dysfunctions, in three areas of family functioning: marital conflict, dysfunction in one of the spouses, or disorders in one or more of the children.

García Badaracco

García Badaracco (1978) assumed that healthy development requires a family structure based on the interplay of maternal and paternal functions, able to offer the children an appropriate emotional climate, where they can experience attachments that will conform their ego structure. The result would be a rich variety of ego resources, and an integration of the personality that would lead to achieving individualisation and autonomy through the ability to overcome life crises and the conflicts inherent in them. If this structure is inadequate, it can create different pathologies.

From this perspective, for a psychosis-inducing family situation to arise, there must formerly be a structural weakness in the *family psychic apparatus*, with different modalities in each one of the family members. According to García Badaracco, this psychosis-inducing conditioning comprises multiple factors: 1) certain pathological traits in the personality of the parental figures; 2) lack of parental capacity to empathise with primitive anxieties and sexuality, to give appropriate help to the subject in the vicissitudes of ego growth; 3) difficulty on the part of the parent to permit and favour aggressiveness and other elements involved in the process of undoing the original symbiosis, and the impossibility of establishing a rule of exogamy; 4) a certain pathology in the family constellation, which determines a particular, specific systemic phenomenon; 5) ideological family problematics functioning as barriers; 6) the pathogenic nature of some kinds of traumatic life events.

García Badaracco, therefore, advocates diagnosing a pathology based on what has not been given, and what has not been experienced, insofar as requirements for a healthy, individual development within the family matrix are concerned. The concept of *lack of ego resources development* is not the same as an affective deficiency; rather, it is a deficiency of positive structural identifications. This is a basic idea in conceptualising the process of mental illness and the process of its cure, conceived as what is necessary to provide in order to generate health.

Social Network Diagnosis

Over the last few decades, various attempts have been made to diagnose psychiatric patients' social support systems, describing their structure and function in the general population (Guimón, Ruiz, Apodaca, de Ros, and Sota, 1985).

Regarding the social network, certain quantitative characteristics have been described (size, density, degree of openness and interconnection), as well as qualitative ones (e.g., support and gratification capacity, facilitation of tasks, initiatives and confidences), measured with instruments such as those described in Chapter 8 .

Schematically, a network is similar to a communicative circuit. Different aspects of such networks have been defined (Cohen and Sokolovsky, 1978), such as size, density, and degree of social networks (see chapter 9). Two major types of networks have been differentiated according to their capacity to activate connections outside themselves. *Open* social networks present a great deal of cultural heterogeneity. Their members include many people without kinship ties; few of the members are personally acquainted with or have relationships with other members of the network. Such a network is typically expected of Anglo-American, middle-class, 'successful', 'healthy' people. These 'weak' connections can act as bridges towards other networks, providing useful information.

Closed (or dense) networks typically present a small number of members, generally with kinship ties (chapter 9). There is a high degree of cultural homogeneity and face-to-face interaction. There is little dispersion, and a tendency to be located in the same geographical area. This type of networks seems to reinforce a feeling of personal identity, and provides a great deal of emotional support to its members. However, it can also put up barriers to problem resolution, due to the lack of bridges to outside networks.

Different authors have tried to determine which characteristics of patients' social networks enable them to provide protective support. Some epidemiological studies highlight the existence of peculiarities in the structure and function of the social network to explain the psychopathological differences in different populations and geographical areas. Thus, a number of authors have pointed out that the social network of schizophrenic patients is smaller in size and number of contacts. By the same token, social networks able to provide support have been considered protectors against the symptomatology of depression, a disorder in which it has been shown to be especially beneficial for the patient to be able to count on someone to act as a confidant (Brown, Bhrolchain, and Harris, 1976). This is also the case in neuroses, although the symptoms seem to be associated more with the individual's *perception* of his social relationships, than the actual structure of the network.

Mosher and Keith (1980), in a review of the literature on schizophrenics' social networks, found that they tended to be smaller than those of normal individuals, especially in terms of number of members and proportion of non-kin connections. Hammer (1981) reported that schizophrenic patients whose social network was 'asymmetrical', highly protective and interconnected, evolved significantly better than patients without such ties, as shown by their re-hospitalisation rates.

Pattison's work (Pattison and Loy, 1981) found major differences in the structure of the social networks of normal subjects, neurotics, and psychotics. For example, normal subjects listed an average of 25 persons whom they considered 'important' to them (whom they could trust to provide them with emotional and material support), including relatives, friends, neighbours, and colleagues. Psychotics seemed to have a decidedly less gratifying social life, according to these investigators, since they mention only half the number of members in their network as the normal group (an average of 13).

Tolsdorf (1976) also found that schizophrenics' social networks had fewer members. Another study showed that schizophrenics with more severe symptoms had smaller networks (Sokolovsky et al., 1978). Beels (1984) postulated that for schizophrenics, structural considerations–such as task and initiatives facilitation, contact, and proximity–are important in their networks, whereas for a depressed patient, the presence of a confidant would be the most influential qualitative characteristic of a social network.

Miller and Ingham (1976) found that not only the presence of a confidant, but also other, more diffuse social relationships seem to serve as protection against the appearance of neurotic symptoms. Henderson (1983) pointed out that the presence of neurotic symptoms seems to be more associated with the patient's *perception* of his social relationships than with the network's real structure.

A study that we conducted in Geneva explored different support functions of the social network: the *instrumental support* functions correspond to the material assistance given by someone and/or the information provided regarding a problem (e.g., insurance, income tax); the *emotional support* function is related to encouragement, consolation, advice, feedback, and availability offered by someone; the possibility to share interests and ideas with someone, and the fact of feeling at ease with someone, form part of the *friendship* function; the *attachment* function concerns the person with whom the subject has a loving, privileged relationship; a function of *support in crisis* is applied to the other four functions, when they involve a crisis situation.

In the general population, intervention of family and friends predominates strongly. The family also occupies a very important position in the sample of mental patients, but they make less use of friends and acquaintances. Patients tend to recur more to professional help than subjects in the general population. Social workers, in particular, play a decisive, instrumental role in specific help functions. Professionals in general also fulfil an *emotional function*, especially when help is required within a psychiatric context. It is, above all, in instrumental and crisis functions that professionals play a role, whereas the weight carried by families in such situations drops notably.

Diagnosis of Institutions

Psychoanalysis Applied to Institutional Assessment

Nearly 200 years ago, Pinel (1809) stressed that 'we should examine the different types of mental disorders analytically, considering them separately, and deducing from them principles of medical treatment and hospital organisation.' Along the same lines, some modern authors, such as Gruenberg (1968), have stated that the needs of psychiatric epidemiology will not be satisfied only by the classification of mental disorders; it must also be able to classify environmental data, the data under which these disorders do or do not appear.

In the opinion of Herman (1984), if this is done, investigators run the risk of including, in their diagnostic classifications, data that do not characterise the patient, but rather are typical of his environment. These 'peripheral' data are interesting, and can help us to understand the disorder, but they do not characterise the patient *qua* patient. It would probably be better to record them separately, in order to compare them with the diagnosis, if necessary. Some multi-axial classifications represent an attempt at solving this problem.

The truth of the matter is that mental health professionals often carry out their work within the context of institutions such as psychiatric hospitals, general hospitals, prisons, and military installations. Therefore, it is not exceptional for them to have to take on administrative duties, which has led them to become interested in assessing and diagnosing the organisations themselves. Although a knowledge of individual and, occasionally, group psychology has sometimes favoured their understanding of the institutional dynamics, they have often, unfortunately, tried to transpose adjectives and labels from psychiatric nosology to the classification of organisations or their leaders. To classify an organisation as 'paranoid', an administrator as 'narcissistic', or an employee as 'obsessive' may be an approximate metaphor, but it is never an adequate diagnosis. To apply such a 'diagnosis' to the organisation itself can be simply inefficient or pretentious. However, to apply it to individuals is undoubtedly abusive and ethically dubious.

We must be extremely cautious when considering the diagnosis of a pathology or character traits of a colleague, and even more cautious in stating it. A mental health professional is only able to make a diagnosis when he has collected data under very precise circumstances, and it is only appropriate to make diagnostic pronouncements when asked to do so. When a professional has doubts regarding the mental pathology of a member of the organisation in which he is working, the most appropriate step is to try to convince that person to consult an outside psychiatrist, and not to use a diagnosis against someone as if it were a weapon.

Just as there are wild interpretations, there is also a danger of making wild diagnoses. It is strange that the same professional who claims to be against using diagnoses for their patients, will blithely diagnose organisations or those who work in them, with insufficient data and without a specific contract to do so.

This does not mean that it is never useful to seek outside consultants who are experts in psychodynamic theory, or who have organisational experience. Indeed, there are authors who have published useful work on institutional diagnosis. Others have applied their group assessment experience to diagnosing organisations. For example, Kaplan (1983) proposed a diagnostic method for determining an organisation's stage of evolution, based on his experience in therapeutic groups and systematic data collection on institutions that he had created. Kernberg (1978, 1979) suggested, when diagnosing a syndrome that he dubbed *organisational regression*, establishing a difference between the effects that institutional disorganisation can produce on a leader, and the problems created by the leader's own regression. Foulkes (Foulkes, 1965; Foulkes and Anthony, 1957) proposed, for institutional diagnoses, the use of his own group analytic techniques, in accordance with certain general principles. The Tavistock Institute, in London, enjoys a highly deserved reputation in institutional analysis with an analytical orientation.

In spite of the indisputable utility of these psychoanalytically oriented approaches, it is noteworthy that the most fruitful advances in institutional assessment are due, undoubtedly, to the modern science of institutional organisation. Everything points to a future in which, although it will be useful to have a taxonomy of organisational pathology, taxonomy will be very different from the typologies derived from psychiatric diagnosis.

TOWARDS A RELATIONAL CLASSIFICATION

The popularisation of new psychopathological findings has led to a high degree of confusion in the labelling of different psychiatric disorders, because the classical terms, established over centuries of use, are co-existing with recent ones, not only in the language of the general public, but in that of medicine, as well. For example, we frequently hear the term 'psychosis' used to designate a fashion or a trend; or 'psychopath' used as if it were synonymous with 'psychotic'; and 'neurosis' is now applied to an infinite number of conditions, or even mere attitudes. Mental health professionals are not exempt from this confusion: the reigning nosological chaos, only partially rectified by the classification efforts of the American Psychiatric Association (APA) and the World Health Organization (WHO), is only one aspect of the problem.

The DSM-IV (as the latest edition of the APA's *Diagnostic and Statistical Manual* is known), includes different principal diagnoses, and the WHO's ICD-10 features similar, although not identical, categories. Although both classifications aim to be atheoretical, they include, without openly admitting it, biological aetiological criteria.

As we noted at the beginning of this chapter, a single classification of reference cannot satisfy all needs, because the type of classification that should be used depends on the objectives of a given study. For a relational approach to psychiatry, a somewhat different grouping of disorders is necessary.

For studies of disorders, we prefer to use a typology of extreme types. At one extreme, we situate the most genuinely relational psychiatric disorders, i.e., the stress-related disorders. At the opposite end are those psychological alterations due to the effect of toxic substances on the brain. This will be, therefore, the order in which the different disorders will be discussed in this book.

REFERENCES

Ackerman, N. (1982). *Diagnóstico y tratamiento de las relaciones familiares*. Buenos Aires: Horné.

Bellak, L., Hurvich, M., & Gedimen, K. (1973). *Ego Functions in Schizophrenics Neurotics, and Normals: A Systematic Study of Conceptual. Diagnostic, and Therapeutic Aspects*. New York: John Wiley & Sons.

Bowen, M. (1961). Family psychotherapy. *American Journal of Orthopsychiatry*, 31, 40–60.
Bowen, M. (1976). Psicoterapia familiar de la esquizofrenia en el hospital y en la práctica privada. In I. Boszormengy-Nagy and J. Framo (Eds.), *Terapia familiar intensiva*. Mexico City: Trillas.
Brown, G. W., Bhrolchain, M. N., and Harris, T. (1976). Social class and psychiatric disturbance among women in an urban population. *Sociol. Rev.*, 9, 225–242.
Cohen, C., & Sokolovsky J. (1978). Schizophrenia and social networks. Expatients in the inner city. *Schizophrenia Bulletin*, 4(4), 546–560.
Fleck, S. (1976). A general system's approach to family pathology. *American Journal of Psychiatry*, 13, 669–673.
Fonagy, P. (2000). *An Open Door Review of Outcome Studies in Psychoanalysis* (www.ipa.org.uk/research/complete.htm). London: IPA.
Foulkes, S. H. (1965). *Therapeutic group analysis*. New York: International Universities Press.
Foulkes, S. H., and Anthony, E. J. (1957). *Group psychotherapy. The psychoanalytic approach*. London: Penguin Books.
García Badaracco, J. (1978). La familia como contexto real de todo proceso terapéutico. *Rev. Ter. Fam.*, 1, 9–16.
Guimón, J., J. E. Mezzich and G. E. Berrios (EAS.) (1988) *Diagnóstico en Psiquiatría*. Barcelona: Salvat.
Guimón, J. (1989). The biases of psychiatric diagnosis. In J. Guimón, G. E. Berrios, and J. E. Mezzich (Eds.), Psychiatric diagnosis (vol. 155, pp: 33–38). *British Journal of Psychiatry*.
Guimón, J., Ruiz, A., Apodaca, P., de Ros, P., and Sota, E. (1985). Red social en la población de Guecho. *Psiquis*, VI (126), 9–22.
Haley, J. (1979). *Nouvelles stratégies en thérapie de famille: le problem-solving en thérapie familiale*. Paris: J. P. Delarge.
Hammer, M. (1981). Social supports, social networks and schizophrenia. *Schizophrenia Bulletin*, 7(1), 45–58.
Herman, P. (1984). *Classification et épidémiologie* (Vol. 24). Cambridge: Cambridge University Press.
Kaplan, S. R. (1983). Phases of development in psychiatric institutions. In J. A. Talbott and S. R. Kaplan (Eds.), *Psychiatric administration*. New York: Grune and Stratton.
Kernberg, O. (1978). Leadership and organizational functioning: organizational regression. *International Journal of Group Psychotherapy*, 28, 3–25.
Kernberg, O. (1979). Regression in organizational leadership. *Psychiatry*, 42, 24–39.
Kernberg, O. (1980a). *Internal World and external reality*. New York: Jason Aronson.
Kernberg, O. F. (1980b). Neurosis, psyhoses and the borderline states. In A. M. Kaplan & F. A. M. & J. Sadock (Eds.), *Comprehensive Textbook of Psychiatry*. Baltimore: Williams & Wilkins.
Minuchin, S. (1982). *Familias y terapia familiar*. Buenos Aires: Gedisa.
Mosher, L. R., and Keith, J. (1980). Psychosocial treatment, individual, group, family and community support approaches. *Schizophrenia Bulletin*, 6, 10–41.
Pattison, E. M., and Loy, M. (1981). Analysis of a schizophrenic psychosocial network. *Schizophrenia Bulletin*, 7, 135–144.
Pinel, P. (1809). *Traité médico-philosophique sur l'aliénation mentale* (2nd ed.). Paris: Brosson.
Tolsdorf, C. C. (1976). Social networks, support, and coping: an exploratory study. *Fam. Process*, 15(4), 407–417.
Widlocher, D. (1984). *Le psychanalyste devant les problèmes de classification. Confrontations Psychiatriques*, 24, 141–157.

11

Organic, Including Symptomatic, Mental Disorders (F00–F09)

DSM-IV entitles this section 'Delirium, Dementia, and Amnestic and Other Cognitive Disorders'. Both this classification and that of the ICD-10 propose a list of agents able to produce delirium (intoxication, abstinence, metabolic and endocrinological alterations, infections, tumours, physical trauma, avitaminosis, epilepsy) and dementia (Alzheimer's and Pick's disorders, tumours, physical trauma, avitaminosis, chronic intoxication, and vascular, metabolic and endocrinal disorders).

RELATIONAL ASPECTS

Some authors have been interested in studying to what extent pre-existing personality traits exercise a pathoplastic action on the symptomatology of these disorders.

Acute Syndromes

The acute syndromes (delirium) show disorientation, agitation, and visual hallucinations. Willi (1968) focused on the influence of the patient's previous personality on the symptoms of acute exogenous reactions. His main sources were studies on 'model' psychoses, and his own experience with patients suffering from acute organic syndromes and dying patients.

His primary question was, to what extent do the symptoms of acute organic psychoses express the idiosyncrasies of the patient's personality. He quotes a paper by Stoll (1974) proposing that aspects of the personality that may become apparent after the administration of LSD are not useful in defining the subject's usual personality, since in daily life they may be controlled by inhibition mechanisms, which are also part of the personality. Referring to his own experiences with patients presenting acute exogenous reactions, Willi agrees that 'what a person can become under different conditions than usual turns out to be very different from what this person has in fact become under normal conditions. These aspects represent something typical of this personality, without embracing its totality.'

The role that an individual's unconscious plays in conditioning the symptomatology of delirium remains controversial. Whereas authors like Leuner (1962) maintain that there is always relational material created from unconscious content, others, such as Beringer (1932), have concluded that only a small amount of repressed material appears in these cases, and that their content bears little resemblance to the patient's personality. Willi (1968), based on his personal experience, says that the disagreement between the two authors cited above is due to their different methodologies. In his own patients, there is relatively little symptoms related to previously unconscious material. A good proportion of these hallucinations and other experiences refer to trivial content, often relational (occupational, 23% of the time). Occasionally, these psychological manifestations are related to a previous anxious or depressed state. However (in a study on 30 patients who presented exogenous reactions after attempting suicide with hypnotics), he more often found calm, lucid states of mood. Therefore, concludes Willi, an acute illness that sets of psychological symptoms does not necessarily intensify previous anxious or depressed situations; rather, it often produces the effect of dampening these symptoms.

Chronic Syndromes

Neuropsychological Aspects

In chronic cerebral syndromes, the behavioral phenomena observed are not explainable merely by the alternation of a function due to a certain anatomical-pathological legion. The chronic syndromes show dementia, with dissemination, amnesia, disturbances in symbolic recognition (gnosias) and gestures (praxias). According to Goldstein (1975), to understand this symptomatology we have to take into consideration all of the patient's behaviour at a given moment. Goldstein believes that the complexity and inconsistency of the symptomatology in brain-damaged patients is due to the alteration of what he calls 'abstract attitude'. This alteration leads to difficulties in: resolving certain mental tasks; considering different aspects of the same situation; comprehending the essential aspects of a totality;

abstracting common properties from a situation; symbolising; voluntarily evoking complex experiences; and separating the self from the outside world and from internal experiences. The difficulty in abstract attitudes is not only present in new situations, but also in familiar ones.

Patients often encounter difficulties at some times and not others with what seems to be the same test. However, says Goldstein, they are, in fact, being confronted with different ones. For example, if we show a patient an angle made out of two sticks, open towards the bottom of the page, and we ask him to copy it after taking away the model, he can do so correctly; but if we show him the same angle facing towards the top, the patient, once we have taken the model away, cannot repeat it because, for him this angle has nothing to do with the one that he was previously able to copy. When he is asked why this is so, he might say that the figure with the angle open towards the bottom reminded him of a roof, whereas the other figure means nothing. The first angle can be related to a concrete experience, whereas the second cannot be reproduced because the patient does not have the necessary abstract capacity to do so. By the same token, the patient fails when we confront him with ideas, thoughts and feelings involving abstract attitudes. For example, he may be unable, after reciting the days of the week, to then recite a series of numbers; or he may be able to converse on a familiar theme, but then be unable to change to another theme, even though it may also be familiar.

Different tasks require different degrees of abstraction. The highest degree of abstraction is required for conscious acts of forming general concepts and thinking in terms of a general principle and verbalising its subordinate acts. A lower level of abstraction is required by voluntarily planning an act or series of acts without stopping to understand each step of the mental process. The loss of the capacity for abstraction cannot be recovered by re-learning; only the improvement of the brain damage can facilitate its recovery.

Patients with chronic brain damage present alterations in automatic reactions (e.g., counting by fours or by fifteens) which are very simple under normal conditions. According to Goldstein (1975), this can only be explained by alterations in the relationship between figure and ground, with *figure* here referring to excitation in the stimulated brain area, and *ground* to excitation in the rest of the body. When there is a cerebral alteration, this can lead to responses related to the entire body (the ground) in reaction to localised cerebral excitations. Likewise, emotional reactions are also altered by brain damage, in a way that is similar, although not identical, to automatisms.

Apart from the behavioural alternations caused by damage to the abstract function, we can, of course, also find disorders stemming from direct damage to the so-called instrumentalities, defined by Goldstein as the sensory and motor functions whereby functions at a higher level are carried out.

These symptoms can represent direct sequalae of damage in a specific area of the brain. Generally, we can observe an increase in the threshold of, and therefore a delay in, the affected area's excitation. One way to detect such an alteration is to check whether the patient can successfully complete a task related to the affected zone if he is given plenty of time, but fails when given little time. In addition, when the affected area is excited, it expands abnormally and acts during an excessive period of time. In examining language reception, for example, a patient may show difficulty in perceiving a word, but once it has been understood and repeated, he may present, in relation to it, a perseveration that may make later examinations more difficult.

Besides the alterations due to damage in a specific area of the brain, symptoms can occur due to the isolation (anatomical or functional) of the damaged area with regard to other, undamaged ones to which it was formerly related. Consequently, stimulus reactions can be abnormally intense or lasting, or excessively influenced by inadequate stimuli. All of this can make the patient appear distracted.

Psychodynamic Aspects

Aside from the impairment in abstract capacity, and behavioural alterations due to specific lesions or the isolation of different cerebral areas, a particular patient's reaction to brain damage depends to a large extent on the totality of his personality.

The general appearance of a patient who is unable to complete a simple task may change completely: his face falls, he may become nervous, irritable, and aggressive or evasive in a reaction similar to that of intense anxiety. Such a state can be produced experimentally in some patients by giving them tasks that we know they are incapable of doing. Goldstein (1975) employed the term *ordered condition* to the describe the state of a patient who has successfully completed a test, and *disordered or catastrophic reaction* to his state when faced with failure on tests which he would have been able to carry out before suffering from brain damage.

This catastrophic condition is frequently seen in patients with a diminished abstract capacity. Goldstein assumed that the patient is unable to realise that he has failed, so that the catastrophic condition is not a conscious reaction to failure, but rather represents the body's real reaction to failure. Individuals develop protective mechanisms to eliminate or reduce the probability of the presentation of catastrophic reaction. After a certain time, patients with brain damage are able to confront failure without catastrophic reactions, in part due to these protective mechanisms and in part to the modification of their environment to avoid having to deal with tasks that lead to failure.

A special mechanism is to not realise that the defect exists, what Anton (1899) called *anosognosia* and which is frequently seen in severe hemiplegias, particularly due to right-hemisphere damage. Many authors consider it an unconscious denial mechanism, although Goldstein does not agree with this interpretation. Patients can, in any case, have any number of unconscious defence mechanisms, the same ones that appear in neurosis, to eliminate the dangers that their self-realisation faces.

An interesting mechanism that is sometimes seen in patients with brain damage having various symptoms of bodily alteration is what Goldstein calls the *preferred condition*. For example, a brain-damaged patient suffering from motor symptoms and balance disorders will over time adjust to his disorders, but will also present a new symptom (e.g., abnormal inclination of the head) not attributable to his brain damage. Should attempts be made to eliminate this new alteration, the patient, despite having already adjusted to his disorder, may again present a catastrophic reaction and in addition, soon go back to adopting the *preferred condition* (in this case, inclining his head).

Besides these mechanisms, another factor decisively conditions the manner of presentation of chronic brain-damaged patients' symptomatology: the doctor-patient relationship, which, if it is adequate, will lessen catastrophic reactions. The development of a good relationship between the doctor and the patient is of the utmost importance in the examination process, in order to properly assess symptoms and put into practice an appropriate therapeutic approach.

The process of personality involution tends to begin with a phase of opposition, and end with a heightened self-consciousness. If no unfavourable events intervene, the patient will eventually begin a new social life, which will involve accepting his limitations based on his own changes and those of his environment. Ties with the patient's surroundings are maintained, although they weaken progressively according to his interests or the circumstances. The demented patient tends to isolate himself, not always because others isolate him, but because he himself needs to do so. His adaptation mechanisms sometime enable him to retire within himself and continue to pay attention to everything that is an object of interest to him, rather than to use the defence mechanisms necessary for emotionally accepting the real situation. The ego tends to control both external and internal stimuli, but the failure in achieving internal dominance causes a loss of confidence in the ego system.

This loss is compensated by changes at the bodily level, such as muscular hypertonia, which takes on the role of containing anxieties and masochistic fantasies. Likewise, behaviours such as incessantly drumming the fingers, or constantly making rhythmic movements with the lips and tongue or rocking the trunk and legs, acquire the same meaning when they stem from a limitation or loss of the capacity to relate, to communicate affectively, or to move about. Sensory-motor and social deprivations play an important role in this regard.

Psychosocial Aspects

Dementia creates many problems for the family and for society as a whole. In such a clinical picture, affective motivations and social conditioning factors are mixed together which involve not only the patient, but also his environment. It is not only a matter of more or less deformed, exalted, or repressed emotional phenomena, of distorted relationships, or unsatisfactory communication. When an individual's autonomy is weakened, his behaviour depends not so much on his environment as on his own personality. The demented person knows (at least, in the early stages of his deterioration) that he has stopped being like other people, and he wants others to understand this. A demented person is deprived of a great many pieces of information due to his sensorial limitations and the monotony of the environment in which he finds himself (limitation of relationships through verbal and eye contact). He can easily fall into a disorganisation of his sense of time and space, accompanied by a quasi-oneiric state, in which the subject experiences an intense imaginary life. If deprivation persists, the demented person progressively becomes distrustful, irritable, quarrelsome, spiteful, suspicious, aggressive, and sometimes expresses persecutory feelings and ideas.

In most cases, the characteristic affective state is one of floating anxiety, and demented patients often become excited and dominated by feelings of insecurity that push them into avoiding social life. If their environment does not react appropriately, and generally as a consequence of life events involving fundamental change (the death of a loved one, change of residence, loss of employment), a discompensation may arise.

Social deprivation is multifaceted, and when the inter-relational system is altered, sooner or later this is going to have an impact on other systems, and on the overall organisation of the personality, severely compromising cognoscitive functions, which are essential to interpersonal relationships. Many symptoms of demented patients are consequence of the social privations that they inevitably suffer. If the affective stimulus of the environment is not adequate in quantity and quality, then simultaneous vindication and rejection constitute the basis of a distorted social relationship.

As Bleuler says, in spite of the frustration that it implies, the demented patient tries to defend and reconstruct his ego, thus constructing a peculiar relationship with the real object.

Psychosocial Interventions

Banerjee and Dickinson (Banerjee & Dickinson, 1997) reviewed the literature on evidence-based health care in geriatric psychiatry, concluding that control studies are scarce and that their results are not encouraging.

In the field of psychotherapy Spector et al. (Spector, Orrell, Davies, & Woods, 2000) have shown the uncertain effects of 'reminiscence therapy' for patients with dementia. However, Ians et al. (Iahns, Haupt M, Karger A, & M, 2000) found an improvement of agitation and anxiety in demented patients after psycho-educational group intervention with their caregivers. This underscores the importance of nonpharmacological strategies in the treatment of dementia.

Draper (Draper, 2000) discussed the factors playing a role in the effectiveness of geriatric psychiatry services, while Cole (Cole, 2001) has stressed the impact of adequate post-discharge geriatric services on the mental state of these patients.

Postconcussional Syndrome

In the literature on psychological syndromes resulting from brain trauma, such terms as *post-traumatic syndrome*, *subjective trauma syndrome*, and *postconcussional syndrome* are used. Much of this work highlights the possible impact of small brain lesions (e.g., micro-alterations in the white matter), undetectable with the usual examination techniques, in the genesis of psychological symptoms after a head injury. Such microlesions could, from a cognitive viewpoint, produce a reduction in the capacity to process information, needed to meet the demands of daily life. In any case, the existence of organic lesions does not automatically exclude the presence of independent psychopathological disorders, provoked not by the brain trauma itself, but by the 'traumatising situation' (Naville). There are some data implying the possibility that postconcussional syndrome has a psychogenous cause (Long, 1986), among them, that the symptoms tend to develop and worsen various weeks or months after the head trauma; that some symptoms (such as anxiety and depression) are not easily explainable by organic causes; and that various somatic complaints (vomiting, nausea, blurred version) disappear before others.

There is little proof that the severity of postconcussional syndrome (as measured by severity and duration, or post-traumatic amnesia) is more intense after more severe head injuries. On the other hand, sociological and psychogenetic factors are often involved in the prognosis. Some authors (including Von Monakow, Minkowski, Grinker and Spiegel, Alexandra Adler, Mittelmann, and Futterman) have suggested that there are cases in which regression to an infantile state plays a primordial role, producing a regression aimed at avoiding confronting daily struggles, and which leads some patients to try to get a disability pension or vindicate the right to special treatment. Glover interpreted these symptoms as the expression of a modelling, on the part of the psychic apparatus, of the inhibition and distribution system of instinctive discharges, in the face of adapting to the imbalance induced by psychological stress.

Other authors have also highlighted the importance of the relational and situational aspects of post-traumatic syndromes. Lamman considered, together with a true traumatic neurosis, a 'compensation neurosis' (not directly related to malingering aimed at obtaining a favourable settlement), whose origin would be an unconscious desire to take advantage of the situation, derived from a conflictive external situation. He believed that other emotional attitudes and disorders could arise, as a result of secondary personality and environmental reactions.

An even more markedly sociological line of thought is found in the work of Allodi, who, after studying 50 post-traumatic patients with hysterical symptoms, without a previous psychiatric history, proposed that the cause for their lack of response to treatment was that the compensation they would receive for the accident had yet to be definitively settled. By the same token, Raskin proposed that the common denominator for all of the functional psychopathological phenomena of post-traumatic neuroses was the existence of an insufficiency in normal ego functioning.

Other authors take an even more radical stance and deny that there is any neurological or neurotic influence on the genesis of post-traumatic symptoms, attributing their appearance to the desire to attain a settlement, expressed in a more or less simulated manner. Probably, as Hécaen and Ajuriaguerra propose, a multidimensional approach would be the most appropriate. Post-traumatic neurosis, therefore, would not be simply a phenomenon of affective regression, nor simply a phenomenon of rationalised vindication. Brain damage could intervene not only directly, but also through a general diminishing in resistance, which would enable the subject to clearly express certain features of his previous personality: 'conflicts and difficulties ignored up to that point would appear on a conscious level; the neurological deficit would crystallise around neurotic elements, ensuring their "reality"... A new biological personality would thus be created, and a neurosis could arise in the face of the slightest social or affective conflict'.

REFERENCES

Ajuriaguerra, J. d., and Angelergues, R. (1962). De la psychomotricité au corps dans la relation avec autrui, à propos de l'oeuvre de Wallon. *L'Evolution Psychiatrique*, 27, 3–25.

Ajuriaguerra, J. d., Rego, A., Richard, J., and Tissot, R. (1970). Psychologie et psychométrie du vieillard. *Confront: Psychiat.*, 5, 27–37.

Ajuriaguerra, J., Rego, A., and Tissot, R. (1963). Activités motrices stereotypées dans les démences du grand age. *Ann. Med. Psychol.*, 5, 641–664.

Alonso Fernández, F. (1977). *Fundamentos de la psiquiatría actual.* Madrid: Paz Montalvo.

Banerjee, S., & Dickinson, E. (1997). Evidence based health care in old age psychiatry. *Int J Psychiatry Med*, 27(3), 283–292.

Barraquer Bordas, L., Grau Veciana, J. M., Guimón, J., Fernández Martín, F., & Sabido, F. (1974). Apraxias and agnosias in the dementias of later life. Paper presented at the X International Congress of Neurology, Amsterdam.

Bleuler, E. (1924). Tratado de Psiquiatría. Madrid: Calpe.

Bleuler, M., Willi, J., & Buhler, H. R. (1968). Síndromes psíquicos agudos en las enfermedades somáticas. Madrid: Morata.

Bonhoeffer, K. (1917). Die exogenen Reaktionstypen. *Arch. F. Psychiatr. Nervenkr.*, 58, 58–69.

Cole, M. (2001). The impact of geriatric post-discharge services on mental state. *Age Ageing*, 30(5), 415–418.

Draper, B. (2000). The effectiveness of old age psychiatry services. *Int J Geriatr Psychiatry*, 15(8), 687–703.

Goldstein, K. (1975). Functional Disturbances in brain damage. In S. Arieti (Ed.), American Handbook of Psychiatry (20 ed., pp. 182–207). New York: Basic Books.

Guimón, J. Las psicosis orgánicas.

Guimón, J. (1971a). Apraxia y agnosia. Bilbao: Elexpuru.

Guimón, J. (1971b). La apraxia ideatoria. *Revista de Psicología y Psiquiatría*, 4 (189–220).

Iahns, J. F., Haupt M, Karger A, & M, J. (2000). Improvement of agitation and anxiety in demented patients after psychoeducative group intervention with their caregivers. *Int J Geriatr Psychiatry*, 15(12), 1125–1129.

Rego, A., Guimón, J., & Sánchez de Vega, J. (1969). Evolución del tono muscular en el curso de la desintegración senil. Paper presented at the X Congreso Nacional de Neuropsiquiatría, Barcelona.

Schneider, K. (1942). Problemas de patopsicología y de Psiquiatría clínica. Madrid: Edit. Morata.

Spector, A., Orrell, M., Davies, S., & Woods, R. (2000). Reminiscence therapy for dementia. *Cochrane Database Syst Rev.*, 4(CD001120).

Willi, J. (1968). Delirio, estado crepuscular y confusión en los enfermos somáticos. In W. and B. Bleuler (Eds.), *Síndromes psíquicos agudos en las enfermedades somáticas* (pp. 33–48). Madrid: Morata.

12

Mental and Behavioural Disorders Due to Psychoactive Substances (F10–F19)

CONCEPT AND CLASSIFICATION

The DSM-IV (Frances, First, and Pincus, 1997) includes two types of substance diagnoses: *substance use disorders*, involving a problematic use pattern (dependence and abuse), and *substance-induced disorders*, which include syndromes caused by these substances. However, it is frequently best to diagnose both disorders at once.

Some substances produce physical addiction, and others do not. Twelve substances are cited as the most frequently involved in these disorders: alcohol, hallucinogens, amphetamines, caffeine, cannabis, cocaine, phencyclidine (PCP), inhalants, nicotine, opioids, hypnotic sedatives, and anxiolytics. Other medications (e.g., steroids, anticholinergics) can also become substances of abuse.

There are cultural patterns that differentiate what is acceptable and unacceptable in substance use. Patients often underestimate the amount that they consume, and clinicians must seek collateral information.

Substance dependence is difficult to overcome, and those patients who manage to do so are generally only successful after a number of relapses. Many people are able to maintain a stable pattern of abuse, with pernicious consequences, but without tolerance, abstinence, or compulsive consumption.

AETIOLOGY

The above mentioned substances can produce psychological disorders. Other medications (e.g., steroids, anticholinergics) can also become substances of abuse. In the aetiology of alcoholism, there is a strong genetic factor; in the aetiology of dependence on other substances, this factor is not so clear.

Substance Use in the General Population

In the last few years, a great deal of data has been collected about the use, on the part of the general population, and especially, that of medical and psychiatric patients, of pharmaceuticals, without a medical prescription, and illicit drugs. On the part of the latter group, there is a tendency to believe that this use involves a more or less conscious attempt to diminish their physical or psychological symptomatology.

In this sense, investigators have related the consumption of illicit drugs and psychopharmacological medication in the general population with the presence of inadequately detected psychological suffering, and, among psychiatric patients, with certain syndromes unresolved by their prescribed treatments. It has also been found that illicit drug use is frequently associated with the use of psychopharmacological medication without a prescription (Guimón, 1992).

Attitudinal Profile of Persons Who 'Self-Medicate'

Various researchers have detected a close relationship between substance abuse and certain sociodemographic factors (including sex, age, socio-economic level), both in the general population and in psychiatric patients.

The predominance of males among those who consume alcohol, illicit drugs and psychopharmacological medication, both in the general population and among medical patients, is in accordance with the finding that women present significantly more negative attitudes than men towards the therapeutic use of psychopharmacological medication. The predominance of young people among the self-medicated and consumers of psychotropics is in keeping with our finding (Guimón, 1992) showing that young people report the least fear of psychopharmacological medication. Generally, these results could be interpreted as stemming from the higher cultural level of the younger generations, since our data show that the subjects with higher cultural levels present less prejudices regarding the use of psychopharmacological medication.

Characteristics of Addicts

Kolb set forth the idea that there are different types of addictive individuals, and that their personality characteristics determine which drugs they use and how, and the different subjective effects that they experience. From a psychoanalytical viewpoint, in opiate addiction, authors have postulated the existence of a libidinal fixation with ulterior regression to pregenital levels of development, especially to the oral phase. Later, ego psychology-based explanations were also taken into account, such as the existence of problems in management of affect.

During the following years, research focused on trying to describe the psychological traits of drug addicts, seeking possible underlying psychiatric disorders that would incite them to take opioids: depression, psychopathic tendencies), schizophrenia, and tension and stress. In any case, the general consensus was that once dependence had occurred, abstinence syndrome came into play, and in such a situation the drug produced 'negative euphoria'.

However, in controlled trials with patients enrolled in methadone maintenance programmes, one study mainly found depressive disorders, whereas others found different disorders, including psychoses. One study reported a rise in symptoms when patients self-administered heroin in a controlled setting. Some studies found that the MMPI profile was influenced by such factors as the setting–e.g., whether or not subjects were in hospital–or the duration of hospitalisation .

To avoid such bias, investigators began to carry out studies with drug addicts in their own environment, trying to understand the adaptive use of drugs to deal with anxiety. An study highlighted their difficulties in recognising painful emotions, and their somatisation tendencies an another surmised that patients are inadequately protected against their own feelings of rage and aggression.

Although no clear signs of risk in childhood have been described, there are certain indications that could be taken as warning signs: early health problems, behavioural disorders revolving around food or school, moderate behavioural disorders, lack of self-confidence, a self-centred philosophy of life, and anti-authoritarian attitudes.

In adolescents, a *heroin behavioural syndrome* has been described, which comprises: underlying depression, often of a nervous or anxious type; passive-aggressive impulsivity; fear of failure; low self-esteem; desperation and aggression; low frustration threshold; need for immediate gratification; limited coping strategies. This profile could lead to the use of heroin as self-medication, and soon a relationship would be established between pleasurable feelings and the act of taking drugs: sporadic control of life situations with drugs, interpersonal relationships maintained through drug use, and so on.

Apart from these predisposing symptoms and personality traits, nearly 90% of opiate addicts have a psychiatric disorder, usually depression. The next most frequent are alcoholism, antisocial personality, and anxiety disorders. At least 13% of heroin addicts have tried to commit suicide at least once.

Regarding environmental aspects, there is no clear relationship between substance use and socio-economic status. However, it is common for addicts' parents to be drug or alcohol abusers. In this sense, it has been said that drug use should be taken as a symptom of family dysfunction.

Studies on samples of patients with multiple addictions have reported severe symptoms of depression, anxiety, and psychosis.

Comorbidity

Causality

The literature supports the idea that mental disorders and substance abuse present together with a frequency so high that cannot be attributable to chance. Indeed, a number of studies (Kay et al., 1989; Lehman et al., 1989; Bukstein et al., 1989) found a higher-than-predicted association, or *comorbidity*, between psychiatric disorders and drug abuse.

Some transversal studies have suggested (Bukstein, 1989) that drug abuse plays a major role in the aetiology and prognosis of such alterations as affective disorders, behavioural and antisocial disorders, hyperactivity, panic disorder and schizophrenia. In a sample of cocaine addicts, 47% (Kleinman, 1990) presented a clinical depression (often with comorbid phobic symptoms); on Axis II, the most frequent diagnoses were antisocial (21%), borderline (18%), and self-destructive (18%) personalities. In the ECA project, it was found that the risk of having psychotic symptoms was higher for marijuana users (double) and for users of cocaine and anxiolytics than in those who did not use drugs.

By the same token, those suffering from psychiatric disorders are predisposed to consume drugs. For example, in a study by, 67% of borderline patients were also drug abusers. A study on patients with antisocial personalities (Alterman, 1990) found that the relationship between this disorder and drug use is complex, and that there are probably two different groups of users: true psychopaths, and symptomatic psychopaths, with the latter having psychoneurotic symptomatology and presenting better response to treatment. Subjects with panic attacks (but not anxiety disorder) presented more abuse of opioids and anxiolytics, and first used marijuana (which can induce panic) at an earlier age (Jensen et al., 1993).

RELATIONAL INTERVENTIONS

Alcoholism

In the treatment of alcoholism, the general consensus today is that complete abstinence is the best method, although this is difficult to achieve without first experiencing various relapses. As an aid to achieving abstinence, the patient might take such medications as cyanamide and disulfiram, which produce unpleasant side effects when mixed with alcohol. Less frequently used today is the creation of conditioned reflexes through the simultaneous administration of alcohol and apomorphine.

In these patients, individual and family support are essential, as well as the application of cognitive-behavioural techniques to avoid relapses. Involvement in associations of rehabilitated patients can be a highly important aspect of their treatment.

Analytical psychotherapy, mainly group psychotherapy, has been successfully used to treat abstinent alcoholic patients, but is of little utility in patients who continue to drink.

Other Types of Substance Dependence

Treatment for addiction to opioids has been the most thoroughly developed and is, to certain extent, the standard model for treatment of other types of substance dependence, which is why we shall focus on it in this section.

Treatment of opioid dependence usually involves programmes including phases of detoxification, abstinence maintenance, and reinsertion. The detoxification phase tries to enable the patient to stop taking the substance of abuse without suffering from symptoms of withdrawal, or at least to make the withdrawal experience tolerable, and lasts from 4–21 days, with tapering dosages of prescription opioids (e.g., methadone, dextropropoxyphen, or buprenorphine). Other treatment programmes use alpha-2 adrenergic agonists (especially clonidine). Such measures easily obtain temporary abstinence, but without further subsequent treatment, the relapse rate is 90%.

In the abstinence maintenance phase, there are maintenance programmes using opioid agonists (heroin, methadone) or antagonists (naltrexone). The latter type of medication should only be used with completely detoxified patients. The reinsertion phase is aimed at reintegrating the patient into the community, with or without going through intermediate structures. Morgenstern (2001) has shown the interest of training substance abuse counsellors to deliver cognitive-behavioural treatment (CBT) using treatment manuals in order to enhance treatment adherence.

Different procedures have been proposed for the reduction of cocaine withdrawal symptoms. Findings from a randomised, controlled trial by Margolin did not support the use of acupuncture as a stand-alone treatment for cocaine addiction.

Relational Aspects of Heroin Maintenance

Although experiments using heroin to treat drug addicts who have failed with other, more conventional methods have been going on for many years (for example, the so-called *British system*), defenders of therapeutic heroin prescription tend to cite experiences in Switzerland, whereas its detractors cite those in the United States to back up their arguments. The Swiss experiences of therapeutic prescription of heroin began in 1992, with studies that compared the patients' condition before and after participating in the programme. However, only the study carried out in Geneva had a control group; its results showed that only 1 patient treated with heroin (compared with 10 in the control group) continued to take the drug on his own, on the street, and participants in the heroin programme showed better mental health and social functioning, as well as less criminal behaviour, than the controls.

Be that as it may, even though the results were favourable, treatment with heroin was not a panacea: there were no differences in the two groups' occupational status, somatic condition, or use of other drugs, and only 9 subjects in the control group, at the end of 6 months, asked to take part in the new heroin programme that they had wanted to join at the beginning of the study, and to which they had a right according to the contract they had signed at that time. On the other hand, various patients from the control group also improved according to several measures, which indicates that even the most serious cases could obtain benefits from more conventional methods, such as methadone programmes. After evaluating the results of the different studies, new regulations went into effect regarding the distribution of heroin by medical prescription in Switzerland, after passing a referendum, according to the laws of that country.

In 1998, the United Nations International Drug Control Programme advised against continued clinical trials with heroin. Some commentarists felt that this decision reflected the critical attitude of the influential American medical community, and the general public, towards this type of approach. In fact, it is true that in the United States there is a prevalent puritanical attitude towards the treatment of drug addicts (as there is regarding other medical issues), and although methadone maintenance programmes began in that country (which was, at the time, considered shocking elsewhere) and have at times been in favour, the majority opinion now tends towards complete abstinence as the only recommended approach. However, it would be mistaken to consider this attitude to be solely the result of excessively conservative or naïve attitudes. Indeed, the first experiments treating heroin addicts with heroin in the United States were already published in the early 1970s (Koran, 1973), followed by a study with a control group (Hartnoll, 1980).

Critics of these programmes point out that heroin has a marked tendency to create tolerance, so that the dosage must be increased over time in order for the patient to obtain the same effect. They also say that heroin is not an innocuous substance, as some would have us believe, but that it can produce organic problems, which does seem likely. With García Sevilla (1997), we have published data obtained from heroin addicts who died of overdose, which suggest that chronic heroin abuse can produce certain cerebral alterations in humans. These data should make us cautious when administering heroin over large periods of time for therapeutic purposes. The defenders of therapeutic use point out, however, and with reasons, that other types of medication, such as those used to treat cancer, can also be harmful to health, but they are used if the benefits that they produce outweigh the potential damage. This would seem to be the conclusion drawn by the many governments that have already decided to accept these kinds of experimental programmes.

Group Therapy

Groups are largely used throughout the world for patients who abuse substances, or in outpatient, halfway programmes, or in hospitals for short or medium stays.

Fisher (Fisher and Bentley, 1996) studied two models of group therapy for patients presenting a double diagnosis of substance abuse and personality disorder. This semi-experimental study was led in a facility treating substance abuse, both on a outpatient and hospital basis. They developed three groups in each context: two groups were formed for the integral treatment of patients with a double diagnosis (substance abuse and personality disorder) and the third was used as a control group, with standard treatment.

One of the experimental groups was developed in accordance with the "illness-and-cure" approach. Its objective was the acceptance of substance abuse as a chronic illness, progressive and possibly fatal. In a similar fashion, although mental illness (personality disorder, for example) is not necessarily fatal, its evolution is typically considered to be chronic and progressive. This approach is based on the assumption that patients have an underlying biological vulnerability, characterised by a loss of control over substance abuse and mental disorders. After the start of treatment, the number of patients per group was set at 7 or 8 members. The groups were led in co-therapy by a principal investigator and another clinician. The immediate objectives in the illness-and-cure treatment model include the development of an identity as an 'alcoholic' or an 'addict', recognition of a loss of control over substance abuse and the effects of personality disorder, acceptance of abstinence as a treatment objective, and participation in group self-help activities such as Alcoholics Anonymous. They also developed a second experimental group in each location, with a cognitive-behavioral approach, which they compared with the other described above.

Therapeutic Communities

There are, in addition, long-stay programmes which are more or less structured, sufficiently specific for substance abuse patients, offering an approach that ranges from very firm restriction on freedom to a progressive autonomy leading to total freedom acquired over successive steps during periods ranging from a few months to several years. Some of these programmes are carried out in centres that are directed in accordance with therapeutic community principles. Such programmes are often sidelined from global psychiatric care.

The "Concept-Based" Model

Psychotherapeutic approaches to treating drug addiction have, above all, followed the therapeutic communities concept, which began in the United States in the 1950s with the Synanon programme, followed by others along the same lines, such as Daytop. These were programmes led, in an authoritarian manner, by former addicts, with little participation from physicians or professionals in general. In Europe, this format integrated professionals trained in community management, who were required to have certain abilities such as flexibility and emotional distance. Interesting programmes came out of these efforts, such as the Proyecto Hombre in Italy and Spain, and in some countries they were supported by the government or the Roman Catholic Church.

The majority of these demanded a total abstinence from drugs, and rejected the use of medication. However, as drug abuse rose in 1980s, many communities became oriented towards accepting patients in treatment with methadone or psychotropics, featuring a more intensive role for professionals, and a shorter stay for the patients.

Technically, these programmes revolved around the idea of the 'encounter', which was proposed by behaviourists as an alternative to the psychoanalytically oriented groups used in therapeutic communities for mental patients, since they believed that, in the case of addicts, insight might constitute an excuse for not changing. In Synanon, the encounter group was called 'the game' or 'reality-attack therapy', and included direct confrontation (sometimes exaggerated) without fear of retaliation. In recent years, these groups have become less intensive and more sensitive, evolving towards a form of intense dialogue, in which 'confronting is as important as being confronted'. With all of this, it is more difficult to direct these activities without specific training, although the former addicts resent this, since they feel they have lost power and influence. On the other hand, more scientific concepts have been introduced gradually, with psychiatric diagnosis and assessment.

Broekaert (2001) pointed out that a drug-free therapeutic community defines itself according to various parameters: it should try to become integrated into the community at large; and offer a sufficiently lengthy stay; both the patients and personnel should be open to questioning; and former addicts should have a high profile as role models. As to the clients, they should be called 'residents' (as opposed to 'patients', who need treatment to which they submit passively); it should be accepted that they are immature, innate manipulators, who suffer from fears and anxieties, and that they use violence to hide their weaknesses; above all, there must be a prevailing belief that they can be educated through a therapeutic programme.

In sum, this therapeutic philosophy springs from a number of different sources (Christian doctrine, Alcoholics Anonymous, Synanon, the humanist theories of Maslow and Rogers), all based on the possibility of personal growth and change.

The treatment phases include: crisis intervention (for detoxification in a few days); out-patient (living outside several times a week); reception (admission in a non-demanding regime), in order to prepare for the community during a few weeks; induction, during which motivation is tested; hospitalisation, in which the community is used as treatment during one year in a hierarchically structured environment; phase of acceptance and security, learning to express emotions and modify behaviour in encounter groups and other therapeutic contexts; and social reintegration, through a halfway house or return to the client's own home.

Recent modifications have included the development of more complex networks involving more flexible programmes and customised treatment, e.g., for those with a dual diagnosis, or for chronic patients who need medication. Among the new therapeutic communities, noteworthy are those specialised in other groups, such as the children of addicts, homeless persons, patients suffering from post-traumatic stress disorder, prisoners, immigrants, prostitutes, and AIDS patients.

The "Democratic" Model

When we discuss democratic therapeutic communities, we are generally referring to a model developed by psychiatrists with a participatory focus, although they have never been truly democratic: the roles were allotted, and a patient could be cured, but not form part of the staff; they never aimed for equity in the parcelling out of power or responsibility. In any cases, these programmes allow all of their members to have a very high level of participation in decision making, with a high degree of information sharing, and a great deal of emphasis on listening to others.

The Differences between These Two Models Today

Over the years, different countries have adopted these two community therapy models, tailoring them to their needs and cultural particularities. For example, in Italy the democratic community therapy model is particularly prevalent in the treatment of mental illness, whereas in England it is mainly used in treating personality disorders. It seems that in Italy, there is more open communication and overlapping between democratic therapeutic communities and concept-based ones, particularly at the management level, with their directors and staff psychiatrists taking part in the same congresses and belonging to the same professional organisations.

However, two important differences can be observed. First, is the fact that the concept-based community is nearly always aimed at those whose primary problem is drug addiction, independent of their 'secondary' problems or incidents that may arise over the course of treatment. On the other hand, democratic therapeutic communities are nearly always aimed at those diagnosed with personality disorders or who are mentally ill. These persons may also be addicted to drugs, but not necessarily. The second major difference is that the staff of democratic therapeutic communities comprises professionals only, whereas that of a concept community may include former residents.

Although outside of Europe, the majority of therapeutic communities for drug addicts are highly structured with a strict staff hierarchy, many European therapeutic communities use a more egalitarian model. These are more similar to therapeutic communities in the psychiatric field using a democratic structure (Jones, 1952). However, therapeutic communities with more than 25 residents have usually adopted the hierarchic structure of American programmes. European therapeutic communities are now, in turn, also influencing their American counterparts – for example, their emphasis on introducing creative activities into programming. In addition, they have shown that the residents can learn new skills, such as gardening, agriculture, and printing, during their stay in the programme. In Europe, as in the United States, detoxification centres have been created that are linked to certain therapeutic communities, and in some cases, day centres and evening programmes have been developed based on the drug-free therapeutic community concept.

Therapeutic communities in Europe have also begun to expand their range of patients to self-destructive behaviours other than drug addiction. Moreover, the concept of hierarchic therapeutic communities has been successfully used in treating alcoholics.

Although research has shown that the time spent in a programme is the main predictor of success, these programmes have recently tended to become shorter, a trend seen in many countries during the 1990s. Relatively inexpensive psychosocial self-help programmes are being transformed into short-stay programmes following a medical model. Indeed, methadone maintenance programmes are being considered in various countries, by politicians and by doctors (aided and abetted by the pharmaceutical industry) as the solution to the problem of heroin addiction. Due to all of these and other factors, the future of the traditional therapeutic communities is in doubt.

In any case, drop out is a frequent problem in these programmes and, for example, Keen et al. (2001) found low levels of completion and high levels of unplanned departure in a residential rehabilitation centre in a 1-year programme for chronic heroin users

Good results have been reported in a special programme created for the integrated treatment of a dual diagnosis involving schizophrenia and substance abuse (Hellerstein et al., 2001). However, Ley (2002), evaluating the effectiveness of six relevant studies, concluded that there is no clear evidence supporting an advantage of special programmes for people with problems of both substance misuse and serious mental illness, and ends saying that 'implementation of new specialist substance misuse services for those with serious mental illnesses should be within the context of simple, well designed controlled clinical trials'.

REFERENCES

Alterman, A. J., et al. (1982). Effect of illicit drugs use in inpatient psychiatric population. *Addictive Behaviour*, 7, 231–242.

Broekaert, E. (2001). Therapeutic communities for drug users: description and overview. In B. Rawlings & R. Yates (Eds.), *Therapeutic Communities for the Treatment of Drug Users* (pp. 29–42). London: Jessica Kingsley Publishers, London.

Bukstein, O., and Kaminer, Y. (1989). Comorbility of substance abuse and other psychiatric disorders in adolescents. *American Journal of Psychiatry*, 146 (9).

Fisher Sr., M. S., & Bentley, K. J. (1996). Two group therapy models for clients with a dual diagnosis of substance abuse and personality disorder. *Psychiatric Services, 47*(11), 1244–1250.

Frances, A., First, M. B., and Pincus, H. A. (Eds.). (1997). *DSM-IV, Guía de uso*. Barcelona: Masson, Barcelona.

García Sevilla, J., Ventayol, P., Busquets, X., La Harpe, R., Walzer, C., & Guimón, J. (1997). Marked decrease of immunolabelled 68kDa neurofilament (NF-L) proteins in brains of opiate addicts. *NeuroReport, 8*, 1561–1570.

Guimón, J., et al. (1992). Automedicacion en poblacion general y en pacientes médicos. In M. Casas (Ed.), *Trastornos psiquicos en las toxicomanias*. Barcelona: Ediciones en Neurociencias.

Jenson, J., Wells, E., Plotnick, R., Hawkins, D., & Catalano, R. (1993). The effects of skills and intentions to use drugs on posttreatment drug use of adolescents. *American Journal of Drug and Alcohol Abuse, 19*(1), 1–18.

Jones, M. S. (1952). *Social Psychiatry: A Study of Therapeutic Communities*. London: Tavistock Publications.

Kay, S. R., Kalathara, M., and Meinzer, A. E. (1989). Diagnostic and behavioral characteristics of psychiatric patients who abuse substances. *Hospital and Community Psychiatry*, 40(10).

Kleinman, P. H., Woody, G. E., Todd, T. C., Millman, R. B., Kang, S. Y., Kemp, J., & Lipton, D. S. (1990). Crack and cocaine abusers in outpatient psychotherapy. *NIDA Research Monographs Series*, 24–35.

Lehman, A. F., Myers, C. P., and Corty, E. (1989). Assessment and classification of patients with psychiatric and substance abuse syndromes. *Hospital and Community Psychiatry*, 40(10).

Morgenstern, J., Morgan, T., McCrady, B., Keller, D., & Carroll, K. (2001). Manual-guided cognitive-behavioral therapy training: a promising method for disseminating empirically supported substance abuse treatments to the practice in community. *Psychol Addict Behav, 15*(2),

Hellerstein, D., Rosenthal, R., & Miner, C. (2001). Integrating services for schizophrenia and substance abuse. *Psychiatr Q.*, 72(4)), 291–306.

Keen, J., Oliver, P., Rowse, G., & Mathers, N. (2001). Residential rehabilitation for drug users: a review of 13 months' intake to a therapeutic community. *Fam Pract*, 18(5), 545–548.

Ley, A., Jeffery, D., McLaren, S., & Siegfried, N. (2002). *Treatment programmes for people with both severe mental illness and substance misuse (Cochrane Review)* (Vol. Oxford). Oxford: Update Software.

13

Schizophrenia, Schizotypal, and Delusional Disorders (F20–29)

SCHIZOPHRENIA

Concept

Schizophrenia is the prototype of the psychoses that are considered to have a biological basis (the *functional psychoses*), although as yet it is unknown or poorly understood. Although some authors have tried to describe schizophrenia as a genuine illness, the prevailing wisdom today is that we would be better advised to consider it a syndrome or disorder, which can arise from different initial alterations, taking different paths.

Kraepelin (1920) dubbed this disorder *dementia praecox*, and differentiated it from the *affective psychoses* (the other major group of functional psychoses), precisely due to the much higher frequency of the appearance of deterioration or *defect* in the course of schizophrenia.

Various authors have tried to delineate the basic symptoms of the syndrome. Thus, so-called primary (Bleuler, 1924) or first-rank symptoms (Schneider, 1942) have been described, but certainly *no pathognomonic* (or exclusive) symptoms. Since Kraepelin described the three basic clinical forms (*catatonic, hebephrenic, and paranoid*), to which Bleuler added the *simple* form, a number of other authors have proposed many more, although only a few of these terms remain in use (*schizoaffective, schizophreniform, residual, positive* and *negative*).

Relational Aetiopathogeny

There are undoubtedly genetic and biochemical factors in the aetiology of schizophrenia (see Chapter 3), but we will focus here on the relational aspects. There is no single aetiological factor in schizophrenia; rather, it depends on factors affecting both the genotype and the phenotype. In this sense, it is generally accepted that there is a genetic predisposition to acquiring certain alterations in the structure and functioning of the brain and the neuroendocrinal system which condition *vulnerability to stress*. There is also a consensus that the defence mechanisms acquired by small children regarding the significant others in their environment enable them to modulate, more or less adequately, external stimuli. Stressful life events are offset by community support mechanisms (family, social networks, health care systems). Only when these are overcome it is necessary for defence mechanisms to intervene, and if these are insufficient, then biological systems of adaptation are forced into action. When an inherited fragility of these biological systems renders them incapable of counteracting stressful stimuli, then schizophrenia arises. The following is a summary of the findings regarding the factors involved in the maintenance of this delicate *homeostasis*.

In many of the recent studies on the aetiology of schizophrenia, a wide variety of aetiological proposals are assigned the rank of theories worthy of consideration (Guimón, 1977). These theories can be grouped, into the three basic models of psychology: the medical model, the psychological model, and the sociological model. However, cognitive theories and those that postulate a predisposition for poor stress elaboration on the part of subjects diagnosed with schizophrenia can also be included in the medical model. Psychoanalytical theories refer to early interpersonal relations within the family, and therefore they can be included in the social model.

Psychological Factors

General Psychology and Neuropsychology

Different psychological studies have confirmed the classic papers that hypothesised the existence in schizophrenics of alterations involving attention, perception, cognition, and reaction time, as well as the fact that they tend to become distracted by irrelevant stimuli. Other classic observations that have been confirmed include a heightened at-rest psychogalvanic response; excessive response to stress; rapid acquisition of conditioned responses; and excessive stimuli generalisation reaction. All of this led researchers to consider the possibility of an excessive predisposition to stress in schizophrenics. From a clinical standpoint, it was theorised that a certain difficulty in 'stimuli filtering' would lead schizophrenics to try to control them through social isolation.

Recent research has shown the existence of neuropsychological alterations in schizophrenics which can be considered 'markers' for the disorder: dysfunction in eye movements; appearance of evoked potentials related to certain events; and alterations observable on attention and information tests.

Regarding these patients' electroencephalogram results, anomalies of evoked potentials are visible. However, these waves are not seen in all schizophrenics, and are not specific to them, since they can also appear in normal subjects.

Eye-movement dysfunction consists of certain alterations in the path that these patients' eyes follow when presented with visual stimuli. These alterations (perhaps cortical in origin), which are independent of the patients' clinical state and neuroleptics that they might be taking, also appear in their non-schizophrenic family members. However, since they can also be seen in normal subjects, bipolar patients, and those with central nervous system disorders, this phenomenon cannot be considered specific to schizophrenia.

Recent research has also shown more specific alterations in schizophrenic patients' information processing. These include such elemental functions as selective attention (directed at stimuli pertinent to the ongoing action) or sustaining attention during longer periods. Also noteworthy are complex alterations at the level of information assimilation and memory management, which are the bases of higher cognitive, deductive, and conceptual activities.

These studies, centred on measuring cognitive deficiencies, have not been able to show a lineal relationship between severity of symptoms and intensity of social dysfunction. This inconsistency has, however, been partially resolved thanks to the development of the vulnerability model of schizophrenia created in the 1970s by Zubin et al. (Zubin, Steinhauser, & Condray, 1992). This author sees in schizophrenia the expression of structural and physiological variations, genetic or acquired, which alter perceptive and cognitive functioning, particularly information processing. Moreover, these alterations interact with environmental factors, and together they can favour an eventual psychotic outbreak.

Psychoanalysis

From a psychoanalytical viewpoint, it has been suggested that certain constitutional disorders in higher nervous functions can alter the child's ego functions (hypersensitivity to sensorial input, increase in aggressive drives), which alter the early mother-child relationship. The literature includes descriptions of schizophrenogenic mothers (aggressive, rejecting, insecure or hyperprotective); inadequate fathers (passive, menacing); bad marital relations between the parents (*'marital schism'*, *'emotional divorce'*); or inadequate communication (*'double-bind'*). However, these data have not been confirmed by rigorously designed studies, or when alterations have been detected, it was impossible to determine whether they were the underlying cause.

Psychoanalysis has focused on the origins of the subjects of patients' delusions. Going beyond Esquirol, who attributed them to excessive passion, some authors preferred the hermeneutic method, analysing them as if they were a text. For Freud, the origin of delusions would have to be found in an earlier stage of infancy than the one that generates neurosis.

The Social Model in the Aetiology of Schizophrenia

Sociocultural Factors

The sociological model of schizophrenia proposes that certain social factors can lead to the presentation in a subject of the psychological disorders that are considered necessary for a diagnosis of schizophrenic psychosis (Guimón, 1977). The defenders of this model base their affirmation on empirical findings that confirm, at least in Western urban society, the existence of different incidence and prevalence indices for schizophrenia in different population groups. Indeed, various studies have highlighted the influence on incidence of socio-economic (poverty, population density, and social disorganisation) and cultural factors (immigration, cultural change, and industrialisation). However, more recent studies have not confirmed that gender, race, educational level, or place of residence play a significant epidemiological role.

This controversy is as yet unresolved, because there are methodological problems in the sociological research carried out on schizophrenia. Most of the studies on the incidence and prevalence of schizophrenia have been carried out by studying the populations in hospital or out-patient psychiatric clinics. However, it is evident that the representation of certain populations in a psychiatric clinic depends to a great extent on such factors as awareness of and ease of access to certain services on the part of the population; the higher or lower tolerance of the subjects' families to psychiatric disorders; or the higher or lower reticence to consult a psychiatrist. These and other factors condition the fact that certain population groups are represented more or less in these samples, so that it is impossible to compare, with a minimal degree of rigour, incidence and prevalence indices in these groups. If the study uses surveys including questionnaires able to detect schizophrenic disorders in the general public, new problems arise. On the one hand, it is reasonable to expect that in this kind of survey, at least 10% of those contacted will refuse to answer. On the other, since the prevalence of schizophrenia is relatively low, and those affected by the disorder are usually suspicious and withdrawn, the schizophrenics themselves are among those who are most likely to be non-responders.

Some studies have tried to overcome these and other difficulties (Hollingshead & Redlich, 1958). Even so, the data they provide cannot be considered unreservedly aetiologically valid. Is the observed higher predisposition to schizophrenia in the lower classes in any way attributable to the higher percentage of foetal damage due to lower quality care during childbirth? Is the higher percentage of schizophrenic outbreaks seen in immigrants possibly due to the socialisation difficulties that they encounter, or on the contrary, are subjects with a schizophrenic predisposition, and therefore with adaptation problems in their countries of origin, more likely to emigrate in the first place?

In spite of these reservations, there is sufficient proof that psychosocial factors do contribute to the appearance of schizophrenia. Even when we consider genetic studies that show concordances of up to 70% in the presentation of schizophrenia in identical twins, their importance is clear. As Arieti puts it (Arieti, 1974), even more noteworthy than this high concordance is the presence of the 30% of twins who, despite being genetically identical to their siblings, never develop the illness.

In the face of such data, there is no other choice than to recur to psychosocial arguments. It seems that we should accept that in the aetiology of schizophrenia there is both a 'sufficient' inherited condition and other 'necessary' conditions of a psychosocial nature.

The General Public's View of Schizophrenia

Angermeyer et al. (Angermeyer & Matschinger, 1999) have discussed why the social representation of schizophrenia is so strongly dominated by the belief that to be schizophrenic means to have a split personality, in the sense of multiple personality disorder. The term *schizophrenia* was first introduced in 1911, by Eugen Bleuler (Bleuler, 1924), to replace the term *dementia praecox* chosen by Emil Kraepelin (Kraeplin, 1920); it comes from the Greek *schizein*, meaning 'to split', and *phren*, which can mean 'soul', 'mind', or 'diaphragm'. As Bleuler put it at the time, 'I call dementia praecox *schizophrenia*, since I hope to show that the splitting of the different mental functions is one of its defining traits.'

After the popularisation of Bleuler's concept of schizophrenia and its incorporation into everyday discourse, the term was configurated as suggested by the 'social representation theory': 'Tangible' persons who appear alternatively and successively, dominating the scene, are replaced by the psychological 'complexes' that are quite difficult for the general public to understand. The psychological phenomenon that originally only 'existed' in theory was transformed, therefore, into a concrete entity.

Relational Interventions

In this section, we include the treatments used, at different dosages and with different combinations, both for schizophrenic and schizophreniform patients, and for those who present schizoaffective disorders, brief psychotic reactions, and severe schizotypic disorders. We exclude from this group paranoid patients and schizoid personalities requiring different approaches.

In the case of schizophrenic patients, many studies have noted that certain paranoid syndromes have a better prognosis compared with other, 'non-paranoid' ones, as well as the fact that patients who present 'positive' symptoms have a better prognosis and better response to phenothiazines than those whose symptoms are mostly 'negative'.

The treatment of schizophrenia, as in most psychiatric disorders, demands a balance between biological and psychosocial measures.

Biological Treatment

Today, lobotomies are no longer practised on schizophrenic patients, and electroshock is used only in neuroleptic-resistent cases of catatonia. After the discovery of the phenothiazines, many other medications have been used from different chemical families (thioxanthenes, butyrophenones, dibenzodiazepines, dihydroindolones) in treating schizophrenia. Although studies are beginning to appear affirming that certain medications are more efficacious than others for positive or negative symptoms, there is still not an irrefutable profile of specific activity for the different neuroleptics regarding different symptoms. The efficacy of neuroleptic medication in the treatment of schizophrenia is now unquestionable, as proved by various studies. Consequently, over the last few decades hopes have arisen both regarding the prognosis of the illness and the patients' quality of life. In fact, admissions to psychiatric institutions have dropped significantly, as shown by the so-called deinstitutionalisation process.

Since side affects are frequent, and the patient is often not even aware of his illness, long-acting (2 weeks–1 month) injectable neuroleptics are very useful for improving treatment compliance.

Among the negative side effects of such medication, some of the most noteworthy are neurological: parkinsonian and dystonic (acute and late onset) side effects, dyskinesia (acute and late onset), akathisia (restlessness, with difficulty remaining seated), malignant neuroleptic syndrome, convulsions, and cognitive dysfunction.

Since a certain proportion of patients does not benefit from chronic neuroleptic treatment, the standard procedure is to try to taper off the medication after one year; treatment can then be resumed after an appropriate time, if the clinician considers that the benefits are greater than possible disadvantages.

Some studies report that minimal doses of neuroleptics produce sufficient saturation of the dopaminergic receptors; in that case, it would not be advisable to give larger doses which could increase extrapyramidal side effects.

However, every day we still face a very disturbing statistical fact: 50% of all schizophrenic patients suffer a relapse in the first year after their latest psychotic episode. These patients are also institutionalised 15–20% of their lives as a result of their frequent relapses. Although there are many factors that influence the development of these relapses, a detailed analysis falls outside of the realm of the present work.

Psychosocial Treatments

Studies that are already decades old report spectacular psychotic episodes with a sudden onset and which evolve positively with psychotherapeutic treatment. To designate them, certain authors have used the term *hysterical psychosis* (Pankow, 1969). With this group of patients it is not, of course, possible to follow the same guidelines as in psychotherapy with other schizophrenic patients.

In spite of all the efforts made to avoid it, schizophrenic deterioration (not necessarily present in schizotypic or schizoaffective disorders) is frequent; it is not only a difficulty on an intellectual level, but also a lack of interest and energy that leads the patient to avoid the efforts of everyday life. Under the name of *absence of social competence*, a series of characteristics has been described which make the chronic schizophrenic less able to live in the community, at least in Western society.

Among the most important factors aggravating social ineptitude, the role played by hospitalisation has been widely discussed (Guimón & Ozamiz, 1982; Guimón, Villasana, Totorika, & Ozamiz, 1981). Therefore, some authors tend to differentiate between the concepts of *clinical remission* and *social remission* (Brown, Monck, Carstairs, & Wing, 1958; Seva Diaz, 1979).

Psychoanalytically Oriented Psychotherapy

Psychoanalytically oriented psychotherapy has, until recently, been shown to be only slightly useful in treating schizophrenia, except in a subgroup of patients with sufficient ego strength, and who remain as in-patients for long periods in special therapeutic settings. However, there was a general consensus that a dynamic understanding of the patient's psychopathology and relationships with family and social networks could be very helpful (Fenton & Schooler, 2000). A recent, randomised study showed that analytical psychotherapy could produce improvement in the social and professional functioning of some schizophrenics that was unattainable any other way (Hogarty, Kornblith, & Greenwald, 1997).

Gabbard (Gabbard, 1995) proposes some general guidelines for psychotherapy with schizophrenia: the main goal should be to establish a relationship; flexibility is necessary regarding therapeutic approach and content; an optimal distance between the therapist and the patient should be established; the therapist must create a setting (*holding*) that serves as a 'container'; he should set himself up as an *'auxiliary ego'*, showing himself to be open, respectful, and candid; and he should postpone making any kind of interpretation until a good relationship has been established.

However, Malmberg et al. (Malmberg & Fenton, 2002), reviewing the effects of individual psychodynamic psychotherapy for people with schizophrenia, concluded that, although the psychodynamic approach may be more acceptable to people than a more cognitive reality-adaptive therapy, current data do not support the use of psychodynamic psychotherapy techniques for hospitalised people with schizophrenia.

Cognitive-Behavioural Therapy

As Roder et al. ((Roder, Zorn, Muller, & Brenner, 2001) pointed out, we have seen three eras in the development and refinement of social skills training for individuals with schizophrenia. In the 1960s, skills training relied on the use of operant conditioning, as exemplified by the token economy, which is still used to motivate anergic individuals to participate actively in community-based programmes. In the 1970s, social learning was introduced to improve nonverbal skills, as well as conversational skills, assertiveness, and emotional expressiveness. Tsang (2001) claimed that a social skills training module, together with appropriate professional support afterward, is effective in enhancing the social competence and vocational outcomes of persons with schizophrenia.

In the third and current era, cognitive methods for training social and independent living skills (Liberman, 1986) and techniques to improve attention, memory, and verbal learning have been introduced. Thanks to better knowledge of deficit symptoms, it has been observed that even simple learning activities are often difficult, due to certain patients' cognitive deficits. Therefore, it has been decided to improve this deficit with cognitive rehabilitation modules. Thus Hans Brenner (Brenner & Pfammatter, 2000), Roder, and others have developed an integrated psychological therapy

(IPT) addressing deficits in the residential, vocational, and recreational domains of community functioning, and they believe that it is more effective than other psychosocial treatments, such as supportive group therapy and pure behavioural methods. However, Suslow et al. (Suslow, Schonauer, & Arolt, 2001), in their review of the literature on training in attentional functioning, contended that evidence on attention training's effectiveness in schizophrenia is inconclusive.

In a Cochrane review, Nicol et al. (Nicol, Robertson, & Connaughton, 2002) evaluated all relevant randomised or quasi-randomised controlled trials on life skills programmes, and found that data are sparse and no clear effects were demonstrated. They concluded, 'If life skills training is to continue as part of rehabilitation programmes a large, well designed, conducted and reported pragmatic randomised trial is an urgent necessity. There may even be an argument for stating that maintenance of current practice, outside of a randomised trial, is unethical.' In another Cochrane study, Cormac et al. (Cormac, Jones, & Campbell, 2002) reviewed the effectiveness of cognitive behavioural therapy for people with schizophrenia, and concluded that it did not significantly reduce the rate of relapse and readmission to hospital when compared with standard care alone. A significant difference was observed, however, favouring cognitive behavioural therapy over standard care alone, in terms of being able to discharge patients from hospital; however, after one year the difference was no longer significant. A cognitive-behavioural therapy approach focusing on compliance may have some effects on insight and attitudes to medication, but the clinical meaning of these data is unclear. When compared with supportive psychotherapy, cognitive behavioural therapy had no effects on relapse rate or clinically meaningful improvements in mental state. A recent trial of Cognitive-Behavioural Therapy delivered by nurse specialists gave a significant improvement of medication resistant psychotic symptoms (Durham et al, 2003).

A modification of cognitive-behavioural therapy, 'Assertive Community Treatment' (ACT), has been shown in a Cochrane review (Marshall & Lockwood, 2002) to facilitate that patients remain in contact with services. People allocated to ACT were less likely to be admitted to hospital than those receiving standard community care, and spent less time in hospital. In terms of clinical and social outcome, significant and robust differences between ACT and standard community care were found on some social variables, but not on mental state or social functioning or quality of life. Present evidence suggests that case management increases health care costs, perhaps substantially, although this is uncertain. In summary, this study's authors say that 'case management is an intervention of questionable value, to the extent that it is doubtful whether it should be offered by community psychiatric services. It is hard to see how policy makers who subscribe to an evidence-based approach can justify retaining case management as "the cornerstone" of community mental health care.'

Psycho-Educational Therapy

Psycho-educational techniques enhance medication compliance, also improving attitudes to treatment, substance misuse and insight (Thornicroft, 2001). Thus, Amenson and Liberman (Amenson & Liberman, 2001) underline the need to overcome the barriers to the incorporation of family psycho-education into the routine care provided at community mental health centres.

However, in a Cochane review, Henderson et al. (Henderson & Laugharne, 2002) warn about the need for tactfully informing patients, because it cannot be assumed that patient-held information is beneficial or cost-effective without evidence from well planned, conducted and reported randomised trials, still lacking.

Personal Therapy

'Personal therapy' (Hogarty et al., 1997) and 'cognitive enhancement therapy' (CET) are long-term interventions for individuals with schizophrenia designed to increase the accurate appraisal of emotional states through psycho-educational and behavioural therapy techniques. It seems that personal therapy improves social adjustment, but can increase the rate of psychotic relapse for some patients living independently from their families.

Family Therapy

Family therapy has been useful for treating the patient in his own environment, and reducing relapse. The techniques are not based so much on the so-called systemic model (which assumes that alterations in family communication can produce schizophrenia) as on psycho-educational techniques (explaining symptoms and therapeutic options to the family). They are based on the finding that the patient's presence produces alterations within the family, especially in those families that tend to adopt excessively emotional attitudes ('high emotional expression') (Guimón & Cuperman, 1982). These psychosocial family interventions tend to improve the alliance with relatives, reducing the adverse expressions of anger and guilt by the family, encouraging the relatives to stay within appropriate limits (Thornicroft, 2001).

Family interventions (Dixon, Adams, & Lucksted, 2000) seem to be of help in keeping patients in the community. A Cochrane collaboration systematic review has concluded that families receiving this intervention can expect less frequent relapse and hospital admission in their relatives with schizophrenia, without any additional burden of care. Multiple family models seem to be more effective than interventions for single families (McFarlane, 2000) in terms of reduced relapse rates and offering an expanded social network. Dixon (Dixon et al., 2000), in a review, contended that the data supporting the efficacy of family psycho-education remain compelling.

However, Pharoah et al. (Pharoah, Mari, & Streiner, 2002), in a Cochrane review, examined randomised or quasi-randomised studies and found that family intervention may decrease hospitalisation and encourage compliance with medication, but does not obviously affect the tendency of individuals/families to drop out of care. It may improve general social impairment and the levels of expressed emotion within the family, although professionals 'cannot be confident of the effects of family intervention from the findings of this review.'

On the other hand, there is a poor availability of these treatments in ordinary clinical settings (Penn, Kommana, Mansfield, & Link, 1999) and a substantial proportion of relatives refuse to attend a group and need sessions in the home (Leff, 2000).

Group Psychotherapy

Even now, in certain developed countries (Sultenfuss & Geczy, 1996), schizophrenics who remain in long-stay units at psychiatric hospitals receive only pharmacological treatment.

Group psychotherapy, above all when the therapist actively tries to develop social abilities and strategies for coping with stress, has been supposed to be useful, especially once florid symptoms are under control. The results seem to be better than those obtained with individual psychotherapy, which can be explained by the fact that the group offers socialisation experiences, behavioural models, and a more shared transference which is less dependent on the therapist (Guimón & Totorika, 1983). However, the treatment of chronic schizophrenics using analytical group psychotherapy has often been an exasperating, fruitless experience (Frankel, 1993), creating a strong emotional response in the therapists which also reinforces a spiral of repeated failures.

Overall, the relatively few controlled trials of group psychotherapy present major methodological problems which limit their generalisability. Scott and Dixon (Scott & Dixon, 1995), in a review of the literature on the clinical outcomes obtained by support and dynamic psychotherapy (both group and individual) and psychosocial skills training, found that the reality-oriented approaches seem better than insight-oriented dynamic psychotherapy.

So-called Integrated Psychological Therapy (IPT) is a group-therapy modality intended to re-establish basic neurocognitive functions (Spaulding, Reed, Sullivan, Richardson, & Weiler, 1999) which has shown incrementally greater gains, compared with controls, on the primary outcome measure, the Assessment of Interpersonal Problem-Solving Skills, after a 6-month intensive trial.

Milieu Therapy

Therapeutic Communities. The use of principles from so-called *milieu therapy*, based on the experiences of therapeutic communities organised into inpatient units, day hospitals, halfway houses and sheltered workshops, have improved the clinical prognosis and socio-occupational adaptation of chronic schizophrenics.

Several studies, of variable methodological quality, have reported a favourable result with this type of approach in psychotic patients. Thus, De Hert et al. ((De Hert, Thys, Vercruyssen, & Peuskens, 1996), who followed up 120 young, chronic patients taking part in the rehabilitation programme at the Night Hospital in Brussels, showed that most of them maintained the level of adaptation obtained and continued to live in the community, engaged in useful pursuits. Dauwalder and Ciompi (Dauwalder & Ciompi, 1995) proved the long-term efficacy of a community-based programme for chronic mental patients which resulted in a great number of them having jobs and independent lives, even if most patients still needed professional help. Jin and Li (1994) observed that the number of suicides decreased and active participation increased at Yanbian Community Psychiatric Hospital, after its transformation from a residential facility for chronic psychiatric patients into a therapeutic community. Coombe (Coombe, 1996), in an account of principles and treatment practices given to the therapeutic community at London's Cassel Hospital, noted the ability of the therapeutic network to render possible the successful treatment of families and individuals suffering from serious disorders.

Mosher (Mosher & Feinsilver, 1971) compared the treatment programme for young schizophrenic patients in the Soteria project with that of a small social environment, generally without neuroleptics. The atmospheres of treatment settings were evaluated using the Moos (Moos, 1997), COPES, or WAS scales. The two systems managed to reduce, in a similar fashion, the serious psychotic symptomatology in six weeks, generally without anti-psychotic medication, as effectively as the normal hospital treatment which included the routine utilisation of neuroleptics. Shepherd (Shepherd & Murray, 2001) presented benefits and limitations of a new type of institutional solution–the 'unit in a home'–for patients suffering from severe disorders recruited in Cambridge, England. Another study (Nieminen, Isohanni, & Winblad, 1994) carried out in a therapeutic community unit for severely affected patients, with an average hospital stay of 40 days, reported that the patients who had obtained a better immediate result stayed 10 to 20 days longer in the hospital than those who had an inferior result. A longer stay was associated with a younger age, a diagnosis of psychosis, and active and motivated participation.

Ward Atmosphere in Short-Stay Units . In short-stay psychiatric units, the patients have to deal with a high degree of stress, arising from short stays, acute symptomatology, auto- and hetero-aggression, rapid turnover of patients, and limited space.

During the last 25 years, we have organised programmes of milieu therapy in a certain number of short-stay units through the organisation of a variety of groups of patients and staff (Guimón, Luna, Totorika, Diez, & Puertas, 1983). Group analysis, with its particular emphasis on the 'here and now' and on inter-member cohesiveness, has shown itself to be, in our experience, a useful stabilising (*'buffer'*) tool, through fostering involvement and support and allowing a controlled expression of anger and aggressiveness.

The patient-staff group is the key holding element of our group analytic programme, due to its basic contribution to creating a *'container'* for the anxieties arising in the ward. It is also of invaluable help because of the information it provides concerning each patient. The other groups also provide the patient with orientation and emotional support. On the staff side, tensions among the therapeutic team are reduced and incoming nursing personnel notice how their previous fears and apprehensions diminish.

Overall, we had the impression that, despite a personnel shortage, a pleasant and supportive atmosphere was created in the wards, constituting a group-analytical network that makes for more harmonious communications among the various units of the hospital. This systemic vision of the institution provides invaluable help in understanding its organisational problems and internal struggles, which can soon be detected, providing the input for the 'healthy anticipatory paranoia' needed (Kernberg, 1979) in the management of these organisations.

Relapse Prevention and Avoidance

Relapse can occur at any moment of the evolution of the disorder but there are some specific moments when it is more likely such as the periods of transition from psychiatric institutions to community housing.

'Critically timed' psychosocial interventions (Thornicroft, 2001) have been tested in randomised trials.

Detection of High-Risk Subjects

If, in schizophrenia, we focus on the problem of primary prevention, we have to settle for genetic counselling and some basic mental hygiene, insofar as there is little clinical evidence of any truly effective preventive measures. However, different authors research findings on children at risk have identified some vulnerability markers, so pessimism on this subject has diminished somewhat.

Schizophrenia prevention could work to lessen stressful conditions, or increase defence and coping mechanisms; but mainly, it could focus on actions applicable from birth, or even before, to inhibit the expression of the illness in those prone to it. But these are non-specific and expensive strategies.

Currently, efforts are centred on identifying groups having an attribute that predicts very high risk for schizophrenia. However, until recently, the only reliable marker for schizophrenia was having a schizophrenic parent, since 10–16% of a schizophrenic parent's children develop the illness. However, it would not be justifiable to engage in wide-ranging prevention projects, given that 86–90% of the cohort is not at risk.

Studies on high-risk individuals are based on genetics, developmental psychology, studies on attention and information-processing, and measurements of intra-family processes. They include prospective studies, following a cohort over time to identify attributes of individuals or families existing before onset of the illness. It is possible that such a marker could reflect a pathophysiological or psychopathological process that contributes to the development of schizophrenia, which could possibly have aetiological implications.

There are antecedents and early warning signals of dysfunction able to identify children and adolescents at risk. Various studies, covering conception to two years, have shown that some of these individuals are subject to identifiable stressful circumstances, and show early delusional symptoms.

Regarding whether these markers identify persons with a specific risk of developing schizophrenia, or merely any psychopathology, most studies show little specificity, except for a one that showed higher cognitive and attention deficits in the children of schizophrenics.

The detection of children at risk would make it possible to work with them in order to modify some vulnerability factors. In a prospective study, it was found that in children with schizoid personalities, their psychosocial adjustments was somewhat worse than other children who attended a child psychiatry clinic; as a group, they tended to be more solitary, lacking in empathy, hypersensitive, with odd ways of communicating, and often with limited interests. As adults, fewer of them had had heterosexual experiences, and more of them had sought psychiatric help at some time. Although the majority developed schizophrenic spectrum disorders, the risk of developing schizophrenia was small (Wolff, 1991).

Various studies indicate that the more serious the mother's illness, the worse her interaction with her child; it has also been shown that low socio-economic status is correlated with poor mother-child relations. Stress and the woman's risk behaviours can produce childbirth complications and create neuro-integrative abnormalities, so that the child may have a difficult temperament, and the stressed mother may treat him inadequately.

Prevention Strategies

Possible prevention strategies are partly based on findings (e.g., early signs of neuro-integrative disorder and alteration in parent-child relations) linked to psychiatric disorders in the mother, or problems during pregnancy and childbirth. In these cases, prevention focuses on improving prenatal care, and stimulating a more favourable parent-child relationship.

Another prevention strategy centres on children with attention deficit disorder aiming at detecting families at risk in order to help their children, improving alterations in communication, affective style, and expression of emotions.

It is also known that programmes aimed at lessening negative attitudes towards psychopharmacological medication and those that aim to reduce 'expressed emotion' within the family can lower relapses.

In Scandinavia, Johannessen et al. (Johannessen, Larsen, McGlashan, & Vaglum, 2000) carried out a campaign to inform the public of the early signs of schizophrenia, aimed at increasing early intervention and reducing the duration of untreated psychosis (DUP), which had positive results. Alanen et al. (Alanen, Lehtinen, Lehtinen, Aaltonen, & Räkköläinen, 2000), in Finland, successfully used an integrated model of early treatment of schizophrenia (primarily psychotherapeutic and dynamic-systemic approaches), working intensely with families and making house calls. This programme reduced the country's annual incidence of schizophrenia from 24.6 per 100,000 (in 1985–89) to 10.4 per 100,000 between 1990 and 1994, when the system was in place. Of the patients who had been formerly hospitalised, 40% were treated on an outpatient basis. The rate of long-term schizophrenic patients in hospital fell to zero in a few years and remained there afterwards.

Although there were some pioneers, such as Sullivan (Sullivan, 1927), only in recent years has there been interest in early intervention, and a more optimistic attitude, encouraged by the Scandinavian countries and by the International Society for the Psychological Treatment of the Schizophrenias and other Psychoses (ISPS). The Early Psychoses Prevention and Intervention Centre (EPPIC) Programme, in Australia, proposed a similar programme.

Klosterkotter et al. (2001) reported on the results of the 'Cologne/Bonn Early Recognition—CER' project on schizophrenia, and found that at re-examination an average of 9.6 years later, 79 of 160 patients had subsequently developed a schizophrenic disorder. Best prediction values with a high positive predictive power and a low rate of false-positive predictions were achieved for 10 symptoms and symptom complexes, mainly from the group of thought, speech and perception disturbances.

McGorry (McGorry, 2001) pointed out that until 1960, dynamic psychotherapy dominated the treatment of psychoses, but later fell into disfavour, and personnel were no longer trained as much in these techniques. The trend swung towards a 'dehumanising and inefficient' behaviourism, to which cognitive techniques were later added as a compromise. However, there has recently been resurgence in interest, because the efficacy of a dynamic psychotherapeutic approach has been shown in certain kinds of cases (Hogarty, Kornblith, & Greenwald, 1995; Hogarty et al., 1997).

Birchwood and Spencer (2001) contend that even if the early detection and treatment of the disorder's first signs appears to confer protection from relapse, the active ingredients of these pharmacologically and psychologically based treatment studies are as yet unclear.

PARANOIA

Concept

Although the concept of *paranoia* appears in ancient Greek medicine, it acquired a central role in psychiatry in the late 19th century, and the term's use has become so widespread that in everyday language it is even used for mere suspicions. Therefore, in such classifications as the DSM-IV, the word *delusional* is used for the disorders previously termed *paranoid*. The definition of delusional disorders hinges on the presence of a non-bizarre delusion, i.e., situations that could occur in daily life (such as jealous, erotomanic, and somatic delusions), generally well systematised, which can be subclassified by their dominant themes; all of this in the absence of diagnoses of schizophrenia, affective disorder, or organic disorder, and with a minimum duration of one month. Although there may be hallucinations, they do not present as an important part of the clinical picture.

Aetiopathogeny

Delusional symptoms are seen in a number of psychiatric disorders; for this reason, there is some doubt as to whether these delusional (or paranoid) disorders should be considered atypical forms of the former, or whether they constitute separate clinical entities, as indicated by epidemiological and genetic studies, and by clinical evolution.

Biological Factors

Until recently, it was assumed that certain neurological alterations could favour the appearance of delusions. Studies of normal persons with sensory deprivation, as well as drug addicts, have provided data supporting this hypothesis. Although no concomitant cerebral alterations have been found, delusions have been related to possible sub clinical neurological lesions.

Psychodynamic Factors

From a psychoanalytical viewpoint, delusions (whether persecutory, erotomanic, jealous, or grandiose) represent attempts to control (through denial and projection) unconscious homosexual drives that are struggling to emerge. This hypothesis has been criticised for its excessive generalisation, and so other authors have complemented it with such concepts as the existence of a vulnerability to the formation of delusions related to different factors (insufficient development of the ability to trust others, certain vicissitudes of narcissism) or with constitutional hypersensitivity. Investigators have pointed out the influence of such factors as social isolation and economic want, acting in a way similar to sensory deprivation.

Interventions

Chronic delusional patients respond worse to neuroleptics than other psychotic patients (partly due to their higher resistance to taking medication); however, they can benefit from them. Some studies have indicated that hypochondriac delusions respond in a particularly favourable manner to pimozide.

Support psychotherapy is valuable in the hands of well-trained therapists, who bear in mind the hypersensitivity and low self esteem usually found in these patients. When there are signs of lack of impulse control, agitation, or suicidal ideas, hospitalisation may be indicated.

OTHER PSYCHOTIC DISORDERS

This section of the DSM-IV includes schizoaffective and schizophreniform disorders (subtypes of schizophrenia), and brief psychotic disorder.

Schizoaffective Disorder

These patients present symptoms of depression or euphoria, mixed with delusional ideas or thought alterations, but which do not fully satisfy the criteria for a diagnosis or depressive disorder or major mood disorder.

Schizophreniform Disorder

This category groups together patients with conditions formerly called reactive schizophrenia, acute schizophrenia, and some others, all having characteristics similar to schizophrenia, but in which the symptoms last less than six months.

Brief Psychotic Disorder

Also known as brief reaction psychosis, this psychotic process has an acute onset, without prodromal symptoms, and can last from several hours to one month. It occurs immediately after a major psychosocially stressful event, presenting with incoherence or delusions, hallucinations, or catatonic behaviour.

ATYPICAL PSYCHOSES

The DSM-IV includes in this category disorders presenting with psychotic symptoms that do not fulfill the criteria for other non-organic psychotic disorders. The types described include chronic hallucinatory delusions, transitory psychoses associated with the menstrual cycle or postpartum syndromes, and psychoses with unclear clinical characteristics or about which the clinician has inadequate information. Epileptic psychoses and certain culture-bound psychotic syndromes can also be included in this section.

REFERENCES

Alanen, Y. O., Lehtinen, V., Lehtinen, K., Aaltonen, J., & Räkköläinen, V. (2000). The Finnish integrated model for the early treatment of schizophrenia and related psychoses. In B. Martindale & A. Bateman & M. Crowe & F. Margison (Eds.), *Psychosis. Psychological Approaches and their Effectiveness* (pp. 235–265). London: Gaskell.

Amenson, C., & Liberman, R. (2001). Dissemination of educational classes for families of adults with schizophrenia. *Psychiatr Serv*, 52(5), 589–592.

Angermeyer, M. C., & Matschinger, H. (1999). Lay beliefs about mental disorders: a comparison between the western and the eastern parts of Germany. *Social Psychiatry and Psychiatric Epidemiology*, 34, 275–281.

Arieti, S. (1974). *Interpretation of Schizophrenia*. New York: Basic Books, New York.

Birchwood, M., & Spencer, E. (2001). Early intervention in psychotic relapse. *Clin Psychol Rev, 21*(8), 1211–1226.

Bleuler, E. (1924). *Tratado de psiquiatria*. Madrid: Calpe.

Brenner, H., & Pfammatter, M. (2000). Psychological therapy in schizophrenia: what is the evidence? *Acta Psychiatr Scand*, 102(sup 407), 74–77.

Brown, G. W., Monck, E. M., Carstairs, G. M., & Wing, J. K. (1958). The posthospital adjustment of chronic mental patients. *Lancet*, 2, 658–659.

Coombe, P. (1996). The Cassel Hospital, London. *Australian and New Zealand Journal of Psychiatry*, 30(5), 672–680.

Cormac, I., Jones, C., & Campbell, C. (2002). *Cognitive behaviour therapy for schizophrenia (Cochrane Review)* (Vol. 1). Oxford: Update Software.

Dauwalder, J. P., & Ciompi, L. (1995). Cost-effectiveness over 10 years. A study of community-based social psychiatric care in the 1980s. *Social Psychiatry and Psychiatric Epidemiology*, 30(4), 171–184.

De Hert, M., Thys, E., Vercruyssen, V., & Peuskens, J. (1996). Partial hospitalisation at night: the Brussels Night Hospital. *Psychiatric Services*, 47(5), 527–528.

Dixon, L., Adams, C., & Lucksted, A. (2000). Update on family psychoeducation for schizophrenia. *Schizophr Bull*, 26(1), 5–20.

Durham, R. C., Guthrie, M., Morton, R. V., Reid, D. A., Treliving, L. R., Fowler, S., & Macdonald, R. R. (2003). Tayside-Fife clinical Trial of cognitive-behavioural therapy for medication-resistant psychotic symptoms. Results to 3-months follow-up. *Br J Psychiatry, 182*, 303–311.

Fenton, W., & Schooler, N. (2000). Evidence-based psychosocial treatment for schizophrenia. *Schizophr Bull*, 26(1), 1–3.

Frankel, B. (1993). Groups for the chronic mental patient and the legacy of failure. *International Journal Of Group Psychotherapy*, 43(2), 157–172.

Gabbard, G. O. (1995). Psychodynamic Psychotherapies. In G. O. Gabbard (Ed.), *Treatments of Psychiatric Disorders* (Vol. 2). Washington: American Psychiatric Press, Inc.

Guimón, J. (1977). Requerimientos ménimos para formulacones etiológicas en la Esquizofrenia. *Gaceta Médica de Bilbao*, 74(6), 507–514.

Guimón, J., Luna, D., Totorika, K., Diez, L., & Puertas, P. (1983). Group Psychotherapy as a basic therapeutic resource in psychiatric community care from the General Hospital. In J. J. L. Ibor & J. M. L. Ibor (Eds.), *General Hospital Psychiatry*. Amsterdam: Excerpta Medica.

Guimón, J., & Ozamiz, A. (1982). Diferencias clinicas y sociológicas entre esquizofrénicos agudos y crónicos hospitalizados. *Actas Luso-Esp. de Neurol, Psiquiatría y Ciencias Afines*, X(1), 3–10.

Guimón, J., & Totorika, K. (1983). Psicoterapia grupal para la de la competencia social del esquizofrénico. *Psiquis*, IV(2), 35–46.

Guimón, J., Villasana, A., Totorika, K., & Ozamiz, A. (1981). Variables sociológicas y clinicas diferenciales en esquizofrénicos crónicos con estancias hospitalarias cortas y prolongadas. *Actas Luso-Esp. de Neurol., Psiquiatria y Ciencias Afines*, IX(6), 441–452.

Guimón, U. J., & Cuperman, P. (1982). Terapia familiar: historia y sistema. *Psicopatologia*, 2(1), 13–20.

Henderson, C., & Laugharne, R. (2002). *Patient held clinical information for people with psychotic illnesses (Cochrane Review)*. (Vol. 1). Oxford: Update Software.

Hogarty, G. E., Kornblith, S. J., & Greenwald, D. (1995). Personal Therapy: a disorder-relevant psychotherapy for schizophrenia. *Schizophrenia Bulletin*, 21, 379–393.

Hogarty, G. E., Kornblith, S. J., & Greenwald, D. (1997). Three-year trials of personal therapy among schizophrenic patients living with or independent of family, I: Description of study and effects on relapse rates. *American Journal of Psychiatry*, 154, 1504–1513.

Hollingshead, A. B., & Redlich, F. C. (1958). *Social Class and Mental Illness*. New York: John Wiley and Sons.

Johannessen, J. O., Larsen, T. K., McGlashan, T., & Vaglum, P. (2000). Early intervention in psychosis: the TIPS project, a multi-centre study in Scandinavia. In B. Martindale & A. Bateman & M. Crowe & F. Margison (Eds.), *Psychosis. Psychological Approaches and their Effectiveness* (pp. 210–234). London: Gaskell.

Kernberg, O. (1979). Regression in organizational leadership. *Psychiatry*, 42, 24–39.

Klosterkotter, J., & Schultze-Lutter, F. (2001). Is there a primary prevention of schizophrenic psychosis? *Fortschr Neurol Psychiatr*, *69*(Suppl 2), 104–112.

Kraeplin, E. (1920). *Psyhiatrie, ein Lehrbuch für Studierende und Aertze*. Leipzig: A. Label.

Leff, J. (2000). Family work for schizophrenia: practical application. *Acta Psychiatr Scand*, 102 Suppl(407)), 78–82.

Liberman, R. P. (1986). *Social and Independent Lliving Skills: Medication-Management Module-Trainer's Manual*. Los Angeles: Mc Neil Pharmaceutical.

Malmberg, L., & Fenton, M. (2002). *Individual psychodynamic psychotherapy and psychoanalysis for schizophrenia and severe mental illness (Cochrane Review)*. Oxford: Update Software.

Margison, F., & Mace, C. (1997). *Psychotherapy of Psychosis*. London: Gaskell, London.

Marshall, M., & Lockwood, A. (2002). *Assertive community treatment for people with severe mental disorders (Cochrane Review)* (Vol. 1). Oxford: Update Software.

McFarlane, W. R. (2000). Psychoeducation multi-family groups: adaptations and outcomes. In B. Martindale & A. Bateman & M. Crowe & F. Margison (Eds.), *Psychosis. Psychological Approaches and their Effectiveness* (pp. 68–95). London: Gaskell.

McGorry, P. (2001). Secondary prevention of mental disorders. In G. Thornicroft & G. Szmukler (Eds.), *Textbook of Community Psychiatry* (pp. 495–508). New York: Oxford University Press.

Moos, R. H. (1997). *Evaluating treatment environments. The quality of psychiatric and substance abuse programs*. New Brunswick: Transaction.

Mosher, L., & Feinsilver, D. (1971). *Special report on schizophrenia*. Bethesda: National Institute of Mental Health.

Nicol, M., Robertson, L., & Connaughton, J. (2002). *Life skills programmes for chronic mental illnesses (Cochrane Review)* (Vol. 1). Oxford: Update Software.

Nieminen, P., Isohanni, M., & Winblad, I. (1994). Length of hospitalization in an acute patients' therapeutic community ward. *Acta Psychiatrica Scandinavica*, 90(6), 466–472.

Pankow, G. (1969). L'homme et sa psychose. Paris.

Penn, D. L., Kommana, S., Mansfield, M., & Link, B. G. (1999). Dispelling the stigma of schizophrenia: II. The impact of information on dangerousness. *Schizophr Bull*, 25(3), 437–446.

Pharoah, F., Mari, J., & Streiner, D. (2002). *Family intervention for schizophrenia (Cochrane Review)* (Vol. 1). Oxford: Update Software.

Roder, V., Zorn, P., Muller, D., & Brenner, H. (2001). Improving recreational, residential, and vocational outcomes for patients with schizophrenia. *Psychiatr Serv*, 52(11), 1439–1441.

Schneider, K. (1942). *Problemas de patopsicología y de Psiquiatría clínica*. Madrid: Edit. Morata.

Scott, J. E., & Dixon, L. B. (1995). Psychological interventions for schizophrenia. *Schizophrenia Bulletin*, 21(4), 621–630.

Shepherd, G., & Murray, A. (2001). Residential care. In G. Thornicroft & G. Szmukler (Eds.), *Textbook of Community Psychiatry* (pp. 309–320). New York: Oxford University Press.

Spaulding, W., Reed, D., Sullivan, M., Richardson, C., & Weiler, M. (1999). Effects of cognitive treatment in psychiatric rehabilitation. *Schizophr Bull*, 25(4), 657–676.

Sullivan, H. S. (1927). The onset of schizophrenia. *American Journal of Psychiatry*, 105, 135–139.

Sultenfuss, J., & Geczy, B. J. (1996). Group therapy on State hospital chronic wards: some guidelines. *International Journal of Group Psychotherapy*, 46(2), 163–176.

Suslow, T., Schonauer, K., & Arolt, V. (2001). Attention training in the cognitive rehabilitation of schizophrenic patients: a review of efficacy studies. *Acta Psychiatr Scand*, 103(1), 15–23.

Thornicroft , G., & Susser, E. (2001). Evidence-based psychotherapeutic interventions in the community care of schizophrenia. *Br J Psychiatry*, 178(1), 2–4.

Tsang, H. (2001). Applying social skills training in the context of vocational rehabilitation for people with schizophrenia. *189*(2), 90–98.

Wolff, S. (1991). Schizoid" Personality in Childhood and Adult Life I: The Vagaries of Diagnostic Labelling. *British Journal of Psychiatry*, 159, 615–620.

Zubin, L., Steinhauser, S., & Condray, R. (1992). Vulnerability to Relapse in Schizophrenia. *British Journal of Psychiatry*, 161, (suppl 18), 13–18.

14

Mood (Affective) Disorders (F30–39)

As far as research in mood disorders is concerned, many authors prefer such instruments as the Research Diagnostic Criteria (RDC) and the Present State Examination (PSE) to the ICD-10 and DSM-IV classification systems. Indeed, for daily clinical practice, it is generally better to describe disorders systematically rather than to classify them. These preferred instruments take into account descriptions of the severity of the episode (mild, moderate or severe), its course (depressive, manic, or mixed) and special clinical characteristics (principally neurotic or psychotic symptoms, agitation, retardation, or stupor). They also describe its course as unipolar or bipolar, and, insofar as aetiology is concerned, refer to the existence of mainly endogenous or reactive factors.

SUBCATEGORIES IN THE CURRENT CLASSIFICATIONS

Subcategories of Depression in ICD-10

The ICD-10 maintains the classic distinction between psychotic and neurotic depressions (Akiskal, 1978), and classifies them, according to their course, into manic disorder, depressive disorder, or bipolar disorder. It subdivides the latter into manic, depressive, or mixed, according to the predominant presenting symptoms. Neurotic depressions are defined using descriptive criteria.

Subcategories of Depression in the Research Diagnostic Criteria

The RDC (based on criteria drawn up by Feighner, 1972) maintains a restrictive definition of depression, and explains norms for inclusion and exclusion from its different subcategories. It includes the categories of *manic, hypomanic,* and *bipolar disorders,* and introduces that of *major depression.* It also incorporates the division into *bipolar I* and *bipolar II,* and divides *major depression* into 10 subtypes: *primary, secondary, recurrent unipolar, psychotic, incapacitating, endogenous, agitated, retarded, situational, and simple.*

Subcategories of Depression in DSM-IV

The concept of *endogenous* depression is included in the DSM-IV under the subcategories of *depression with melancholic features,* and *major depression with psychotic symptoms.* Both have good diagnostic reliability, and have been validated by clinical and biological data, which has led many investigators to use them in their samples.

We can assume that the DSM-IV approach to depressive disorders is based on the *unitary* theory of depression. Only the subcategories of major depression with melancholic features *and major depression with psychotic symptoms* are reliable. Contrariwise, it has not been possible to validate *major depression.*

AETIOLOGY: ENDOGENOUS AND REACTIVE

Depression can be considered a rupture of homeostasis. Certain external occurrences (life events) overcome the subject's support factors, and force into action certain coping and defense mechanisms. When these fail, the biochemical equilibrium in the synapses is altered, and depression appears. Therefore, there are biological (that we will not discuss here, [see Chapter 3]), psychological, and social factors implied in the aetiology of depression.

Psychological Factors

Cognitive-Behavioural Theories

Cognitive theories propose that depression results from a mode of anomalous thought (triad of symptoms) which, in vulnerable subjects, leads to breakdown.

Dynamic Theories

After Freud's proposals in his paper *'Mourning and Melancholia'*, the most important contributions to the psychoanalytic understanding of depression are those of the Kleinian school. Melanie Klein (Klein, 1948) believed that the early onset of guilt is one of the consequences of excessive envy. If this premature guilt is experienced by an ego that is not yet in a position to deal with it, then it is felt as persecution, and the object that arouses it becomes a persecutor; some months later, when the depressive position arises, the ego has a greater capacity to deal with the pain of guilt, and to develop the corresponding defences, above all the tendency to repair. This affirmation regarding the appearance of early guilt turns out to be contradictory to Klein's statement that in order to experience guilt, the child must have a sufficiently integrated ego.

Grinberg (1981) explains this contradiction by accepting two kinds of guilt: depressive guilt, which requires an integrated ego and which has reparatory effects, and persecutory guilt, which is seen early on in a weak, immature ego, and which increases in the face of any frustration or failure, evolving into a depressive phase, determining all kinds of inhibitions or extreme masochistic attitudes, practically condemning the patient to a paralysis of healthy or normal activities. This leads him to introject the lost object (the shadow of the object falls across the ego, in Freud's sense) as a recourse to control or placate it. Persecutory guilt coexists with the persecutory anxiety defined by Klein as the perception of the death instinct in the body. In persecutory guilt, there is also the sense of a damage that has already been inflicted on the ego or the object. The essence of guilt, in this view, resides in the feeling that the damage done to the loved object is caused by the subject's aggressive impulses. The need to repair this damage comes out of the feeling of guilt.

In the first months of life, persecutory anxiety delays the process of integration and experiences of depressive anxiety, guilt, and reparation are able to attain only a fleeting, transitory nature. Therefore, says Klein, the damaged loved object can quickly become transformed into a persecutor, and the need to repair or revive the loved object can become a need to pacify and propitiate the persecutor. Here, persecutory guilt has its origin in pacifying a feared and persecuting object, and not in repairing a loved object. Under such circumstances, regression occurs, and other defences are used, including that of projecting guilt and accusing the object.

All of these mechanisms can be explained by an instinctive duality (persecutory guilt depends on the death instinct, and depressive guilt on the life instinct). The main emotions that intervene in persecutory guilt are resentment, pain, desperation, fear, and self-reproach. The ego, dominated by the death instinct, acts masochistically. In depressive guilt, the most important feelings are worry about the object and about the ego, sorrow, nostalgia, and responsibility. This is especially manifest in normal mourning, with sublimatory and reparation activities, and falls within the realm of the life instinct.

The intensity with which guilt intervenes after a loss, and the persecutory or depressive quality of the loss, will determine the type of reaction that the subject feels. In some clinical situations, mostly in melancholy, patients carry to extreme lengths their self-punishing tendencies as determined by persecutory guilt, to the point of actually mutilating themselves or even committing suicide.

Depressive and persecutory guilt can coexist throughout life, and one or the other can predominate according to whether the love instinct or the destructive instinct predominates. What essentially characterises depressive guilt is the desire to repair the object, which the subject feels to be damaged by his own destructive impulses.

It is well known that in the depressive position, there is mourning for the mother's breast and what it has come to represent in the child's mind: love, goodness, security. The feeling of pain for having destroyed objects in fantasy, and anxiety about preserving them, with the corresponding defences, constitute the basis for this depressive position. The child now recognises the complete object, the mother. The projective mechanisms diminish. Ambivalence increases. There is memory, nostalgia, and guilt revolving around the lost object; in the latter case, there is mourning, during which the child has feelings that Klein calls *paining* about the loved objects, about the fear of losing them, and anxiety to reconquer them. Hatred, to a certain point, is mitigated by love, while the feelings of love are to a certain extent controlled by the hate; the result is a change in the quality of the infant's feelings about his objects. In synthesis, the depressive position is a series of processes that lead to an ambivalent configuration, with a feeling of loss in the face of the ambivalent destruction of good objects and the restoration of objects, and also a series of normal processes that involve ambivalence and reparation in the form of projective identification.

In order for sublimation to be possible, the direct expression of sexual and aggressive instincts must be inhibited. The inhibition of these instincts depends on the capacity to deprive oneself of the object, which occurs when it is possible to install it within oneself. But the previous condition for the successful development of sublimations is that the love for the primitive objects can be maintained, because, if not, it disturbs the capacity to repair and sublimate; there is a failure to overcome the depressive position, and the subject recurs to manic defences and the guilt becomes transformed into the persecutory variety.

Reactive Aspects

Brown (1978) believes that we already have sufficiently strong aetiological models of psychosocial factors contributing to unipolar depression, and expresses the hope that these will eventually be applicable to other psychiatric situations. He points out that in his studies, he has been able to confirm, as other authors have also done, that during the year before a depressive episode, the subject has frequently experienced various crises or difficult life events. There is an age-old opposition between the concept of a 'reactive' aetiology in depression, involving an outside event, and an 'endogenous' aetiology, depending on internal biological factors. The clinical factors classically considered as defining an endogenous syndrome are, according to some authors (Kiloh et al., 1972): 1) absence of a precipitating factor; 2) early wakening; 3) abrupt onset; 4) autonomous course of mood (i.e., once depression is present, mood is not alleviated by pleasant changes in the situation); 5) the 'distinct' quality of the experience, including a feeling on the part of the patient that no one can understand the pain he is suffering; 6) inhibition, which can affect different areas (cognitive, motivational, motor); 7) premorbid personality with a low level of neuroticism.

The reactive category is phenomenologically determined as opposite to the endogenous one, without any kind of specificity. On the contrary, other authors have tried to defend the need to describe positive criteria for this category, among which they include: 1) reactiveness of mood to the outside world; 2) insidious onset of the depressive episode; 3) normal sadness; 4) hypochondriasis; 5) verbal aggression against the patient's environment.

However, some of the symptoms considered classic within the realm of endogenous depression have been questioned by the latest psychopathological research: 1) the absence of a precipitating factor has been discussed by various authors (Paykel and Priest, 1992), who have found many cases of endogenous depression with clear antecedents of stressful situations; 2) early awakening, circadian rhythms, and appetite disorders are questioned as defining one or the other type of depression (Craig, Nelson, and Chamey, 1981), and are perhaps an expression of a non-specific general reaction to the illness; 3) the existence of a premorbid personality with a low level of neuroticism has also been called into question by many authors.

In any case, there is a general consensus in the contemporary literature that in any depression, endogenous and environmental factors have an impact, so that neither the ICD-10 nor the DSM-IV mention this dichotomy.

TREATMENTS

There are now increasingly effective treatments for depression, using both biological and relational approaches. In moderate depression, cognitive and interpersonal psychotherapies are as useful as antidepressants, and analytical psychotherapy is also useful, but less than the other two types. In more severe cases of depression, medication is more useful than psychotherapy. In any case, the combination of antidepressants and psychotherapy has better results than the use of only one of these techniques. However expert-estimated effectiveness for "usual care" for major depression has recently shown an excessive rate of ineffective care (Horvitz-Lennon, 2003).

Biological Treatments

In mania, lithium salts are useful, but since it takes some time for their effects to be noticed, treatment is often initiated with neuroleptics (e.g., haloperidol). Some earlier reports of severe side effects associated with combining lithium and haloperidol have not been confirmed in later studies.

In the preventive treatment of bipolar disorders, lithium has been confirmed to be the most effective medication (Burgess, 2001). Carbamazepine and valproic acid have lower efficacy rates. In treatment-resistant cases, two of these products can be associated, and sometimes a neuroleptic can be added in the long run. Rapid-cyclers respond better to treatment with valproic acid (Macritchie, 2001). Other drugs are currently under study as mood stabilisers.

The effectiveness of antidepressants has been assessed using active placebos (Moncrieff, 2001); it has also been specifically assessed in older patients (Wilson, 2001), and in children and adolescents (Hazell et al., 2000). Drug adherence has been shown to be better with selective serotonin reuptake inhibitors versus tricyclic and heterocyclic antidepressants (Barbui et al., 2000).

In treatment-resistant depression, it is important for the clinician to verify whether the patient has taken antidepressants at a high enough dose for a long enough time, at least 6–8 weeks. If this is the case and there has been no response to the medication, the patient can be switched to another antidepressant from the same chemical family (tricyclics, MAOI, serotonin reuptake inhibitors, and atypical antidepressant). If there is still no response, then the clinician can try changing to an antidepressant from another chemical family. In case of failure, thyroid hormones, tryptophan (Shaw, 2001), lithium, amphetamines, another antidepressant or atypical antipsychotics can be added to the medication being taken, exercising caution (Shelton, 2003). Data suggest that these combinations are underutilized.

Electroshock therapy is still considered useful for resistant depression, depression with melancholic features, stuporous depression, and cases in which comorbidity with physical illness (prostatic hypertrophy, glaucoma, cardiovascular disorders) makes its use less risky than medication. In spite of every effort, there is a certain number of severe depressions that do not respond to medication or to psychotherapy, leading to disability, chronic psychological suffering, or suicide.

Relational Aspects: Individual Psychotherapy

There is evidence of the effectiveness of cognitive and interpersonal therapy and, to a lesser degree, of psychoanalytically oriented and behavioural therapy in the treatment of mild to moderate depression, but not of severe depression. Teasdale et al. (2001) found that cognitive therapy reduced relapse in patients with residual depression through reductions in dichotomous thinking style. No studies have documented a preventive effect of psychotherapy on future recurrent depressive episodes (Balslev Jorgensen et al., 1999).

Clinical guidelines for psychiatrists for the treatment of depressive disorders have been proposed (Segal et al., 2001), and many studies have compared the efficacy of pharmacotherapy, cognitive psychotherapy, and psychoanalytically-oriented psychotherapy in depressive disorders. Both analytical psychotherapy and cognitive psychotherapy have been shown to be as effective as tricyclic antidepressants in patients with major depressive disorders (Elkin et al., 1988). When the intensity of depression is severe, antidepressants are more effective and act faster than psychotherapy; of the psychotherapeutic approaches, Klerman's interpersonal psychotherapy (IPT, 1984) has been shown to be more effective than cognitive psychotherapy (Rousaville et al., 1984). DeRubeis et al. (1999), comparing antidepressant medication and cognitive-behavioural therapy in severely depressed outpatients, found that cognitive-behavioural therapy has fared as well as antidepressant medication with severely depressed outpatients.

Psychotherapeutic treatments have a greater impact on social adaptation and the risk of relapse than pharmacological products. Specifically,

IPT has been shown to be highly effective in avoiding relapse in cases of unipolar depression.

Results with pharmacotherapy are more consistent than those of psychotherapy. In the latter, it is important to remember that the therapist's personality plays a relatively important role. In the case of patients with mixed anxiety and depressive disorders, psychotherapy's effects are as beneficial as those of pharmacotherapy.

Combining psychotherapy and pharmacotherapy sometimes (but not always) results in better results, and clinical guidelines have been proposed for its correct indications (Segal et al., 2001). In a major clinical study, 1356 patients with depressive symptoms were enrolled in a randomised controlled trial for depression (Unutzer et al., 2001). Patients were randomised to usual care or to one of two different quality improvement programmes that involved training local experts, who worked with patients' regular primary care providers (physicians and nurse practitioners) to improve care for depression through patient education assessment, and referral to study-trained psychotherapists. The quality improvement programmes substantially increased the success rates of antidepressant treatment. 16 sessions of Psychodynamic Supportive Psychotherapy in addition to pharmacotherapy produced a significant reduction in personality pathology (mostly in cluster C psychopathology) in depressive patients (Koll, 2003).

Several studies (Gitlin, 2001; Miklowitz et al., 2000; Rothbaum et al., 2000) have reviewed the efficacy of in individual and group (Colom et al., 2003) psycho-education, individual cognitive-behavioural therapy (Lam et al., 2003), marital and family interventions, and individual interpersonal therapy in treatment-resistant bipolar disorder. Family-focused psycho-educational treatment appears to be the most efficacious adjunct to pharmacotherapy for bipolar disorder (Miklowitz et al., 2003).

There is little evidence of the efficacy of suicide-prevention activities, although some general measures (public awareness, optimising primary care, restricting the presentation of suicides in the mass media, and restricting the access to means for suicide) may help (Althaus et al., 2001).

Relational Aspects: Group Psychotherapy

Brief Group Treatments in Depressive Patients

In a controlled clinical trial, Piper et al. (1994) studied the capacity of seven characteristics of patients to predict their success in an intensive psychodynamic group therapy programme aimed at patients with affective and personality disorders. Among them, two personality characteristics (psychological sophistication and the quality of object relations) were shown to be the strongest success predictors. Recently, specific intensive groups have been aimed at helping to elaborate mourning, obtaining good results.

McCallum et al. (1993) compared the results of two dynamically-oriented group therapy programmes, one brief, the other of long duration. Both were aimed at outpatients who presented difficulty in managing personal losses due to death or separation. The post-sessions assessments of positive and negative affect were carried out by the patients themselves, their therapists, and the other patients in their groups. The psychodynamic work was independently assessed, using the content analysis system. Patients who had suffered a separation presented more affective inhibition. Positive affect increased over time, and a direct relationship was found between positive affect and favourable results.

In earlier work along the same lines, Lieberman et al. (1972) created a brief group format–eight 80-minute sessions–in which the therapists were particularly aware of the need to discuss, with those undergoing mourning, certain issues, such as the meaning of life and loneliness. Other authors have developed analytical group psychotherapy programmes for depressive patients with or without personality disorders (Rosie et al., 1995). In any case, it is noteworthy that the majority of papers reporting on the results of brief group psychotherapy programmes with depressive patients highlight that the results are more favourable with cognitive techniques or interpersonal therapy than with dynamically-oriented techniques. The interpersonal approach has been used in groups aimed at patients who have had episodes of major depression or dysthimia, but not in bipolar patients, those who suffered from a psychotic depression, or who were considered at risk for suicide.

McKenzie (1997) explored, in his groups, each patient's type of depression, interpersonal relationships, and the disorder's impact on their lives. The psychotherapy was centred on current and future problems, rather than on past experiences. The 16 sessions lasted 90 minutes each, and no medication was used. No new patients were allowed to join the group after the third session. This format was adapted from Klerman and Weissman (*interpersonal therapy*, 1984) and has been shown to be as effective as cognitive-behavioural therapy, and with perhaps more lasting effects. Interpersonal therapy has been shown to have effects similar to those of antidepressant medication, even in severe cases with marked endogenous symptoms. Interpersonal group therapy is useful for all patients, including those who present a double diagnosis (major depression/dysthimia).

Interpersonal therapy strategies are halfway between psychodynamic therapies and cognitive-behavioural techniques, and focus on relationships and their alteration, using models similar to those of cognitive-behavioural therapy. Different categories of life stress are discussed (loss, mourning, interpersonal disputes, role transitions, loneliness and social isolation). The therapist works more with support techniques than with interpretations, trying to reinforce patients' coping and resource-mobilisation strategies. This model can also be used in a wider range of patients, such as those presenting simultaneously with anxiety disorders and depressive syndromes.

Regarding the cognitive-behavioural approach, Stravynski et al. (1994) reported good results in a study in which outpatients suffering from major depression were assigned to 15-session programme of cognitive-behavioural group therapy.

Bright et al. (1999) compared the relative efficacy of professional and paraprofessional therapists in providing group cognitive-behavioural therapy and mutual support group therapy, and found clinically significant improvement, although more patients in the professionally-led cognitive-behavioural therapy groups were classified as non-depressed than in the paraprofessionally-led groups.

Groups with Bipolar Patients

Contrary to the former pessimistic reports in the literature, Graves (1993) described a study conducted with bipolar outpatients, showing that dynamic group therapy improved their compliance with medication and lowered their denial mechanisms, facilitating a higher consciousness of internal and external stress factors.

For this type of patients, simple cognitive or psycho-educational techniques have been found to be very effective. Honig et al. (1997) described a controlled study using a multifamily psycho-educational intervention in bipolar disorder. The parents showed a significant change from a high to a low level of expressed emotion, compared with a control group. In addition, the patients who had parents with a low level of expressed emotion were hospitalised less frequently than those who lived with parents having a high level of expressed emotion. The multifamily groups were well received by the participants, and there were only a few dropouts.

Weiner (1992) showed the positive impact of group therapy on bipolar outpatients who attended at least 12 sessions over the course of a year. Kanas (1993), in a review of the literature, suggested that bipolar patients could be treated in homogenous group therapy programmes, in conjunction with lithium treatment. Interpersonal and psychodynamic techniques were used. The groups' objectives included educating the patients regarding the nature of their illness, helping them to learn how to manage their symptoms, and encouraging them to discuss important interpersonal and psychodynamic issues. To reach these objectives, therapists used techniques that included education and support, facilitating group discussion.

Group Programs for Hospitalised Depressive Patients

In a study we have conducted for the past 6 years at the University Hospital of Geneva, a 10-bed unit for suffering from resistant or recurrent depression had registered an average length of hospitalisation of 28.78 days, with a median of 15 days (Guimón, 2001). The patients' average age was 44, and 42 was the median.

Care of patients was articulated in individual and group moments, with each staff category taking part in both. Most of these patients had been hospitalised more than once before, so it is important that their pharmacological treatment be well evaluated. In this context, crisis intervention had to be associated with a more in-depth assessment of the incidence of depression on cognitive and relational skills.

At the arrival of each patient, a brochure was distributed stipulating ward rules. The programme of the group included a daily 15-minute staff meeting for all personnel, except for weekends. A social skills group, led by a nurse and a psychologist, meets during two hours per week, and a verbal group, led by two physicians, during one hour per week. The medication group, led by a resident and two nurses, met once a week for 30 minutes. A family group, led by a physician, with the participation of each professional category, met monthly during an hour and 30 minutes. Three recreational-occupational groups, led by occupational therapists and nurses, also meet for several hours a week.

The results of this programme were highly satisfactory and they have been reported elsewhere (Guimón, 2001, 2002).

REFERENCES

Akiskal, N. S., Bitar, A. A., Puzantian, V. R., Rosenthal, T. L., and Walker, P. N. (1978). The nosological status of neurotic depression. *Archives of General Psychiatry*, 35, 756–766.

Althaus, D., and Hegerl, U. (2001). Evaluation of suicide prevention measures. Current state of research and resulting implications (in German). *Nervenarzt*, 72(9), 677–684.

Balslev Jorgensen, M., Dam, H., and Bolwig, T. (1999). The efficacy of psychotherapy in non-bipolar depression: a review. *Acta Psychiatrica Scandinavia*, 99(5), 394–396.

Barbui, C., Hotopf, M., Freemantle, N., Boynton, J., Churchill, R., Eccles, M., Geddes, J., Hardy, R., Lewis, G., and Mason, J. (2000). Selective serotonin reuptake inhibitors versus tricyclic and heterocyclic antidepressants.

Bright, J., Baker, K., and Neimeyer, R. (1999). Professional and paraprofessional group treatments for depression: a comparison of cognitive-behavioral and mutual support interventions. *J. Consult. Clin. Psychol.*, 67(4), 491–501.

Brown, G. W., and Harris, T. D. (1978). *Social origins of depression*. London: Tavistock.

Burgess, S., Geddes, J., Hawton, K., Townsend, E., Jamison, K., and Goodwin, G. (2001). Lithium for maintenance treatment of mood disorders (Cochrane Review). *Cochrane Database Syst Rev.*, 3 (CD003013).

Colom, F., Vieta, E., Martinez-Aran, A., Reinares, M., Goikolea, J. M., Benabarre, A. T. C., Corbella, B., Parramon, G., & Corominas, J. (2003). A randomized trial on the efficay of group psychoeducation in the profilaxis of recurrences in bipolar patients whose disease is in remision. *Arch Gen Psychiatry, 60*(4), 402–407.

Craig Nelson, J., and Chamey, D. S. (1981). The symptoms of major depressive illness. *American Journal of Psychiatry*, 138, 138–141.

DeRubeis, R., Gelfand, L., Tang, T., and Simons, A. (1999). Medications versus cognitive behavior therapy for severely depressed outpatients: mega-analysis of four randomized comparisons. *American Journal of Psychiatry*, 156 (7), 1007–1013.

Elkin, I., Pikonis, P. A., Docherty, J. P., and Sotsky, S. M. (1988). Conceptual and methodological issues in comparative studies of psychotherapy and pharmacotherapy. I: Active ingredients and mechanisms of change. *American Journal of Psychiatry*, 145 (8), 909–917.

Feighner, J. P., Robins, E., Guze, S. B., Woodruff, R. A., Winokur, G., & Muñoz, R. (1972). Diagnostic criteria for use in psychiatric research. *Archives of General Psychiatry, 26*, 57–63.

Freud, S. (1957). Mourning and Melancholia, *Standard Edition of the Complete Psychological Works of Sigmund Freud*, (Vol. 14, pp. 243). London.: Hogarth Press.

Gitlin, M. (2001). Treatment-resistant bipolar disorder. *Bull. Menninger Clin.*, 65 (1), 26–40.

Graves, J. S. (1993). Living with mania: a study of outpatient group psychotherapy for bipolar patients. *American Journal of Psychotherapy*, 47 (1), 113–126.

Grinberg, L. (1981). Observaciones Psicoanalíticas sobre la creatividad, *Psicoanálisis*. Buenos Aires: Paidos.

Guimón, J. (2001). *Introduction aux thérapies de groupe*. Paris: Masson.

Guimón, J., & Weber, B. (Eds.). (2002). *Thérapies groupales Brèves*. Paris: Masson.

Hazell, P., O'Connell, D., Heathcote, D., and Henry, D. (2000). Tricyclic drugs for depression in children and adolescents. *Cochrane Database Syst Rev.*, 3 (CD002317).

Honig, A., Hofman, A., Rozendaal, N., & Dingemans, P. (1997). Psycho-education in bipolar disorder: effect on expressed emotion. *Psychological Research, 72*(1), 17–22.

Horvitz-Lennon, M. (2003). "Usual care" for major depression in the 1990's: caracteristics and expert-estimated outcomes. *Am J Psychiatry, 160*(4), 720–726.

Kanas, N. I. (1993). Group psychotherapy with bipolar patients: a review and synthesis. *International Journal of Group Psychotherapy*, 43 (3), 321–333.

Kiloh, L. G., Andrews, G., Nelson, M., and Bianchi, G. N. (1972). The relationships of the syndromes called endogenous and neurotic depressions. *British Journal of Psychiatry*, 121, 183–196.

Klein, M. (1948). Mourning and its relation to manic-depresive states. In M. Klein (Ed.), *Contributions to 1921–1945*. London: Hogarth Press.

Klermann, G. L., Weissman, M. M., Rounsaville, B. J., & cols. (Eds.). (1984). *Interpersonal Psychotherapy of Depression*. New York: Basic Books.

Kool, S., Dekker, J., Duijsens, I. J., deJonghe, F., & Puite, B. (2003). Changes in Personality Pathology after Pharmacotherapy and Combined Therapy for Depressed Patients. *J Personal Disord, 17*(1), 60–72.

Lam, D., Watkins, E., Hayward, P., Bright, J., Wright, K., Kerr, N., Park Davis, G., & Sham, P. (2003). A randomized controlled study of cognitive therapy for relapse prevention for bipolar affective disorders. *Arch Gen Psychiatry, 60*(2), 145–152.

Lieberman, M. A., Yalom, I. D., and Miles, M. D. (1972). Encounters groups: First facts. New York: Basic Books.

López-Ibor Aliño, J. J. (1972). Masked depressions. *British Journal of Psychiatry*, 120, 289–292.

Macritchie, K., Geddes, J., Scott, J., Haslam, D., and Goodwin, G. (2001). Valproic acid, valproate and divalproex in the maintenance treatment of bipolar disorder (Cochrane Review). *Cochrane Database Syst Rev.*, 3 (CD003196).

McCallum, M., Piper, W. E., and Morin, H. (1993). Affect and outcome in short-term group therapy for loss. *International Journal of Group Psychotherapy*, 43 (3), 303–319.

MacKenzie, R. (1997). *Time-Managed Group psychotherapy: effective clinical applications.* Washington: American Psychiatric Press.

Miklowitz, D., Simoneau, T., George, E., Richards, J., Kalbag, A., Sachs-Ericsson, N., & Suddath, R. (2000). Family-focused treatment of bipolar disorder: 1-year effects of a psychoeducational program in conjunction with pharmacotherapy. *Biol Psychiatry, 15*(48), 582–592.

Miklowitz, D. J., Richards, J. A., George, E. L., Frank, E., Suddath, R. L., Powell, K. B., & Sacher, J. A. (2003). Integrated family and individual therapy for bipolar disorders:results of s treatment development study. *J Clin Psychiatry, 64*(2), 182–191.

Moncrieff, J., Wessely, S., and Hardy, R. (2001). Antidepressants using active placebos. *Cochrane Database Syst Rev.*, 2 (CD003012).

Paykel, E. S., and Priest, R. G. (1992). Recognition and Management of Depression in General Practice: Consensus Statement. *British Medical Journal*, 305, 1198–1202.

Piper, W., Joyce A. S., Azim H. F., and Rosie, J. (1994). Patient characteristics and success in day treatment. *Journal of Nervous Mental Disorders*, 182 (7), 381–386.

Rosie, J. S., Azim, H. F., Piper, W. E., and Joyce, A. S. (1995). Effective psychiatric day treatment. Historical lessons. *Psychiatric Services*, 46, 1019–1026.

Rothbaum, J., & al, e. (2000). Integration of pharmacotherapy and psychotherapy for bipolar disorder. *J Clin Psychiatry, 61*(Suppl 9), 68–75.

Rousaville, B. J., Chevron, E. S., and Weissman, M. M. (1984). Specification of techniques in interpersonal psychotherapy. In J. B. W. Williams and R. L. Spitzer. (Eds.), *Psychotherapy research: Where are we and where should we go?* New York: Guilford Press.

Segal , Z., Whitney, D., and Lam, R. (2001). Clinical guidelines for the treatment of depressive disorders. III. Psychotherapy. *Canadian Journal of Psychiatry*, 46 (Suppl. 1), 29S–37S.

Segal, Z., Kennedy, S., and Cohen, N. (2001). Clinical guidelines for the treatment of depressive disorders. V. Combining psychotherapy and pharmacotherapy. *Canadian Journal of Psychiatry*, 46 (Suppl. 1), 59–62.

Shaw, K., Turner, J., and Del, M. (2001). Tryptophan and 5-hydroxytryptophan for depression (Cochrane review). *Cochrane Database Syst Rev.*, 3 (CD003198).

Shelton, R. C. (2003). The use of antidepressants in novel combination therapies. *J Clin Psychiatry, 64*(Suppl 2), 14–18.

Stravynski, A., Verreault, R., Gaudette, G., Langlois, R., Gagnier, S., and Larose, M. (1994). The treatment of depression with group behavioural-cognitive therapy and imipramine. *Canadian Journal of Psychiatry*, 39 (7), 387–390.

Teasdale, J., Scott, J., Moore, R., Hayhurst, H., Pope, M., and Paykel, E. (2001). How does cognitive therapy prevent relapse in residual depression? Evidence from a controlled trial. *J. Consult. Clin. Psychol.*, 69 (3), 347–357.

Unutzer, J., Rubenstein, L., Katon, W., et al. (2001). Two-year effects of quality improvement programs on medication management for depression. *Archives of General Psychiatry*, 58(10), 935–942.

Weiner, M. F. (1992). Group therapy reduces medical and psychiatric hospitalization. *International Journal of Group Psychotherapy*, 42(2), 267–276.

Wilson, K., Mottram, P., Sivanranthan, A., and Nightingale, A. (2001). Antidepressant versus placebo for depressed elderly. *Cochrane Database Syst Rev.*, 2 (CD000561).

15

Neurotic Disorders (F40–49)

The DSM-IV splits this category in two, under the names of *anxiety disorders* and *dissociative disorders*. We prefer to maintain here the ICD-10 classification, which maintains the concept of *neurosis*.

The most convincing model to explain these kinds of disorders is based on the relationship between stress and anxiety, in the context of the maintenance of homeostasis. The importance of life events from infancy and early childhood, and certain specific defense mechanisms, make it possible to incorporate psychoanalytical concepts into this model.

AETIOPATHOGENY

There is a general consensus regarding biological relational factors in the aetiology of neurotic disorders.

The Biological Substrate

A great deal of recent research has studied the evolution, over the course of the history of medicine, of the biological conception of neurological phenomena.

Is the Current Concept of Anxiety Disorder More Valid Than That of Neurosis?

Although the reliability of the new classifications is noteworthy, their validity is not always as clear. Moreover, response to different treatments has not been established as specifically as would be desirable. These are, at any rate, the conclusions to be drawn from recent investigation in this field that tries to focus the classification of anxiety disorder based on biological parameters, which we shall summarise below.

Recently, a group of investigators has found a genetic alteration in subjects with different anxiety disorders. The duplication of an extensive zone of chromosome 15 (where 20–60 genes are found) is responsible for the heightening the cerebral mechanisms that regulate alert processes. This region, called DUP25, is flanked by long, repetitive DNA sequences, 13,000–60,000 nucleotides long. This genetic predisposition would mean that such subjects would have a higher number of neuronal connections involved in warning mechanisms, or that such mechanisms would be more sensitive. Under these conditions, certain environmental factors, as well as some personality traits, would accentuate the possibility of suffering from panic disorders, agoraphobia, social phobia, and other forms of anxiety.

A series of neuroimaging studies has shown structural anomalies in patient with different anxiety disorders. Overall, the data proposed for validating new anxiety syndromes are insufficient, because such laboratory results have not always been confirmed. In addition, the sensitivity and specificity of the different tests involved are insufficient.

In conclusion, although the new classifications of anxiety disorders have been validated to a certain extent in therapeutic practice, due to the different responses of panic disorders and generalised anxiety disorders to imipramine and benzodiacepines, these results are not conclusive. Indeed, it has been confirmed that certain benzodiacepines, such as alprazolam, are in fact effective in panic disorders, and that generalized anxiety can respond to certain antidepressants.

Relational Aspects: Psychological Conception

Current Psychoanalytical Conceptions of Anxiety

The recent descriptive classifications of anxiety disorders represent an undoubted advance in their reliable delimitation. However, our understanding of a patient with anxiety is impoverished when we exclusively use these diagnostic criteria, insofar as they strip the symptom or the syndrome of its meaning. Without examining the meaning of the symptoms, the clinician can act like an expert neuroendocrinologist, but not as a competent psychiatrist. Psychoanalytical theory and practice have played a basic role in describing and understanding anxiety. Their contributions have, unfortunately, been ignored by a psychiatric school that aims to be biological, but which forget that biologists can never stop asking about the origin, the meaning, and the finality of the behavioural acts that they observe.

Psychoanalytical concepts link anxiety to a biological predisposition, to life events from infancy, to external stressors, and to specific defence mechanisms. However, research in this area suffers from a noteworthy methodological restraint, due to the variety and complexity of the forms of anxiety currently differentiated by the psychoanalytical literature (Rycroft, 1968; Guimón, 1997a).

Other Dynamic Conceptions

Freud quickly abandoned his theory that the persistence of a painful memory about a traumatic situation could later produce disorders, given the existence of subjects without any psychological difficulties who reported accurate memories of traumatic experiences. Later psychoanalysts have arrived at the conclusion that a trauma's pathogenic effect was due to an inadequate reorganisation of ego functions, necessary to restore the 'barrier' that we have discussed previously. This purely quantitative view of trauma, however, does not explain many aspects of the syndromes seen in clinical practice; to do this, according to Titchener and Ross (1974), the following should be taken into account: the meaning of a traumatic experiences for the person (at both conscious and unconscious levels), the nature of the individual's relationship with his environment (adaptive viewpoint), and the effects of past experiences on response to trauma (psychodynamic approach).

Relational Aspects: Environmentalist Conceptions

The concept of *trauma*, when discussing neuroses, should refer both to physical aggressions and to psychologically important events in the subject's life. American authors tend to use the term *stress* instead, because it has less mechanical connotations.

The importance attributed to trauma in the genesis of neuroses has diminished in the post-Freudian literature. Many psychoanalysts invoke less striking 'traumas', while others are markedly inclined to assign greater importance to the subject's biographical factors that could have an impact on his personality, and make him more vulnerable to certain events.

Consequently, in recent decades the idea has been gaining ground that, in the aetiology of neuroses, 'persistent traumas' play a more important role than a single trauma.

TREATMENT

In the treatment of anxiety featuring panic attacks (panic disorders), imipramine has generally been shown to be useful in avoiding the appearance of new crises, and improving the depressive symptoms frequently associated with this condition. Anxiolytics can lessen anticipatory anxiety and also panic attacks, but not make them disappear. A multicentric study showed the efficacy of high doses of alprazolam, an atypical benzodiacepine, in controlling panic attacks. However, its clinical use has been on the downturn, due to the dependency that these dosages produce.

Freud always maintained that a physiological factor was behind the development of panic attacks, which he believed that future investigators would find. Nemiah (1961) assumed that in patients with such a biological predisposition, psychological conflicts would take the form of panic attacks, whereas in those not having such a predisposition, they would present as 'signal anxiety'.

In any case, psychotherapy can also be useful for panic attacks, and it is always advisable to investigate the attack's catalysing circumstances, and take a detailed history of each patient to see what the psychodynamic factors are. Indeed, it has been shown that there is a relationship between the latter and separation anxiety, because its onset frequently comes after stressful events, such as loss of a loved one (Klein, 1948). Moreover, the placebo effect in these patients has been well documented, which also indicates the importance of psychological factors. Psychotherapy can help patients to face the world again, or simply help them to accept taking medication.

In panic attacks, a cognitive-behavioural approach, based on *anxiety management techniques*, is useful, including desensitisation, exposure, cognitive management of anxiety, and relaxation. In agoraphobia, which is frequently associated with panic attacks, *exposure techniques* are useful, with or without a *therapeutic companion*.

For generalised anxiety antidepressants (serotonin reuptake inhibitors, serotonin-norepinephrine reuptake inhibitors, and nonsedating tricyclic antidepressants) are generally the most useful. Anxiolytics are useful, but their use in clinical practice is limited by the risk of producing dependency. However, in principal, the patient should learn how to control his anxiety with relaxation and stress management techniques. Cognitive-behavioural therapy is the preferred form of psychotherapy (Ballenger et al., 2001).

Although *generalised anxiety disorder* is something of a hotchpotch category, different research findings have made manifest the role played in its genesis and maintenance by psychodynamic mechanisms. Although we should remember that anxiety is a symptom that can have many causes, generalised anxiety can be improved by studying the constellations of internal and external object relations that evoke it. Some patients respond well to brief educational techniques; others, with sufficient ego strength, to brief dynamic psychotherapy, or to psychoanalysis. Analytical psychotherapy improves phobic neuroses, sometimes strikingly so, as well as obsessive disorders, although not as successfully. Dynamically oriented support psychotherapy, as well as psychoanalysis, can also be useful for these conditions in the medium- and long-term.

In phobic disorders, antidepressants and anxiolytics often improve the symptomatology, but psychotherapeutic techniques (exposure, desensitisation, flooding) are also necessary in order to modify these symptoms in the long run (Guimón, 1973).

Cognitive-behavioural group therapy has been found effective in reducing social and general anxiety (Durham et al., 2003). However, patients participating in social skills training experienced a significantly greater reduction of social anxiety and a greater increase in social skills than those in CBT in a control trial (Van Dam-Baggen et al., 2000). Analytical psychotherapy has also good medium- and long-term results.

For obsessive-compulsive neurosis, the most useful medication is chlorimipramine at medium or high doses, either orally or endovenously. Some studies suggest that the good results obtained with its endovenous administration depend more on the relationship with the professionals providing the treatment, with a maternal attitude, than with the actual pharmacokinetics. In hysteria, small doses of anxiolytics can be useful, but the most appropriate treatment is support psychotherapy with family intervention. Analytical psychotherapy and psychoanalysis produce good results in the so-called 'good' hysterias.

Muscular relaxation techniques offer symptomatic relief, and are used in conjunction with cognitive-behavioural techniques. Although some authors have reported good results with psychosurgery in some highly disabling cases of obsession and anxiety, ethical impediments rule against such an approach.

REFERENCES

Ballenger, J., Davidson, J., Lecrubier, Y., et al. (2001). Consensus statement on generalized anxiety disorder from the International Consensus Group on Depression and Anxiety. *J. Clin. Psychiatry*, 62 (Suppl. 11), 53–58.

Durhan, R. C., Chambers, J. A., Macdonald, R. R., Power, K. G., & Major, K. (2003). Does cognitive-behavioural therapy influence the long-term outcome of generalized anxiety disorder? An 8–14 year follow-up of twoclinical trials. *Psychol Med*, *33*(3), 499–509.

Guimón, J. (1997). La névrose est-elle morte? Archives Suisses de Neurologie et de Psychiatrie, 148 (suppl. III), 19–23.

Klein, M. (1948). Mourning and its relation to manic-depressive states. In M. Klein (Ed.), *Contributions to Psychoanalysis 1921–1945*. London: Hogarth Press.

Rycroft, C. (1968). *A critical dictionary of Psychoanalysis*. Harmondsworth: Penguin Books.
Titchener, J. L., and Ross, W. A. (1974). In S. A. and E. B. Brody (Ed.), *American handbook of psychiatry* (Vol. III). New York: Basic Books.
Van Dam-Baggen, R., and Kraaimaat, F. (2000). Group social skills training or cognitive group therapy as the clinical treatment of choice for generalized social phobia? *J. Anxiety Disord.*, 14 (5), 437–451.

16

Stress-Related Disorders

The American Psychiatric Association's DSM-IV scatters somewhat post-traumatic stress, adaptive disorders, factitious disorders, and malingering. We believe that it is preferable, as does the World Health Organization's ICD-10, to group them under a single category, one highlighting the importance of stress in their genesis.

STRESS AND RELATIONS

The role of external circumstances (physical or psychological trauma) in the genesis of neuroses has been the object of a discussion ranging from the old *traumatic neuroses* to *today's post-traumatic stress* syndromes (Gonzalez de Rivera, 2001).

In the diagnosis of stress disorders, the DSM-IV includes the aetiological factor (i.e., stress) among its inclusion criteria, excluding such a diagnosis when the stress factor is not found on the list of accepted trauma. The ICD-10 classifies these disorders in a similar manner, including the factors on the DSM-IV, adding 'change of personality after a catastrophic experience'. We include here acute stress disorder, post-traumatic stress disorder, and adaptation disorders.

Biological Aspects: Post-Traumatic Neuroses

Since the 1950s, there has been a tendency to group together, under the name of *traumatic neuroses,* those functional nervous disorders of a psychological origen suffered by subjects who had previously suffered a 'trauma', regardless of whether it involved bodily harm. In this context, little importance is laid on the distinction, frequently proposed, between *traumatic neuroses* and *post-traumatic neuroses* (the latter commonly used to designate psychological disorders stemming from physical aggression). However, the psychiatric literature contains numerous references to the latter type.

Aetiopathogeny

Pathogenic interpretations can be divided into three types: those considering the symptoms to be a direct result of neurological alterations (Oppenheimer, 1889); those giving preferential attention to a vindicative attitude, bordering on malingering; and those emphasising the overall modifications in the personality integrated into a syndrome of disadaptation to the social group, which involve a regression to an infantile attitude (Miller, 1966).

Other authors have looked at the relational factors involved in this problem, both psychogenetic and situational (Schilder, 1979). Hécaen and Ajuriaguerra (1952) preferred a homeostasic, multidimensional approach.

DYNAMIC ASPECTS: TRAUMATIC NEUROSES

At the beginning of his work, Freud maintained the notion that human beings strive primarily to reduce sexual and aggressive drives and that neuroses were the consequences of early traumatic events. Later on, Freud reacted with an overemphasis on inner phantasies and drive discharge. Later object-relation theories disorders emphasised the need to seek objects, assign meanings, test previous beliefs and assimilate new schemes (Migone et al., 1998).

Laplanche and Pontalis (in their *Dictionary of Psychoanalysis*, 1996) described the traumatic neuroses as types of neuroses in which the appearance of symptoms is the consequence of an emotional shock, of a situation in which the subject has felt his life to be threatened. According to this view, from the moment of the first shock, these neuroses become manifest through a paroxystic anxious crisis, which can produce states of agitation, stupor, or mental confusion. In their later evolution, usually after a symptom-free period, two kinds can be differentiated: 1) the trauma acts as a catalyst, revealing a pre-existing neurotic structure; 2) the trauma plays a determining role in the content of the symptoms (e.g., recurrent dreams), which appear as an attempt to take shelter in the trauma—this fixation on the trauma is accompanied by a more or less generalised inhibition of the subject's activity. It is for the latter clinical picture that psychoanalysts usually reserve the term *traumatic neurosis.*

Aetiopathogeny

The importance of trauma in the theory of neuroses is evident, in spite of the fact that it has been losing ground in recent years, due to the influence of object relation theories and to the idea of the role played in the aetiology of neurosis by a *persistent trauma* rather than a *single trauma* (Totorika et al., 1976).

After World War I, many papers were published in which the role of emotions was progressively recognised as an aetiological factor. With the rise of the psychoanalytical movement, psychoanalytical treatment centres were created to treat war-induced neuroses, but they were soon closed after the end of the conflict. However, the resulting experience led to a modification in the conception of traumatic neuroses: that predisposing factors had to be taken into account as much as the catalysing trauma itself, and the trauma should only be considered within the context of the subject's particular biography and psychological organisation. Titchener and Ross (1974), in a review of the literature, stressed the 'strength' and 'weakness' of the ego to confront stress, which depends on the first formative infantile experiences. These experiences, united with constitutional factors, would condition the subject's resistance to the 'stimuli barrier' discussed earlier, as well as explain why some subjects are able to endure certain traumatic aggressions, but not others. They also believed that the state of a greater or lesser feeling of *hopelessness* would condition subjects' reaction to stress. Indeed, this state of hopelessness, produced, for example, by being wounded and immobilised, would revive similar situations from infancy. The capacity for basic trust, acquired in the earliest mother-child relationship, would diminish the hopelessness of a traumatic situation. They also highlighted the fact that the traumatic experience could also act as a screen onto which subjects could project conflict and defences existing prior to the traumatic situation.

Siebeck (1975), discussing the social pathogenesis of psychiatric illness, included these disorders among those that he called *social neuroses.* This author insisted on the clinicians overriding need to acquire a true understanding and accurate knowledge regarding insured persons seeking help under the pretext of exercising their legal rights, although he may suspect that their complaints lack an organic justification.

The so-called *compensation neuroses* present symptomatology of a type particularly similar to that seen in the *traumatic neuroses* (Guimón, 1975). However, they are characterised by behaviour seeking some kind of compensation or benefit, which can sometimes lead the clinician to consider the possibility of malingering. Therefore, when making a differential diagnosis, it is important to take into account other conditions included in the same classification group.

It should be considered normal for patients to exhibit a certain tendency to try to obtain 'secondary gains' from their illness. When these 'gains' are economic, it can be extraordinarily difficult to distinguish these subjects from malingerers and 'gain-seekers'.

Ganser's syndrome would seem, today, to be classified more within the hysteric neuroses than the disassociative psychoses.

In any case, malingering is a common behaviour. However, showing that a patient is malingering does not necessarily mean that he does not have some kind of psychological disorder. Psychoanalysis relates these syndromes with the secondary gains that neurotic patients (especially hysterics) obtain from their disorders, e.g., special attention from their families, justification for avoiding responsibilities. The development of psychosomatic medicine has shown that many of their symptoms can be interpreted as involving, for the patient, transactions with significant subjects, in the form of a dialogue; sometimes an aggressive one, other times, seeking affection and help.

Any physical illness can originate an attitude of seeking secondary gains, but especially a neurosis: in the psychological regression of a prostrate patient, his attitude towards significant others (e.g., mother, spouse, physician, nurse) becoming one of imploring affection and attention; the subject who has survived major surgery will, once recovered, seek the admiration of his friends by narrating the event; the individual who is little able to inspire affect or compete aggressively will, after an illness, utilise a supposed consequent weakness to downplay his insufficiencies. Along these same lines, patients often seek additional remunerated sick leave.

The reduction of tension and conflict through a neurotic illness is the first proposition, or primary gain, of the disorder. However, the individual can try, more or less consciously, to obtain other advantages from the outside world through the illness, by provoking pity to get attention and sympathy, and even compensations he feels are due to him.

There are, indeed, few aspects of medicine as controversial as those referring to malingering, and every physician has had the experience of suspecting at some time that a certain patient was simulating his presenting symptoms.

It is commonly accepted that malingering consists of the voluntary and conscious invention of an illness. The DSM-III-R suggests considering the possibility of malingering in the presence of any combination of the following: 1) the patient presents outside of a clinical context, as when a person is referred to the physician by a lawyer for examination; 2) a large discrepancy between the reported discomfort and objective findings; 3) a lack of co-operation in the diagnostic evaluation and of compliance in following the treatment prescribed; 4) the existence of an antisocial personality disorder. In reality, these criteria are too wide: the second is also frequent in functional disorders and cases of diffuse brain damage; the fourth is symptomatic of frontal and temporal brain damage.

What is especially interesting, from the viewpoint of mental health, is the attitude of the professional in such situations. Regarding this aspect, Rosenhan's work (1973) has been widely cited, in which psychiatrists and psychologists were shown to be susceptible to error in assessing filmed interviews in which incorrect information was given; however, both the method, analysis, and conclusions of this paper have been severely criticised (Spitzer, 1976). It is not infrequent in forensic psychiatry to see patients who, after having legally obtained their objectives, then admit that they had faked their disorders. However, faked psychoses are infrequent in practice, and can evolve towards a true psychosis.

In this regard, we should mention the concepts expressed in a paper by Szasz (1957), in which he comments that psychiatrists have accepted malingering as a clinical entity, but in doing so have intruded into fields which are not strictly theirs. In reality, according to Szasz, in *malingering* it is possible to distinguish: 1) a diagnosis, 2) a violation of certain social rules, and 3) a psychopathological syndrome characterised by certain psychological characteristics. For Szasz, in sum, the term malingering expresses condemnation for a behaviour on the part of the psychiatrist, and such an attitude can only be understood within a psychosocial context.

Based on this last point of view, we consider it clinically impracticable to clearly differentiate between some cases of malingering, and others of opportunistic neuroses. Our attitude is not original. Bleuler (Bleuler, 1924) said that subjects who persistently and skillfully simulated an illness were, in part, truly mentally ill. And he added 'proving that there is simulation does not indicate that the subject examined is mentally healthy and responsible for his acts.'

PSYCHOSOCIAL INTERVENTIONS IN STRESS-RELATED DISORDERS

The efficacy of selective serotonin reuptake inhibitors in the treatment of post-traumatic stress disorder has been confirmed in a meta-analysis of randomised controlled trials (Stein et al., 2000) On the other hand, Adshead (Adshead, 2000) review the the effectiveness of different psychological therapies and suggests that psychotherapeutic treatments are effective in the therapy of reactions based on fear, and may increase the effectiveness of pharmacological therapy.

Lubin et al. (1998) contend that the so-called 'Interactive Psychoeducational Group Therapy', a form of 16-week cognitive-behavioural group therapy, may provide more targeted treatment of core symptoms of chronic PTSD.

On the contrary, Rose et al. (Rose et al., 2002) evaluate all randomized studies assessing the effectiveness of brief psychological debriefing for the management of psychological distress after trauma, and the prevention of post-traumatic stress disorder. Single session individual debriefing did not reduce psychological distress nor prevent the onset of post-traumatic stress disorder (PTSD). Those who received the intervention showed no significant short term (3–5 months) reduction in the risk of PTSD. At one year one trial reported that there was a significantly increased risk of PTSD in those receiving debriefing. There was also no evidence that debriefing reduced general psychological morbidity, depression or anxiety. They conclude that there is no current evidence that psychological debriefing is a useful treatment for the prevention of post-traumatic stress disorder after traumatic incidents. Compulsory debriefing of victims of trauma should cease.

REFERENCES

Adshead, G. (2000). Psychological therapies for post-traumatic stress disorder. *British Journal of Psychiatry*, 177, 144–148.

Bleuler, E. (1924). *Tratado de Psiquiatría*. Madrid: Calpe.

González de Rivera, J. L. (2001). Clasificación de los síndromes de Estrés. *Psiquis*, 22(1), 1–7.

Guimón, J. (1975). *Revisión crítica del concepto de neurosis de renta*. Madrid: Instituto de España. Real Academia Nacional de Medicina.

Hecaen, H., & Ajuriaguerra de, J. (1952). *Méconnaissances et hallucinations corporelles*. Paris: Masson.

Laplanche, J., and Pontalis, J. B. (1996). *Diccionario de psicoanálisis*. Barcelona: Paidos.

Lubin, H., Loris, M., Burt, J., and Johnson, D. (1998). Efficacy of psychoeducational group therapy in reducing symptoms of posttraumatic stress disorder among multiply traumatized women. *American Journal of Psychiatry*, 155 (9), 1172–1177.

Migone, P., and Liotti, G. (1998). Psychoanalysis and cognitive-evolutionary psychology: an attempt at integration. *Int. J. Psychoanal.*, 79(6), 1071–1095.

Miller, H. (1966). Mental after-effects of head injury. *Proceedings of the Royal Society of Medicine*, 59, 257–261.

Oppenheimer, D. R.(1889) Microscopic Lesions in the Brain Following Head Injury. Journal of Neurology, *Neurosurgery and Psychiatry* 31, 299–306.

Rose, S., Bisson, J., and Wessely, S. (2002). Psychological debriefing for preventing post-traumatic stress disorder (PTSD) (Cochrane Review). *The Cochrane Library*, 1.

Schilder, P. (1979). Neuroses following head and brain injuries. In L. Bender (Ed.), Paul
Siebeck, R. (1975). *Medicina en movimiento.* Madrid: Ed. C. Med.
Spitzer, R. L., & Klein, D. F. (1978). *Critical Issues in Psychiatric Diagnosis.* New York: Raven Press.
Stein, D., Seedat, S., van der Linden, G., & Zungu-Dirwayi, N. (2000). Selective serotonin reuptake inhibitors in the treatment of post-traumatic stress disorder: a meta-analysis of randomized controlled trials. *Int Clin Psychopharmacol, 15*(Suppl 2), S31–39.
Szasz, T. S. (1957). *Pain and pleasure.* New York. : Basic Books.
Stein, D., Seedat, S., van der Linden, G., and Zungu-Dirwayi, N. (2000). Selective serotonin reuptake inhibitors in the treatment of post-traumatic stress disorder: A meta-analysis of randomized controlled trials. *Int. Clin. Psychopharmacol.*, 15 (Suppl. 2), S31–39.
Titchener, J. L., and Ross, W. A. (1974). In S. A. and. E. B. Brody (Eds.), *American handbook of psychiatry* (Vol. III). New York: Basic Books.
Totorika, J. L., Guimón, J., Cortina, C., and De la Herrán, J. (1976). Síndromes psíquicos crónicos tras traumatismos craneales: A propósito de una investigación personal. *Informaciones Psiquiátricas*, 64, 6–16.

17

Somatoform Disorders (F45)

Behavioural Syndromes Associated with Physiological Disturbances and Physical Factors (F50–59)

NOSOLOGICAL UNCERTAINTIES

The DSM-IV scatters about this set of disorders, which have to do with what were formerly called 'psychophysiological disorders' or 'psychosomatic disorders': mental disorders due to a medical illness, somatoform disorders, sexual and sexual identity disorders, eating disorders, sleep disorders. It also includes a new section: other problems that can be the object of clinical attention.

We prefer the category used as this chapter's title, which is the one proposed by the WHO in its ICD-10 classification.

In these disorders, appropriate processing of information is altered, so that a discrepancy is produced between the patient's subjective and objective health: there are physically healthy subjects who believe themselves ill, or who have mild disorders which they experience in an exaggerated manner. On the other hand, there are patients who do suffer from illnesses, including serious ones, but who consider themselves healthy. There are also alterations of some physiological functions (eating, sexuality) which have deep psychological implications. In addition, many patients with physical illnesses present psychological alterations (e.g., anxiety, loss of self-esteem, depression). Finally, there can be alterations in the behaviour of some patients regarding the fact of being ill.

All of these conditions are discussed together (with criteria that is, of course, open to debate) in the present chapter.

The 'psycho-somatic' concept comes from the American work of Hallyday (1930), and Dunbar. Alexander (1968) tried to find a specific meaning for each psychosomatic symptom, interpreting them according to the co-ordinates of the symbolism of the unconscious. Various illnesses where then considered psychosomatic, and grouped together in this new discipline: first, bronchial asthma, duodenal ulcer, and arterial hypertension; and later many other symptoms, syndromes, and disorders.

The aetiological idea was that some frustrating infantile situations could leave, from early childhood, certain traces susceptible to being reactivated at an adult age by different events. This idea of a 'trace' evokes that of 'trauma', and has been severely questioned in much subsequent work. Another idea from this era was that of 'somatic weak points', or 'calling' places, which would be used by future unconscious affective investments, which could disturb the functions or organs. This idea is similar to that of 'somatic fixation', which would later be used by Pierre Marty (1990).

Marty introduced a new view of somatisation, in which he included a defect of expression of the symptom, and an inadequate utilisation of anxiety close to that of today's neuroses. He also described the use of language deprived of affect: 'the neurotic's thought associates words with things; that of the psychotic treats words as if they were things, and the "operational" (*opératoire*) thought says the words without the things.' He also mentioned 'over-investment in the factual', which signals the preference for acting instead of fantasising.

The *Paris psychosomatic school* (Smadja, 2001), founded by Marty, also described a certain variety of depression termed "essential depression", which features an absence of symptomatic expression, without guilt or self-accusatory phantasies and which proceeds from a deep, lasting loss of libido. It also described a certain quality of thought, called 'operational thinking', and a more or less generalised absence of 'phantasmatic formations' in thought. Marty (1990) said that the unconscious in what he called *operational life* 'receives but does not emit'.

In sum, operational life is thus a psychopathological group that associates essential depression, operational thinking, and operational behaviour.

SOMATOFORM DISORDERS

Clinical Varieties

The DSM-III coined the term *somatoform* to designate these disorders, and the DSM-IV also includes, under this heading, various disorders: bodily dysmorphophobia, conversion disorder, somatisation, somatoform pain, non-specific somatoform disorder, and undifferentiated somatoform disorder. The *Chronic fatigue syndrome* could be included in this group of disorders (Afari et al., 2003).

The designation *anosognosia* is used for the opposite behaviour, in which the patient does not accept the existence of an illness that has been medically confirmed by his physician. Such a situation can be seen, with different degrees of intensity, in the context of many clinical conditions, such as organic brain disorders, but they have greater relational interest when they present without brain damage, such as denial of having a serious illness.

The commentaries of classical authors regarding the denial of illness tended to centre on the consideration of the *phantom limb* phenomenon. The feeling, in these cases, of the presence of a limb that had been previously amputated was usually explained by peripheral (appearance of a neurinoma in the damaged section of the nerve) or central neurological factors (alterations in the body representation). More recent work tends to highlight the importance of concomitant psychological factors, in which denial phenomena play an important role. This explanation has been proposed for the persistent feelings in the chest felt by some patients after a mastectomy, feelings which, as an extension of the previous concept, have been labelled a 'phantom breast'.

Sometimes, different degrees of denial are used to ignore certain bodily deformations. Nathan (1978), in a study of 25 young people who were about to undergo corrective surgery for idopathic scoliosis, found that those who showed a tendency to deny their deformity were significantly differentiated from the others in their capacity to face the stress involved in undergoing the operation. Those who showed a tendency to deny their deformity presented more feelings of vulnerability, and experienced the surgery as an aggressive attack on the self.

Interpretations

Disorders involving the patient's own experience of health can be considered a particular case of psychopathology of the body, which can be included within the more general context of consciousness disorders. It is interesting to remember that 'consciousness' in the psychological sense, and 'conscience', in the moral sense, derive from the same Latin *cognate, conscire*; indeed, in some contexts, the word 'conscience' is used for both concepts. Therefore it makes sense to say that a certain patient is 'conscious' of his illness, bringing in both the meaning of 'awareness of his own knowledge', while not excluding that of possible feelings of guilt about that illness.

From a neuropsychological viewpoint, these disorders have been attributed to alterations in perceptive *filtering*. From a psychoanalytical viewpoint, the literature cites the intervention in these conditions of denial, projection, and introjection mechanisms, and alternations of object relations in infancy or early childhood.

Neuropsychological Explanations

As we have discussed elsewhere (Guimón, 1999), everyone perceives only certain aspects of the surrounding world. We filter a great deal of the information that we do not consider essential for the task on which our attention is focused at a given moment. Indeed, if we are attentively reading these very pages, we pay little heed to perceiving the visual stimuli coming from areas surrounding the book, or the tactile stimuli deriving, for example, from the our skin's contact with the chair on which we are sitting. However, the very fact of mentioning, just now, the existence of these stimuli has surely induced a momentary dip in the attention being paid to the printed letters. Following the concepts of Gestalt psychology, on the backdrop of a heterogeneous set of perceptions, the most noteworthy, when reading, is the part of a sheet of paper filled with printed letter. The perception of the sensations that inform us about our body's state of health is also subject to the action of this filtering.

Not much is known regarding the nature of this filter, which, more or less automatically and unconsciously (although subject in part to the control of our consciousness and our conscience), conditions our perceptions and, to a certain extent, even the flow of our thoughts. Some recent neuropsychological experiments suggest that sophisticated mechanisms are at work, here. In a state of good health, we can acquire a growing consciousness regarding different parts of the body, both internal and external, which usually escape our notice. Certain muscular relaxation exercises, as well as yoga and meditation techniques, can place under our conscious control perceptions that had, until then, escaped us. On the contrary, in certain states of physical illness involving intense pain, we are able to stop perceiving certain stimuli that were formerly very present in our minds. 'One pain kills another', goes the saying; but pain can also distort our perception of pleasure, and diminish our interest in the world around us.

Distortions in the filtering process could explain the perceptive alterations that we have noted in patients with anorexia nervosa and early-onset obesity, and in normal women during adolescence and pregnancy. By the same token, they could explain phenomena such as the fact that more or less accurate knowledge regarding the activity of our organs can modify our consciousness of their disorders; or that knowledge of the anatomical and physiological aspects of childbirth can lessen labour pains; or, contrariwise, that knowledge of organic dysfunctions can lead medical students to interpret minor dysfunctions as being serious.

It could be supposed that, in certain situations, this filter can function with less intensity, enabling the appearance of what Ortega y Gasset (1946) called a *hyperesthesia of the body,* which he considered an explanation for hypochondria. On the contrary, if the filter functions intensively, it would erase our consciousness of certain perceptions. This would be the case in certain traumatic situations, highly freighted with affective content, and in certain dissociative states (e.g., fugues, multiple personality). Ignorance or denial of an illness could be special forms of this filtering activity. Some authors, such as Shakow (1963) have invoked the possibility of a defective functioning of this hypothetical filter in schizophrenic patients, who would therefore find themselves overwhelmed with irrelevant information, which would force them to resort to withdrawal behaviours.

Regarding the place where information about a patient's own health is processed, there is a general consensus regarding the central role played by the parietal lobes. Schilder (Schilder, 1979) pointed out that patients with sensorial aphasia presented an unjustifiable euphoria, whereas those who suffered from motor aphasia were conscious of the disorder, even exaggeratedly so. He attributed the presence of symptoms that mimicked organic illnesses to lesions in the periventricular grey matter, and reported the existence in the girus supramarginalis of a centre whose injury would block perception of pain. He concluded that the experience of health and illness depends on the functioning of specific cerebral areas, among which Wernicke's area is the most important. However, later research does not seem to have confirmed this interesting theory.

Relational Interpretations

Abnormal illness behaviours, including exaggerated worry about illness that is either nonexistent or less serious than the patient believes, have been interpreted from a psychoanalytical standpoint, along the lines of work carried out by Abraham (1966), Freud (1957), and Jacobson (1957) involving psychotic depression. Due to ambivalent object relations, object loss means that the aggressive cathexes formerly deposited therein become deposited in the ego itself. As we have discussed elsewhere (Guimón, 1999), Cotard's syndrome (Cotard, 1882) has been interpreted as the result of the aggressive cathetic energy projected onto the body image: the denial of organs would be a kind of anticipatory death, the destruction of the body image. In hypochondria, the organs, charged with aggressive cathexes, actually become the patient's persecutors.

It was Schilder (1935) who first studied the psychoanalytic aspects of devaluation or minimisation of alterations in bodily health. He pointed out that organic illness and its symptoms do not constitute a personal concern of the individual, because they are not situated at the centre, but rather at the periphery of what he called the 'ego circle'. Our problems, feelings, and attitudes are close to the ego nucleus, especially those involving pain, sexual excitation, and anxiety, which are at the very centre of personality. Perceptions coming from the outside, or from our own bodies, occupy a peripheral place, although certain parts of the body are closer to the ego centre, such as the genitals, breasts, and eyes.

In severe illnesses, as the disease progresses the minimisation mechanism becomes inadequate to deal with the situation, and to conserve the experience of health, the subject needs to recur to a more complex defence, such as regression, which frequently leads patients to adopt attitudes reminiscent of the oral phase of development. In other cases, projection mechanisms are more prominent, whether under the form of feeling persecuted (when the patient projects his anxiety outwards) or when a patient attributes a severe illness to another person, denying his own. In Schilder's opinion, in obviously delusional cases, the patient not only feels cured of his illness, but thinks that he can also cure the illnesses of others, with grandiose, narcissistic ideas coming to the forefront.

Authors after Schilder have stressed the importance of denial mechanisms and early object relations in the genesis of experiences of devaluation of illness.

Denial was described by Freud as a very early mechanism in the child's development, related with 'expelling' the 'bad', which is denied, while 'introjecting' and affirming the 'good'. Melanie Klein (1946) interpreted denial as a defence mechanism of the schizoparanoid position, where the existence of the 'bad object' or the 'persecutor' is denied, as well as the part of the ego that is linked to it. This denial is possible through the infant's own 'sense of omnipotence'. Resnik (Racamier, 1976) approached the problem of denial in relation to Cotard's syndrome and *depersonalisation* (in the sense employed by Pichon Ribiere). He agreed with Cotard that the usual evolution towards denial occurs through intermediate processes of hypochondria: simple at first, and then delusional.

Finally, we should mention that Rosenfeld contends, in commenting on the role of early object relations in hypochondria and psychosomatic illnesses, that many states of mental anxiety can produce physical pain, and by the same token, physical pain can cause mental suffering. He compared the vicissitudes of communicating pain in psychoanalytical treatment with the communication between the mother and child in early infancy, when physical sensations and mental experiences are not clearly differentiated. He pointed out that in hypochondriac patients, vestiges of object relations experienced with painful anxiety are often observed. He related this anxiety with worry about the organs in the body, which would explain that painful hypochondriac anxieties increase during analysis, when the patient tries to relive significant object relations. He also theorised that hypochondriac patients present difficulties in differentiating between depressive and paranoid anxieties. On the contrary, in psychosomatic illnesses, if there is no hypochondria then, in principle, there is no anxiety or mental pain.

EATING DISORDERS

The tendency to keep to strict diets with the object of avoiding excessive weight has been recorded since ancient times, and conditioned by diverse sociocultural factors. These include the sublimation of sexuality; mastering self-control (as in the case of Saint Catherine of Sienna in the 14th century); the search, on the part of women, to meet an ideal of beauty (associated in the West, for centuries, with thinness); and the desire to astound the public, as in the so-called 'living skeletons', usually men, and especially in the 18th and 19th centuries.

Research over the last few decades has shown that there are major alterations in the bodily experience of obese and anorexic subjects, but also in those who present alterations in their eating habits, even while maintaining a normal weight.

Obesity

In our culture, people are anxious about the idea of gaining weight, especially in urban settings. Being fat is considered bad, and the feeling of guilt about gaining weight is as intense as that of a sinner who has broken one of the Ten Commandments. To a certain extent, the social sanction regarding the goodness and virtue of an individual is tied up in the degree to which he is able to control his weight, which means that he has a strong will and leads a healthy life.

This negative view of obesity is not shared by all cultures, and in some, being fat is associated with respectability, and even beauty. It is not clear why fatness has such negative connotations, even from early infancy. There are those who say that it is due to the association with vulnerability to heart disease, but the negative connotations of obesity existed even before such a link was established.

Perhaps fatness is associated with being voracious and narcissistic. Indeed, obesity has been related with unsatisfied unconscious oral desires, immature and regressive tendencies, and a desire to avoid adult responsibilities (including mature sexuality). Some patients, on the other hand, consider their obesity a sign of power, and a way of impressing others. When these persons lose weight after going on a diet, their unconscious impression of vulnerability grows.

Some studies suggest that, on the contrary, certain persons, when their social status rises, tend to gain weight. On the contrary, adolescent girls with anorexia nervosa present an unconscious tendency to remain small, erasing the curves of the breast and hips that they begin to develop at puberty in order to stay like little girls, and avoid the responsibilities of adult life, including sexual activity. With this behaviour they want, unlike obese patients, to reduce the impression of power in their appearance. It has been observed that some patients with *compulsive eating disorders* (DSM IV, Frances et al., 1997) present more psychopathological symptoms. Other research in the same area has established a relationship between compulsive eating and consequent obesity with depression (Baeriswil-Waydelich, 1993).

As for the treatment of these disorders, a systematic review of interventions to improve health professionals' management of obesity has been conducted by Harvey et al. (1999), and a recent Cochrane study evaluated the different psychotherapies that have been shown to be useful for bulimia nervosa and binging (Hay et al., 2002). A manual-based cognitive-behavioural method has been proposed for bulimia nervosa (Tuschen-Caffier et al., 2001).

Anorexia

Some biological characteristics have been described that correlate with anorexia nervosa, but they seem to be more a result than a cause of the disorder. However, it is well known that the body image of anorexic patients is different from the one found in normal subjects (Garner et al., 1976).

In anorexic disorders, when the patient's life is at risk, the treatment approach tends to be medical: hospitalisation and nasogastric feeding. Hospitalisation should be in a setting including 'reward and punishment' cognitive-behavioural techniques involving isolation, visiting times, recreational activities, and so on. In maintaining weight, cognitive-behavioural psychotherapy with pharmacological support and family counseling are useful. Some patients respond well to in-depth psychodynamic techniques.

SEXUAL DISORDERS

Psychosocial Issues

Due to Freud's influence, until the last quarter of the 20th century, sexuality (to a much greater extent than aggression) was considered the energy responsible for personality development, its prime mover. While other biological needs (hunger, thirst, breathing) are usually satisfied easily in daily life, sexual desire (especially pregenital ones) are subjected to constant frustrations, generating many behaviours aimed at satisfying them. Going deeper into this argumentation, psychoanalysts saw in the avatars of the libido (i.e., the mental representation of the sex drive) the fundamental bases of psychopathology, also conditioned—but to a lesser extent—by aggression.

However, beginning in the 1960s, the increase in sexual permissiveness and the ever-wider availability of contraceptives attenuated the air of mystery that had previously surrounded sexuality, which had made it seem more evil and, partly for this reason, more attractive. There was a movement that vindicated, and rightly so, easier access to sexual activity for adolescents, the mentally retarded, chronic psychiatric patients, paraplegics and other severely ill patients, and the elderly. Some studies on sexual activity in the general population (starting with the Kinsey reports of 1948 and 1953) exaggerated the sexual capacity of certain population segments, paradoxically contributing to the creation of a feeling of inadequacy among those who compared their own, more modest, activities with those proclaimed by these statistics.

Meanwhile, the women's liberation movement set off profound changes in sexual relations, contributing to the appearance of new sexual pathologies, or the emergence of previously hidden ones, mainly certain forms of male impotence. Regarding the latter problem, a series of new therapeutic techniques has been developed.

A recent study in the United States showed that young adults in that country were more worried about economic problems than about sexual ones. A review of recent films internationally successful with the general public shows that those with aggressive themes are much more common than sexually oriented ones, especially among young people. Even in those films dealing with sexual themes, the public's preference tends towards scenes in which sexuality is contaminated with violence. Adolescent males today seem more interested in seeking new sensations through such sports as bungee-jumping or hang-gliding, even sometimes lethal experimentation with drugs, than in attaining new sexual experiences. It would not be far from caricature to say that their activities seem to be ruled more by serotonin than testosterone.

During the last quarter of the 20th century, among many sexologists an opposite trend was seen, including the landmark work of Masters and Johnson (1971): one of studying sexuality as just another organic function (such as digestion, excretion, or locomotion) regulated by organs and systems (e.g., respiratory or cardiovascular) which can present specific pathologies.

Many psychiatrists, interested in psychopharmacological and even surgical advances, wound up considering sexuality more as a function whose disorders could be treated medically or through simple behaviouralist procedures, rather than as one of the fundamental bases of human behaviour and psychopathology. This was, therefore, a 'de-libido-ised', or 'de-phantasised' sexology.

However, since those years, new elements have sparked fresh controversy regarding different views of the behaviours and pathologies involving human sexuality.

It would not be fair to settle for criticising a supposed 'Freudian pansexualism' and affirm that in a more sexually tolerant society, the aetiopathogenic theories of psychoanalysis are no longer of the slightest interest. These conclusions are those of a linear type of thinking that ignores that Freud's thought is, according to a sort of circular logic, largely responsible for this new sexual permissiveness.

The reductionist bias of such approaches and attitudes was, however, overcome by certain sexologists with a more holistic view who, after the pioneering work of Helen S. Kaplan, managed to conquer the International Psychoanalytical Association's misgivings about experimental approaches and integrate empirical sexological findings with the tenets of psychoanalysis. The work of Kaplan (1974), a professor at Cornell University, provided a fundamental complement to that of Masters and Johnson (Masters et al., 1971), to which she added the psychoanalytical viewpoint that these authors had neglected. This new approach had an extraordinary impact in the United States and then in Europe, for example, the Geneva school of sexology, led by Abraham (1995) and Passini.

Minority Sexual Orientations

Crowden et al. (1995) studied the influence of the gender and sexual orientation of a sample of volunteers in relation to a number of variables (e.g., body image, sexual guilt). The results indicated that sexual orientation had a significantly higher impact on several of these attitudes towards sex than did gender. Generally, homosexual subjects reported more negative attitudes than heterosexuals.

More research is needed in order to clearly delimit the concept of transsexualism and other related *gender identity disorders*. As highlighted by Money (Money, 1994), a sex change involves surgery that produces alterations which affect different areas and organs of the body that correspond to the body image. These changes can include almost the entire body: face, hair, breasts, external genitals, gonads, penis, prepuce, internal genitals, limbs, and skin. These surgical interventions, therefore, represent an important psychological aggression. Moreover, transsexual patients who request sex-change surgery often present severe psychiatric problems, so that they should be subjected to a complex evaluation process before being accepted for this kind of treatment.

In spite of all the precautions that are taken, the results are sometimes psychologically negative for the patient. Bodlund (1995) studied a group of 19 transsexuals using a semi-structured DSM-III interview, the SCID, with the aim of examining their personality, both dimensionally and categorically. He added other instruments to study psychosocial functioning, self-image, and psychological defence structures, from a psychodynamic perspective, and found that, after surgery, 68% of the subjects had improved, and 16% reported unsatisfactory results. A single patient regretted the sex change. Pathology as measured on the SCID was a significant predictor of a negative result, as were being biologically male, and lacking a stable partner.

Hypoactive Sexual Desire

A certain degree of timidity and avoidance of sexual conduct is frequent in the population, and has a high correlation with difficulties in sexual activity. The concept of *spectating* refers to a cognitive disorder involving excessive self-observation, so that individuals fixate on and carefully examine parts of their body and/or the adequacy of their personal sexual functioning. Excessive self-observation was a significant predictor of sexual avoidance in the sense of presenting a lower frequency of sexual behaviour, in both men and women (Faith, 1993).

Male impotency (or a man's incapacity to obtain or maintain a satisfactory erection during heterosexual intercourse) is often due to organic factors (systemic illnesses, advanced age, diseases of the genital organs, neurological disorders, frequent use of certain medications or toxic substances). However, they occasionally have a predominantly or exclusively psychological aetiology. The most striking characteristic in psychological impotence is its selectivity, e.g., it presents under certain circumstances, but not others; with any sexual object, but the subject has spontaneous morning erections. The degree of impotence can vary from a complete absence of desire and inability to engage in sexual intercourse (what some authors call *sexual aversion*), to diminished desire, insufficient erection, premature or late ejaculation, and infrequent intercourse (*hypoactive sexual desire*). Some authors refer to sexual impotence in cases of manifest timidity and difficulty in establishing social contact with women.

Among the psychological factors that can diminish male potency, the most often cited include: inexperience (with premature ejaculation, it is sometimes interpreted as representing feelings of hostility towards one's partner); inability to identify the loved object with the sexual object due to infantile emotional problems; fear (e.g., of getting one's partner pregnant, of contracting venereal disease, of getting caught in the act, of the moral implications of the act); and sexual object deviancy (usually homosexuality, whether open or hidden). A study of 10 subjects with hypoactive desire and 10 controls using the Thematic Aperception Test (TAT) found a number of significant alterations in those with sexual difficulties (Guimón et al., 1972).

Psychoanalysis considers impotence a form of infantile reaction, with different modalities, including: unconscious desire for revenge on a woman who represents another woman whom the patient previously loved and who treated him badly (the mother); envy of the woman's pleasure; homosexuality; anxiety due to a castration complex; early libidinal fixations; *vagina dentata* fantasy (sometimes based on oral sadism, with the projection of a fear of being bitten by the mother). Women's sexual hypoversion varies from frigidity to vagninismus. The efficacy of different interventions have recently been reviewed (McGuire et al., 2001).

PSYCHOLOGICAL FACTORS THAT AFFECT THE PHYSICAL STATE

With the name of *psychophysiological disorders* (i.e., psychosomatic disorders), the DSM-I and DSM-II grouped together as many as 10 conditions affecting different organic systems and organs (e.g., digestive, cardiovascular), specifying that the affected organs tended to be enervated by the autonomous nervous system. The DSM-III changed this heading to *psychological factors affecting a medical condition*, and included them in Axis I, whereas physical illnesses were assigned to Axis III. Psychological factors can affect a medical illness during its course (appearance, exacerbation, remission) or have an impact on its treatment.

NORMAL AND ABNORMAL ILLNESS BEHAVIOURS

Kirmayer (1984) and Lipowski (1976) described the expectations that physicians have in our culture regarding how patients should behave: the patient should complain, to a reasonable extent, about his condition, as long as it corresponds to demonstrable physical alterations; he should refer to his physical problems with 'body' terminology, and to his emotional ones with psychological terms; he should also meekly accept the physician's opinion and advice.

In recent years, the concept of *illness behaviour* (Liao et al., 1995) has been used in referring to how individuals respond to physical symptoms, how they define them, what value they assign to them, and what actions they take to remedy them.

REFERENCES

Abraham, G., & Vlatkovic, D. (1995). *Douleur et plaisir-Maladie et santé une perception subjective.* Genève: Georg, Collection Janus.

Abraham, K. (1966). Esquisse d'une Histoire du Développement de la libido basée sur la psychanalyse des troubles mentaux, *Oeuvres Complètes de Karl Abraham* (Vol. II). Paris: Payot.

Afari, N., & Buchwald, D. (2003). Chronic fatigue syndrome: a review. *Am J Psychiatry, 160*(2), 221–236.

Alexander, F. (1968). *Psychosomatic specificity.* Chicago: University of Chicago Press.

Baeriswil-Waydelich, D. (1993). *Les troubles alimentaires compulsifs, les boulimiques nerveuses et les "Mangeuses compulsives": Quels rapports entretiennent-elles à leur image du corps et à la dépression* (A propos de 104 patients). Geneva: Université de Genève.

Bodlund, O. K. (1995). *Transsexualism and personality: Methodological and clinical studies on gender idendity disorders.* Umea, Sweden: Umea University.

Cotard, J. (1882). Du délire des négations. *Archives de Neurologie, 4,* 152–170; 282–296.

Crowden, C. R., & Koch, P. B. (1995). Attitudes related to sexual concerns: Gender and orientation comparisons. *Journal of Sex Education & Therapy, 21*(2), 78–87.

Faith, M. S., & Schare, M. L. (1993). The role of body image in sexually avoidant behavior. *Archives Of Sexual Behavior, 22*(4), 345–356.

Frances, A., First, M. B., and Pincus, H. A. (Eds.). (1997). *DSM-IV, Guía de uso.* Barcelona: Masson.

Freud, S. (1957). Mourning and Melancholia, *Standard Edition of the Complete Psychological Works of Sigmund Freud,* (Vol. 14, pp. 243). London.: Hogarth Press.

Garner, D. M., Garginkel, P. E., Stanger, M. C., and Moldofsky, H. (1976). Body image disturbances in anorexia nervosa and obesity. *Psychosomatic Medicine,* 38(327–336).

Guimón, J., Navarro, E., and Delclaux, I. (1972). La vivencia del cuerpo del impotente. *Revista Española de Psicoterapia Analítica,* 3, 25–42.

Guimón, J., (1999). *Los lugares del cuerpo.* Barcelona: Paidos.

Harvey, E., Glenny, A., Kirk, S., and Summerbell, C. (1999). A systematic review of interventions to improve health professionals' management of obesity. *Int. J. Obes. Relat. Metab. Disord.,* 23 (12), 1213–1222.

Hay, P., and Bacaltchuk, J. (2002). Psychotherapy for bulimia nervosa and binging (Cochrane Review). *The Cochrane Library*, 1.
Jacobson, E. (1957). Normal and pathological moods; the nature and functions. *Psychoanalytic Study Of The Child, 12*, 73.
Kinsey, A. C., Pomeroy, W. B., & Martin, C. E. (1948). *Sexual Behaviour in the Human Male.* Philadelphia: Saunders.
Kinsey, A. C., Pomeroy, W. B., & Martin, C. E. (1953). *Sexual Behaviour in the Human Female.* Philadelphia: Saunders.
Kirmayer, L. J. (1984). Culture, affect and somatization. *Transcultural Psychiatric Research Review*, 21, 159–188.
Klein, M. (1946). Notes on some schizoid mechanisms, *The Writings of Melanie Klein* (Vol. 1). London: Hogarth Press.
Lipowski, Z. J. (1976). Psychosomatic medicine. An overview. In O. Hill (Ed.), *Modern Trends in Psychosomatic Medicine* (Vol. 3, pp. 1–20). London: Butterworths.
Liao, K. L. M., Hunter, M., and Weinman, J. (1995). Health related behaviours and their correlates in a general population sample of 45-year old women. *Psychology and Health*, 10(3), 171–184.
Marty, P. (1990). *La Psychosomatique de l'adulte.* Paris: PUF.
Masters, W. H., & Johnson, V. E. (1971). *Les mésententes sexuelles et leur traitement.* Paris: Robert Laffont.
McGuire, H., and Hawton, K. (2001). Interventions for vaginismus. *Cochrane Database Syst. Rev. Review*, 2, CD001760.
Money, J. (1994). Body-image syndromes in sexology: Phenomenology and classification. *Journal of Psychology and Human Sexuality*, 6(3), 31–48.
Ortega y Gasset, J. (1946). Vitalidad, alma y espíritu. Madrid: *Revista de Occidente.*
Resnik, S. (1995). Le corps de la folie. *Revue de Psychotherapie Psychanalytique de Groupe, 25*, 13–18.
Schilder, P. (1935). *The image and appearance of the human body: Studies in the constructive energies of the psyche.* London: Paul Kegan.
Schilder, P. (1979). Neuroses following head and brain injuries. In L. Bender (Ed.), Paul Schilder: *On Neuroses* (pp. 179–219). New York: International Universities Press, Inc.
Shakow, D. (1963). Psychological deficit in schizophrenia. *Behav. Sci.*, 8, 275.
Smadja, C. (2001). *La vie opératoire.* Paris: Presses Universitaires de France.
Tuschen-Caffier, B., Pook, M., and Frank, M. (2001). Evaluation of manual-based cognitive-behavioral therapy for bulimia nervosa in a service setting. *Behav. Res. Ther.*, 39 (3), 299–308.

18

Disorders of Adult Personality and Behaviour (F60–69)

The DSM-IV separates personality disorders and impulse-control disorders not otherwise specified.

CONCEPT

Personality disorders involve maladaptive, invasive, and permanent behaviours, deeply ingrained, and which are not due to any physical illness, nor to cultural particularities. Their traits are behavioural, emotional, cognitive, perceptive, and psychodynamic.

For decades, there has been an ongoing discussion on 'character pathology' (Coderch, 1991), referring to different aspects of an individual; however, the most generalised classification was that of Kurt Schneider (1942), who referred to psychopathic personalities, describing a series of conditions that were included in the standard international classifications, and which later served as a basis for the classifications used today.

AETIOPATHOGENY

Biological Model

The aetiology of these disorders has not been clearly established, and various studies seem to indicate that there is a variety of intervening factors. The genetic component seems important, as certain studies have shown, but it is not always present. The existence of constitutional factors, which condition defects in information processing by the central nervous system, has also been highlighted.

In recent years, empirical psychology has described personality disorders as traits or states. Compared with the 'categorical' diagnosis used in the DSM-IV, 'dimensional' diagnoses have been put forward, an alternative which would enable us to better understand the heterogeneity of the symptoms, and the lack of clear boundaries between the diagnoses. Such a system also enables clinicians to better detect symptoms and subthreshold traits, and to quantify symptoms. Factor analysis then makes it possible to discover these variables' principle underlying dimensions, and identify the personality traits that they involve.

Most research in this area has been carried out using Livesley's personality model, which differentiates among four major factors: emotional dysregulation, antisocial behaviour, inhibition, and compulsiveness. Many studies have also been conducted using Cloninger's Seven Factors Model (SFM) and Five Factors Model (FFM), which seem to show that there is a certain inherited, biological basis for these traits. Various studies relate the FFM to some personality disorders. Both the FFM and the SFM may eventually be incorporated into the official diagnostic systems.

Experimental psychologists have carried out research on the spectrum of the so-called impulsive and compulsive disorders, relating this axis to other psychological and physiological parameters. Their typology features an extreme 'impulsive' group, characterised by sensation seeking and harm avoidance. This extreme includes antisocial disorders and borderline personality disorders. The intermediate area of the spectrum includes sexual compulsions, pathological gambling, trichotillomania, and Tourette's syndrome. The other extreme includes depersonalisation, anorexia nervosa, dysmorphic disorder, hypochondria, and, at the far end, obsessive-compulsive disorder.

Compulsiveness has been related to hyperfrontality, with an increase in 5-HIAA, and to some modifications in serotonin inhibitors, and impulsiveness to hypofrontality and serotoninergic hypofunction.

Within the realm of personality, Cloninger distinguishes between temperament, which contributes 50% and includes such factors as sensation seeking, harm avoidance, reward dependency, persistence; and character, which contributes the other 50% and includes factors such as self-directedness, co-operation, and self-transcendence. Gabbard et al. (1988) tried to make this conception compatible with the psychoanalytical viewpoint, and compared the self-directedness factor with the self-esteem factor; self-coherence with representations of the self and ego functions; co-operation with internal relations of the externalised object in interpersonal relationships; and self-transcendence with sublimation and altruism.

Relational Aspects

Psychoanalytical concepts of personality disorders began with Freud (1905, 1916), who related character with anal eroticism.

Kernberg (1980) related personality disorders to early defence mechanisms against sexual and aggressive drives, and referred to a pathology of the super-ego, an alteration in ego organisation, difficulties in internalised object relations, and a pathological development of narcissistic functions. He highlighted the role played by dysfunctions in object relations established during early infancy. The patient sets into motion pathological defence mechanisms, systematically using dissociation, acting out, projective identification, and so on, which are going to create relational difficulties in adult life.

To assess a personality disorder, it is important to have information on the patient's manner of being and acting over quite a long period of time, and not during a certain, specific moment, since these disorders are characterised above all by an identical, lasting model of functioning. Their evolution and prognosis are variable, and difficult to establish.

In personality disorders, the DSM-IV maintains a categorical system for diagnosing personality traits, that are distributed along a continuum which differentiates among the various abnormal patterns in relationships with others that are characteristic of these patients.

Group A, also known as the 'odd-eccentric' group, includes paranoid, schizoid, and schizotypal personality disorders. Group B (or the 'dramatic-emotional' group) features the antisocial, borderline, histrionic, and narcissistic personality disorders. Group C (the 'anxious-fearful' group) includes avoidant, dependent and obsessive-compulsive personality disorders.

Borderline Disorder

The concept of borderline disorder first appeared in the psychiatric literature to designate patients with neurotic and psychotic symptoms. It was later suggested that they formed part of a spectrum including other disorders. The psychoanalytical school has considered them disorders involving a pathology of character (Kernberg, 1980) or personality (Gunderson, 1994).

It has even been said that the term borderline is inadequate, because it describes, above all, impulsiveness, disordered hostility, self-destructive acts, mood swings, and splitting; i.e., it defines symptoms, not traits.

The validity of this concept is not high because, although it has been similarly described in many countries, the biological findings are doubtful, in spite of some reliable neurophysiological findings.

The instrument most often used to assess this disorder is Gunderson's diagnostic interview for borderline cases.

Different aetiological hypotheses have been proposed to explain this disorder, ranging from constitutional factors (difficulty in regulating affect) to family and psychodynamic factors: perturbations in the establishment of object relations and inadequate processes of identification during early infancy (Herman, 1992). From an anamenesic viewpoint, in women there seems to be a relationship with childhood incest.

TREATMENT

General Orientations

There is not specific treatment for the different personality disorders. The treatments based on drugs are only useful in the presence of such symptoms as anxiety or depression, but have no influence on the underlying personality traits. Thus, in cases of anxiety, anxiolytics can be useful, as can antidepressants, if a depression appears. In certain disorders, such as schizotypic disorder, as well as transitory episodes of borderline disorder, neuroleptics can reduce anxiety. In the case of avoidance personality disorder, MAOIs have been used, with variable results.

In any case, a psychotherapeutic approach is advisable, with the aim of helping the patient to establish a different kind of relationship with his environment. Analytically oriented psychotherapy, with appropriate technical modifications, can be beneficial for many of these patients.

The psychotherapy of personality disorders has been evaluated by Perry et al (Perry et al., 1999) who examined the evidence for the effectiveness of 15 studies, including three randomised, controlled treatment trials. They concerned psychodynamic/interpersonal, cognitive behaviour, mixed, and supportive therapies. All studies reported improvement in personality disorders with psychotherapy. They estimated that 25.8% of personality disorder patients recovered per year of therapy, a rate seven times higher than that in a published model of the natural history of borderline personality disorder.

In the realm of antisocial personality disorder, Dolan et al. (1997) evaluated the impact of psychotherapeutic treatment on the principle symptoms of 137 hospitalised patients with personality disorders. They noted a reduction that was significantly greater in patients who received such treatment than in those in the 'non-hospitalised' control group of patients. The changes were in significantly positive correlation to the length of treatment.

The treatment of sex offenders, who qualify frequently for the diagnosis of personality disorders, has been approached through antilibidinal medication (e.g., medroxyprogesterone acetate) and psychotherapeutic procedures (such as imaginal desensitisation). White et al. (2002) reviewed antilibidinal management of those who have been convicted of sexual offences or who have disorders of sexual preference. A relapse prevention programme has suggested that although there is no discernible effect on the outcome of sex offending, those treated with response prevention do have less non-sexual violent offences. Another single trial (McConaghy, 1988) found that the effect of medication plus desensitisation was no better than imaginal desensitisation for problematic/anomalous sexual behaviour, although those committing both sexual and violent offences also declined in the response prevention group. A large-scale study evaluating the efficacy of group therapy for sex offenders (Romero, 1983) found no effect on recidivism at ten years.

A Cochrane review of all randomised controlled trials on psychological and pharmacological treatments for patients presenting pathological gambling (who also frequently had a diagnoses of personality disorder) revealed a paucity of evidence for effective treatment of this problem (Oakley-Browne et al., 2002), although there was a trend for long-term treatment with BT/CBT to be more efficacious than the control treatments.

Treatment of Borderline Disorders

Overall Results

In patients presenting borderline personality disorders, some fairly specific treatments have been used, including serotonin re-uptake inhibitors, mood stabilisers, and neuroleptics at a low dosage level.

These patients are difficult to manage in individual analytical psychotherapy, due to their instability, which is frequently related to a loss of self-esteem and identity confusion. There is a high percentage of drop-out in these patients. The course of therapy tends to be disturbed by intense transferences and various "actings," such as suicide attempts, attacks of rage, and self-mutilation caused by suicidal thoughts. Kernberg (1968) recommended confronting these patients and interpreting their negative transference early on, whereas other authors (Buie and Adler, 1982) advise therapists to limit themselves to acting as a holding environment for the patient and avoid interpretations. Group therapy, traditionally used in these patients when they are hospitalised, is currently considered of particular interest for outpatients. Springer and Silk (1996) designed an efficient, short programme, and discussed, particularly, the advantages and disadvantages of Linehan's dialectical behaviour therapy (1987). Indeed, group therapy offers the advantages of being less expensive, making transference easier to manage, and producing an improvement in ego functioning (Kretsch, Goren, and Wasserman, 1987) and interpersonal functioning (Schreter, 1970, 1978), and a drop in the patient's regressive tendencies (Horwitz, 1987). Moreover, these patients are more likely to take advice or engage in confrontations with other patients than with the therapist, and they have the possibility to relate with them on an equal level.

Group therapy should be part of a multidimensional programme, and the group should, in principle, be heterogeneous. The orientation of groups tends to be eclectic, and although open psychodynamic groups are the most frequent, others (Klein, 1993) focus on such aspects as acting out, splitting, countertransference and eroticisation of relationships.

Group therapy was found to be as efficient as individual therapy in a program of 'managing emotions' (Dawson, 1988, 1993) and patients who participated in groups showed better treatment compliance. In these programs therapists show themselves as permissive even if they forbid acting out. Regular attendance at meetings was not obligatory, which meant that only 30% of regular participants, forming the nucleus of patients, was more or less constant, while there was also a much larger subset of patients who showed up from time to time at the group meetings, searching for occasional help. A controlled study comparing individual and group psychotherapy (Clarkin et al., 1991) showed better results with this approach.

Significant, positive results have been found with Linehan's cognitive-behavioural approach. This method was first proposed for young women who were parasuicidal, and was then extended to persons with behavioural problems to resolve 'dialectic' failures. Indeed, from a theoretical point of view, Linehan made reference to this dialectic reasoning, which brings into opposition poles such as active passiveness versus competency, demonstrative crises versus emotional inhibition, and so on.

These programmes combine individual and group approaches in problem-solving and in skills training. In the psycho-educational groups, patients are taught a certain number of skills in regulating emotion, interpersonal functioning, and stress tolerance. Patients take part in these groups during at least one year, and then participate in help groups, or groups to reinforce skills application. In individual and concomitant therapy, which lasts at least one year, patients are taught to integrate these skills into daily life. Rules to generalise apprenticeship in the outside world (even using the telephone) are proposed. The group is closed or, at the maximum, slowly opened.

The psychoanalytical approaches are especially based on the theory of object relations. Most of the approaches have been developed in hospital environments or in halfway centres, based principally on the work of Kernberg, who used the psychoanalytical model of object relations. The accent is placed on increasing the strength of the ego and improving the reality testing, with an attempt at internal reconstitution. From a technical point of view, the splitting mechanism is reinforced rather than fought, and they propose open exteriorising of aggression and the realisation of group interpretation based on the 'here and now', which favours cohesion.

Certain authors, in comparing these two approaches, have pointed out that in both of them, the therapist is strongly committed, even if the attitude of Kernberg is neutral and that of Linehan (1987) is active, with attitudes of reinforcement. However, the expression of aggressiveness is encouraged by Kernberg, whereas Linehan does not encourage it, and Linehan is not interested in the here-and-now of the group, nor in group phenomena.

Wood et al. (2001) compared group therapy with routine care in adolescents (most of them borderline) who had deliberately harmed themselves, and found that those who had undergone group therapy were less likely to be 'repeaters', although their global outcome did not differ. Hawton et al. (2002) evaluated all randomised controlled trials regarding the effectiveness of treatments of patients who have deliberately self-harmed, and found reduced rates of further self-harm for depot flupenthixol versus placebo, and for dialectical behaviour therapy versus standard aftercare.

Hospitalisation

Because of the risks of acting out, the therapist must be able to count on a support system offering more holding for these kinds of patients, i.e., a hospital unit (which should be avoided as much as possible in order to not embark on a prolonged and counterproductive relationship with the institution) or a day hospital.

Using a dynamic perspective, recent work by Bateman and Fonagy (Bateman et al., 1999) has shown favourable results with treatment based on dynamic psychotherapy in a day hospital. These authors compared the evolution of 19 patients, whose treatment in hospital was partially oriented from a psychoanalytical point of view, with the same number of patients who had received general psychiatric treatment. Self-mutilating behaviour and suicide attempts decreased during the 18-month programme. Moreover, the average hospital stay was shorter than for those who followed specific treatment.

In the hospital environment (and also in halfway institutions), the treatment is carried out in settings where several caregivers interact. Adshead (1998), in light of attachment theory, reported that the hospital environment provides security only if caregivers are capable of tolerating both the external demands of the system and the internal demands of patients. He pointed out that therapeutic relationships between staff and patients are only repetitions and recreations of internal object relations, and that responses from the team to splitting and to projective identification can sometimes be negative. He further indicated that a certain number of negative reactions can be detected through the patronising and contemptuous way that caregivers may sometimes express themselves to the patient; moreover, that certain excessive reinforcements of the regulation of services, for example the inappropriate use of restriction on movement, may result from this attitude on the part of staff. Adshead also remarked that the conflict between therapist and patient may be exacerbated by the new organisation of cost containment, particularly in a managed-care system, e.g., by the interference of insurance companies. Finally, he pointed out that problems in the unit's structural organisation, such as inadequate accounting practices, lack of leadership, difficulties in communication and violation of boundaries, can seriously aggravate the condition of patients.

The programme developed at the Francis Dixon Lodge is an example of these issues. The patients are generally hospitalised because of their destructive manner of expressing their mental pain. After three weeks of hospitalisation, staff embark on a psychodynamic programme, which includes predictions regarding transferential reactions that they can expect, and which try to cover the self-aggressive behaviour (feelings of abandonment, trigger situations, and so on). Personnel try to forge a therapeutic relationship in which the patient feels sufficiently reassured to explore avenues of new relationships, while allowing him or her access to the horrors of the past, which may carry so much negative emotion that they could even endanger the relationship. In addition, they consider acting out to be an expressive and defensive function and that even more self-destructive behaviour can be an attempt to avoid another catastrophe (psychosis, hetero-aggression, etc.), which can be experienced as more destructive to their own integrity.

These patients, because of their poor self-esteem, do not know how to ask for help in an appropriate manner, and do so by provoking crises, which causes the therapeutic team to counter-react. Staff explains to patients that they must learn to talk about their suicidal feelings or their ideas about self-mutilation, explaining that they try to be tolerant, but that we also expect them to modify their behaviour. They try to avoid patients' feeling of omnipotence when they trigger self-aggressive activities, and pay special attention to phenomena of hostile and envious dependency, by trying to avoid or to manage negative therapeutic reactions.

Springer (Springer and Silk, 1996), based on the existing literature, proposed a framework in which an effective, short-term group treatment can be organised, particularly emphasising the advantages and disadvantages of the adaptation of Linehan's dialectical behaviour therapy by using it in a short-term programme for hospitalised patients. For their part, Dolan et al. (1997) evaluated the impact of psychotherapeutic treatment on the principal symptoms of 137 hospitalised patients with personality disorder. They noted a significantly greater improvement in those treated than in the 'non-admitted' group, as well as a significant, positive correlation with length of treatment. Similarly, Hafner and Holme (1996) conducted a prospective study on 48 residents of a therapeutic community, 34 of whom presented borderline personality disorders in order to determine which elements of the programme were most useful. A reduction in significant symptoms on the Brief Symptoms Inventory took place at discharge after an average stay of 64 days, and the rates of admission to hospital fell significantly during the year after discharge. Patients rated group therapy as the most useful element of the programme. A five-year follow-up study by Sabo et al. (1995) on 37 hospitalised patients presenting borderline personality disorder evaluated the changes in two forms of self-destructiveness. They noted that suicidal conduct diminished significantly, but that self-aggressive conduct, although it presented a certain downward trend, did not drop significantly, nor did aggressive ideation (both suicidal and self-destructive).

Finally, Schimmel (1997) stressed the efficacy of therapeutic community treatment for patients suffering from borderline personality disorder, concluding that it was necessary to carry out further research to evaluate its efficacy for other diagnostic groups because, in principle, this intensive treatment approach can be very appropriate for patients who are resistant to treatment by other means.

REFERENCES

Adshead, G. (1998). Psychiatric staff as attachment figures. *British Journal of Psychiatry, 172*, 64–69.

Bateman, A., and Fonagy, P. (1999). Effectiveness of partial hospitalization in the treatment of borderline personality disorder: a randomized controlled trial. American Journal of Psychiatry, 156 (10), 1563–1569.

Buie, D. H., and Adler, G. (1982). Definitive treatment of the borderline personality. International Journal of Psycho-Analysis and Psychotherapy, 9(51–87).

Clarkin, J. F., Marziali, E., and Munroe-Blum, H. (1991). Group and family treatments for borderline personality disorder. Hospital Community Psychiatry, 42, 1038–1043.

Clonninger

Coderch, J. (1991). *Psiquiatría dinámica* (5 ed.). Barcelona: Herder.

Dawson, D. F., and MacMillan, H. L. (1993). Relationship management of the borderline patient. New York: Brunner/Mazel.

Dolan, B., Warren, F., & Norton, K. (1997). Change in borderline symptoms one year after therapeutic community treatment for severe personality disorder. *British Journal of Psychiatry, 171*, 274–279.

Freud, S. (1905). Psychopathic Characters on the Stage, *S.E.* (Vol. 7, pp. 35).

Freud, S. (1916). *Some charactter-Types met with in psycho-analytical work* (Vol. 14). London: S.E.

Gabbard, G. O., Horwith, L., Frieswyk, S. H., et al. (1988). The effect of therapist interventions on the therapeutic alliance with borderline patients. Journal of the American Psychoanalytic Association, 36, 697–727.

Gunderson, J. G. (1994). Building structure for the borderline construct. Acta Psychiatrica Scandinavica. Supplementum, 379, 12–18.

Hafner, R. J., & Holme, G. (1996). The influence of a therapeutic community on psychiatric disorder. *Journal of Clinical Psychology, 52*(4), 461–468.

Hawton, K., Townsend, E., Arensman, E., et al. (2002). Psychosocial and pharmacological treatments for deliberate self-harm (Cochrane Review) (Vol. 1). Oxford: Update Software.

Herman, J. (1992). *Trauma and recovery*. New York: Basic Books.

Horwitz, L. (1987). Indication for group psychotherapy with borderline and narcissistic patients. *Bulletin of the Menninger Clinic*, 51, 248.

Kernberg, O. (1968). The treatment of patients with borderline personality organization. *International Journal of Psycho-Analysis, 49*(4), 600–619.

Kernberg, O. F. (1980). Neurosis, psychoses and the borderline states. In A. M. Kaplan and F. A. M. and J. Sadock (Eds.), *Comprehensive textbook of psychiatry*. Baltimore: Williams and Wilkins.

Klein, R. H. (1993). Short-term group psychotherapy. In W. Wilkins (Ed.), *Comprehensive group psychotherapy* (pp. 256–270). Baltimore: Williams and Wilkins.

Kretsch, R., Goren, Y., and Wasserman, A. (1987). Change patterns of borderline patients in individual and group therapy. *International Journal of Group Psychotherapy*, 37(1), 95–112.

Linehan, M. M. (1987). Dialectical behavior therapy for borderline personality disorder. Theory and method. *Bulletin of the Menninger Clinic*, 51(3), 261–276.

Livesley

Oakley-Browne, M., Adams, P., and Mobberley, P. (2002). *Interventions for pathological gambling (Cochrane Review)*. The Cochrane Library (1).

Perry, J., Banon, E., and Ianni, F. (1999). Effectiveness of psychotherapy for personality disorders. *American Journal of Psychiatry*, 156(9), 1312–1321.

Sabo, A. N., Gunderson, J. G., Navajavits, L. M., Chauncey, D., & Kisiel, C. (1995). Changes in self-destructiveness of borderline patients in psychotherapy. A prospective follow-up. *Journal of Nervous and Mental Disease, 183*(6), 370–376

Schneider, K. (1942). *Problemas de patopsicología y de Psiquiatría clínica*. Madrid: Edit. Morata.

Schimmel, P. (1997). Swimming against the tide? A review of the therapeutic community. *Australian and New Zealand Journal of Psychiatry, 31*(1), 120–127.

Schreter, R. K. (1970). Treating the untreatable: a group experience with somaticizing borderline patients. *International Journal of Psychiatry in Medicine*, 10, 205.

Springer, T., and Silk, K. R. (1996). A review of inpatient group therapy for borderline personality disorder. *Harvey Review of Psychiatry*, 3(5), 268–278.

White, P., Bradley, C., Ferriter, M. and Hatzipetrou, L. (2002). Managements for people with disorders of sexual preference and for convicted sexual offenders (Cochrane Review). The Cochrane Library, 1.

Wood, A., Trainor, G., Rothwell, J., Moore, A. and Harrington, R. (2001). Randomized trial of group therapy for repeated deliberate self-harm in adolescents. *J. Am. Acad. Child Adolesc. Psychiatry*, 40(11), 1246–1253.

19

Individual Psychotherapy

In this chapter, we shall first try to define the frontiers of psychotherapy, and summarise the classifications that have been proposed for the more than 2000 psychotherapies extant today. We shall then go on to examine what seem to be the original theoretical and technical aspects of the latest procedures, and then discuss which therapeutic aspects are common to these techniques, and which are specific to some of them. All of these reflections will lead to a set of final recommendations for the training of mental health workers.

THE FRONTIERS OF PSYCHOTHERAPY

The term *psychotherapy* was used for the first time by J.E. Reil in 1803, referring to the application of psychological methods to the treatment of mental disturbances. We should try to maintain this original meaning, restricting application of the term to curing mental illnesses. If we accept psychopathology as being the science aimed at the study of the disturbances of human behaviour and experience, then psychotherapies would be approaches to the cure of both behaviour and experience, at the same time. To deserve the name, *psychotherapy* would additionally have to be carried out by professionals adhering to theories concerning not only the genesis of the disturbances, but also the processes implied in their modification. They should, moreover be able to predict and evaluate the results of their interventions. Obviously, certain concepts included in this proposed definition are ambiguous, such as 'psychic abnormality' or 'professionally'. However, this is an inevitable shortcoming when we enter the field of psychopathology. It is not a bad idea, on the other hand, to bear in mind that tolerance of ambiguity is one of the necessary prerequisites of all psychotherapists.

History gives us many examples of attempts at modifying man's experience and behaviour by psychological methods. In Ancient Greece, for example, mental patients had to sleep in Aesklepion's labyrinth in order to be healed by this divinity. Meditation has been fostered by many religions. Education throughout history gives us an idea of man's attempts to modify childish impulses. Penal practices show us how asocial behaviour was handled down the ages; for example, so-called witches, many of whom were mental patients, were tortured and executed during many centuries. In all these practices, charismatic leaders and re-educators played a central role, enhanced by suggestion. Hypnotists and 'magnetisers' have skilfully used, from the beginning of time, the influence that some men have over others.

Freud conceived psychoanalysis as a method aimed at modifying psychic disturbances, which he considered to be rooted in biological abnormalities. Paradoxically, given his pessimistic view of the human condition, he considered that all men have psychic disturbances. Because of this, psychoanalysis became separated from the medical model of therapy, which distinguished between health and illness, and adopted a conception of psychotherapy that bears clear educational connotations. Freud described the psychoanalytic technique as a verbal procedure of resolving unconscious conflicts through the use of transference, and he took great care to keep away from suggestive methods. However, he unwillingly used the power of his personal charisma in the context of an atmosphere prone to suggestion. Moreover, in 1918, in Budapest (Freud, 1918), Freud already acknowledged that, in the future, to make psychoanalysis available to a larger proportion of the population it would be necessary to mix the pure gold of analysis with the copper of suggestion. What seemed in fact to differentiate Freud from his predecessors was his desire to know exactly what he was doing and his interest in increasing the self-awareness of the people he treated.

Freud's disciples in the years to follow continued to juxtapose psychoanalysis with suggestion giving a pejorative connotation to the latter. However, in the 1950s they were bound to accept that other specific techniques, such as those derived from behaviourism, had their place in therapy.

A new conception concerning man's destiny in the world, which is not alien to the cultural movement of the 1960s, has given rise to the emergence of an extensive range of techniques for self-actualisation and personal growth. A common element in all of these techniques is an anti-intellectualism that stresses emotional development. Some of these techniques are based on psychoanalysis; others have a strong oriental flavour. Some psychotherapists have even introduced the use of drugs and sexual contacts in their techniques.

What seemed to have happened, in fact, is parallel to the problem of hunger in the world today. After satisfying chronic hunger, the underdeveloped countries, as they begin to emerge from their poverty, show a growing interest in the delights of the palate and sophisticated cooking. A part of the population that would not normally be considered mentally ill, even though being dissatisfied and unhappy, has sought, in the use of these techniques, to enter an artificial paradise. Still others have sought consolation and hope formerly provided by the traditional religions at moments of crisis. With all of this, the boundaries of psychotherapy have become blurred. Not only encounter groups, but also jogging, aerobics, and even golf could be considered, in this context, psychotherapies. The supporters of these approaches proclaim the renunciation of the concept of therapy due to its medical overtones, equating the search for wellbeing with the force and equilibrium of truth and liberty. Psychotherapy thus claims to be a radical event that modifies our way of life.

It is evident that these concepts assume the proposition of a model for the human being that is as controversial as the one first suggested by Freud. The new psychotherapies smack of an indoctrination much more intense that traditional psychoanalysis. On the other hand, the repercussions of these theories and practices concerning the human ecosystem, are scarcely taken into account by their leaders.

Indeed, it is preferable to not even refer to such procedures as psychotherapy. Let us leave the fostering of utopian felicity to these modern 'gurus'.

CLASSIFICATION OF NEW PSYCHOTHERAPIES

As invariably occurs in nosology, a particular classification cannot cover the whole range of psychotherapy. Moreover, classifications are always reductive, and the use of different classifications in accord with the different aims we have in view is imperative.

If we classify therapies according to their relationship to the psychiatric models from which they derive, we will obtain a typology ranging from behaviourism to milieu therapy. The classification of psychotherapies based on their mechanism of action leads to a typology ranging from those intending to gain insight through verbal communication, to those based on facilitating instruction. In the middle are those based on cognition, behaviour modification, and corporal experiences.

We can also characterise contemporary psychotherapies according to their theoretical derivations. Some novel psychotherapeutic procedures are derived from psychoanalysis and make use of theories very similar to those advocated by Freud. Others propose new theoretical models; for example, behaviourism and systemic family therapy. Many are only techniques in the fruitless search for a theory, such as reality therapy, rational-emotive therapy and primal therapy. Some, like Erhard's seminars training, do not claim to be therapies, nor do they take into account a theoretical base, and only offer experiences of 'personal growth'. In the following, we shall refer only to those therapies that have a more substantial theoretical and technical base.

THEORETICAL AND TECHNICAL NOVELTIES IN MODERN PSYCHOTHERAPY

Psychoanalytic Therapy

Psychoanalysis detects disturbances different from those acknowledged by the patient. Frequently, in trying to cure these disturbances, painful consequences can result in the life of the patient. The analyst, moreover, usually works according to some project about what and how the patient should ideally be in the future. This project is conditioned culturally and often does not coincide with the patient's own ideal of himself. Sometimes, we see the paradoxical situation is arrived in which the patient has to face unexpected problems and live up to an ideal image that, in principle, he does not share. His acceptance of this reframing of his difficulties and this new image requires a good deal of indoctrination. This inevitable ambiguity constitutes one of the most poignant ethical questions confronting the psychoanalyst.

Moreover, it is evident that even our usually compliant patients have learned (as happens in every field) to become very demanding consumers of psychotherapy. Psychoanalytic psychotherapy is costly and frustrating. The realisation of its aims can be delayed over long periods of time. The patient seeks immediate results through more agreeable channels. The faith needed to travel along the difficult road with the analyst has been weakened by public controversy concerning the efficacy of psychoanalysis. However, if we study the proposed therapeutic alternatives, we shall see that they are, for the most part, based on psychoanalysis and have not been able to demonstrate better results. The claim that traditional psychoanalysis is on the decline is quite false. If, for instance, we stop to examine the causes of some recent litigation presented by psychologists in the United States against the American Psychoanalytic Association, we shall see that what they are demanding is in fact to join that powerful organisation.

Classical psychoanalysis has given rise to many forms of psychoanalytic psychotherapy, with major technical implications. These techniques include those based on the theory of ego psychology, self psychology, and the relational drive model. Some forms of short-term dynamic and group psychotherapies should be included here. Ego psychology derives from the work of Anna Freud, Hartman, Spitz, Mahler, and Jacobson. There are two main schools of thought regarding object relationships: the 'drive/structure model', in which relationships are conditioned by the need for drive satisfaction (Freud), and the 'relational/structure model', in which the relationship in itself is the motivating force (Sullivan).

There are mixed models, as well, among which the most influential is the one designed by Kohut (1978). This author proposed the 'psychology of the self', which attempts to replace the Ego/Id model. He stated that narcissism has a different line of development to that of the psychosexual line of Ego development. Another mixed model is the one proposed by Greenberg and Mitchell. They do not consider drive/structure and relational/structure models as incompatible. They combine them in the so-called drive/emotional model, and believe that drive and relational needs exist in all of us, playing different roles at different moments in psychological development. Both needs can be frustrated and subverted and this, in turn, gives rise to different emotional problems.

Following the attempts of Ferenczi (1967), Alexander and French (1946), and Balint (1972), the, establishment of a short dynamic psychotherapy has now become a reality. The names of Malan (1975), Sifneos (1977), and Davanloo (1980) are associated with these new conceptions and practices. Such techniques have been applied successfully not only to circumscribed complaints of selected patients, but also to cases presenting with severe psychopathology.

Psychoanalytic group psychotherapy has seen enormous development in the last decade. Its well-documented efficacy in the treatment of neurotic and character disorders has made it the technique of choice for many patients. After unsuccessful attempts at carrying out techniques based on the analysis of the group, instead of its individual components, an intermediate approach, Foulke's group analytic technique, is gaining ground in Europe.

Behavioural and Cognitive Therapy

Milton (2001) suggested that 'contemporary enthusiasm for cognitive-behavioural therapy reflects our longing for swift, rational help for psychological suffering', and contended that a cognitive model is commonsensical, but with less potential explanatory and therapeutic power. Attempts to 'integrate' cognitive and dynamic treatments have not been very successful to date. Milton stressed that brief psychotherapies of either variety have a similar, moderately good outcome, and that 'there is some evidence that this may be based more on "dynamic" than "cognitive" elements of treatment'.

Indeed, there are subtle ties that link the new techniques to psychoanalytic psychotherapy (Guimón, 2001b); a good example here is the treatment of phobias by means of desensitisation.

It was first thought that systematic desensitisation worked by a mechanism of inhibition of the symptom through muscular relaxation. Soon, however, it became apparent that the efficacy of desensitisation was similar even when muscular relaxation was omitted. On account of this, it was then thought that the technique worked through mechanisms of extinction, through the exposure of the subject to the phobiogenic situation. The technique of flooding the patient with phobiogenic situations, thus proposed, did not seem to have many advantages, and it does not seem to enjoy the support and esteem of specialists today. More complex techniques are preferred; for example, 'anxiety management training', in which anxiety is caused and later reduced by means of relaxation, and through the introduction of some modifications of cognition.

Many subtypes of therapy or specific techniques stem from the cognitive-behavioural model. Psycho-educational approaches are of great benefit in several disorders. A variety of this, bibliotherapy, is widely used (Adams et al., 2000). The most common reason for recommending books was to encourage self-help.

Systemic Family Therapy

The contribution of general systems theory to the modern conceptions of family therapy have made possible the development of a new theoretical frame and some new practices. From a theoretical point of view, the idea of systems having a certain kind of isomorphism and specific operational laws had already been envisaged in Freudian psychoanalysis and in the interpersonal psychiatry of Sullivan. However, there are elements arising from general systems theory that can be considered as original contributions (Durkin, 1975). For example: (1) the principle of 'equifinality'; (2) the concept of 'stable states'; (3) the concept of 'negantropy'.

But the most important contribution of systemic therapy has been in its strategic and tactical approaches. Regarding power strategies, for example, the therapist apparently allies himself with the strongest figure in the family (let us say, a tyrannical father), rather than with the adequate mother. But the possible risk that such opportunist alliances seem to portend is, in reality, minimal, according to these therapists. The family, they claim, has a long history, and therefore is much more resistant to change than a normal psychotherapeutic group.

Starting from this peculiar power situation, the therapist resorts to seemingly original tactics, the basis of which lies in the production of more or less contradictory messages: 'reframing' 'task prescriptions', and so on. All of these techniques produce confusion in the communicative system, which forces the adoption of alternative behaviours. 'Reframing' techniques are used with a view to making the acceptance of an interpretation tolerable through revealing its most positive connotations. 'Prescription' of symptoms has been frequently used in psychoanalysis to combat masochistic defences, and in behavioural psychotherapy in 'flooding' techniques.

There is no doubt that these techniques, even when they have precursors, are an original contribution to psychotherapy and a powerful instrument in producing change. The passing of time, a more rigorous conceptualisation, and the realisation of controlled studies will, in future, reveal their true value.

Indications

Many attempts have been made to define what kind of psychotherapy is useful for which patient, with which symptoms, at what 'dosage', and applied by which therapist. An interesting evidence-based strategy has recently been implemented by the Birmingham Health Authority for the use of psychotherapy services in a population of just under 1 million.

The need for evidence-based psychotherapy services was estimated, and it was found that the demand for psychotherapy exceeded service provision by a factor of four. Interventions were targeted on the basis of objective criteria to ensure that patients were referred for the appropriate level and intensity of psychological intervention, including greater use of brief and cost-effective, focused forms of integrative therapy from a variety of psychotherapeutic schools.

When discussing the integration of psychotherapies, it has been observed that a therapist's function seems essential for the success of any kind of psychotherapy, no matter what its theoretical orientation may be: to provide adequate space for the patient's confiding his or her worries, desires and anguishes to the therapist. The therapist thus becomes a container in which all those affections can be processed and, once modified, taken in again by the patient. This 'container' meets the patient's needs for emotional contact and cognitive information, which lead to passive learning. From that moment, the patient is ready to accept the conceptual framework of the therapist concerning his or her view of the world, of people, of the causes of the patient's disturbances and the means of curing them. At this point, we are dealing with an active learning process in which there is an attempt at modifying the patient's perceptions, feelings, cognitions, and behaviour. All of the above involve psychoanalytical implications, but also existential, philosophic and educational connotations.

SCOPE AND LIMITATIONS OF PSYCHOANALYSIS IN CLINICAL PSYCHIATRY

The Scope of Dynamic Psychiatry

Psychoanalysis, as a science and as an exceptional instrument for self-knowledge, will continue to grow through its institutes and associations. However, its role in clinical psychiatry has diminished. A report sponsored by the International Psychoanalytical Association (Fonagy, 2000) underlines that even if 'classical psychoanalysis' remains a set of defined technical operations different from those expected under 'psychoanalytic psychotherapy', in practice, conceptual and process differences between psychoanalysis and the various forms of psychoanalytic psychotherapy become ambiguous. Furthermore, the report underlines that technique varies considerably among analysts, even those trained at the same institution. In any case, the report, through the review of 50 major research projects (some of them involving a variety of evaluation studies), makes clear the value of psychoanalysis for many persons with mental suffering.

As we said, in our view, however, the only way for psychoanalysis to play a relevant role in the future of public mental health will be through a 'decaffeinated' dynamic psychiatry.

The theoretical orientation of psychiatrists has been substantially modified in the last 20 years. If, from the dawn of the 20th century through the 1970s, dynamic psychiatry prevailed in most Western countries, in the 1980s and 1990s the advance of the biological model was impressive. Spectacular advances in biological research, the presence of psychiatrists in the new short-stay units in general hospitals, and the difficulty in proving the efficacy of community approaches have led to a remedicalisation of the psychiatric profession.

However, many psychiatrists in the West continue to be interested in dynamic psychiatry. Although there is a penury of empirical data, it appears that the intensity of their commitment varies from one country to another. Be that as it may, surveys conducted in North America, Britain, Switzerland, and Spain, have all shown that interest in psychoanalytically

Table 19.1. Activities at the individual level in percentages (several answers possible)

	Switzerland	Spain
Analytically inspired psychotherapy	81.3	28.2
Psychoanalysis	25.8	9.1
Short or focal psychotherapy	69.2	18.2
Relaxation	42.6	49.0
Hypnosis	17.7	
Behavioural therapies	34.3	
Cognitive therapies	35.4	
Systemic therapies	46.8	
Deconditioning	35.9	33.0
Psychotherapy + medication	91.2	71.2
Principally medication	68.1	27.3

oriented models has decreased in the last two decades, although to varying degrees.

Regarding clinical practice, we will mainly refer in this book to data gathered in Spain (Azcúnaga et al, 1986; Guimón et al, 1987; Guimón, 1990) and Switzerland (Guimón et al, 1997a; Guimón et al, 1997b; Guimón et al, 1998a; Guimón et al, 1998b), since they illustrate two opposite tendencies in the ascription of psychiatrists to the psychodynamic model. For example, although the majority of Spanish psychiatrists consider themselves well or very well informed about psychoanalysis, few actually practise psychodynamic psychotherapy (28%) or psychoanalysis (9.1%). In contrast, the profile of Swiss psychiatrists' practices which emerges is characterised by a marked predominance of psychotherapeutic activities: more than 80% use psychoanalytically inspired psychotherapies (Table 19.1), and one-quarter of them mention psychoanalysis.

At the group level, the analytical approach is mentioned by one-third, and systemic therapy by almost half of psychiatrists (Table 19.2). At the individual level, on the other hand, 28.2% of Spanish psychiatrists use analytically oriented psychotherapy, while only 9.1% of them do psychoanalysis and 18.2% mention short psychotherapies.

However, both in Spain and in other Western countries, psychiatrists try to maintain an eclectic attitude, using, to a greater or lesser degree, elements from any of the models of practice. In fact, a predominant characteristic resides in the fact that almost all psychiatrists (91.2% in Switzerland) prescribe medications in association with psychotherapy. We refer later in this chapter to this important issue.

A psychiatrist's degree of information on theoretical issues runs in parallel with his explicit theoretical approach and with the nature of his

Table 19.2. Activities at the couple, family and group level, in percentages (several answers possible)

	Switzerland	Spain
Family, couple interviews	79.7	43.9
Family, couple analytic psychotherapy	38.8	15.2
Family, couple systemic therapy	47.2	14.1
Analytic group therapy	14.8	20.2
Other group therapies	17.4	12.1

practice. Thus, although most Swiss psychiatrists have fairly good information on psychoanalysis, those who declare themselves 'psychoanalysts' appear to be the most selective in their reading, concentrating principally on their specific field. Indeed, almost half of them (47.8%) regularly read psychiatric and psychotherapeutic periodicals, one-third of them (38.7%) read psychoanalysis journals, 16.3% read periodicals regarding family therapy, and 12.0% read child and adolescent psychiatric and psychotherapeutic periodicals. The comparison of information levels about the different theoretical orientations between Swiss and Spanish psychiatrists, in a way, reflects the differences in practices we noted. The latter are appreciably better informed in biology, group psychotherapy and in phenomenology.

The theoretical orientation of psychiatrists depends to a large extent on the kind of training they received during residency and the type of practice they then undertook. Dietz carried out a sociological study on the kind of treatments psychiatrists applied. Those psychiatrists using ECT had received less psychoanalytic training, treated patients of a lower socio-economic status, and used more drugs and less intensive psychotherapy. In Spain, we found a link between the place where psychiatrists work and the theoretical model to which they subscribe. The medical model is backed principally by psychiatrists working in hospitals and those working in centres for alcoholism and drug addiction. On the other hand, those working in community mental health centres are inclined towards the psychodynamic model. All this is, of course, of the utmost importance for the training of future psychiatrists and even for the education of generalists.

The Indications of a Psychodynamic Approach in Psychiatry

Some Limitations

Psychoanalysis detects disturbances different to those acknowledged by the patient. Frequently, in trying to cure these disturbances, painful consequences can result in the life of the patient. Moreover, it is evident that even our usually compliant patients have learned (as happens in every field) to become very demanding consumers of psychotherapy. Psychoanalysis is costly and frustrating. The realisation of its aims can be delayed over long periods of time. The patient seeks immediate results through more agreeable channels. The faith needed to travel along the difficult road with the analyst has been weakened by public controversy concerning the efficacy of psychoanalysis. However, if we study the proposed therapeutic alternatives, we shall see that they are, for the most part, based on psychoanalysis and have not been able to demonstrate better results.

As it has been discussed in this chapter, many psychoanalysts contend that analysing and not 'healing' is their main task, and that one should avoid a megalomaniac *furore curandis*. So, when speaking about treatment, we should restrict ourselves to referring to psychoanalytically oriented psychotherapies rather than to psychoanalysis.

The Problem of Indication

The IPA report cited above (Fonagy, 2000) illustrates the value of psychoanalysis through the review of 50 main research projects (some of them involving a variety of evaluation studies). Indeed, psychoanalysis has been shown to be associated with an improvement in the capacity for work, and can lead to a reduction in health care utilisation and in the use of psychotropic medication. Thus, the report concludes that they are cost beneficial, and perhaps even cost effective. In addition, analytically oriented group therapy has been shown to be even more cost beneficial. Estimates of the percent of patients benefiting clearly and significantly from treatment varies widely across studies, from 55% to 96% of patients.

It appears that 'completed' and more intensive psychoanalytic treatment tends to be associated with greater benefits than less intensive psychoanalytic psychotherapy, especially for more severe disturbances, although this superiority of psychoanalysis over psychotherapy sometimes only becomes apparent some years after the treatment has ended. In any case, such a superiority of psychoanalysis over psychotherapy is not maintained at long-term follow-up.

It appears that psychoanalysis may be an effective treatment for severe psychosomatic disorders and borderline symptomatology. Psychiatric symptom measures show bigger changes than personality or relationship measures. Younger children benefit more from psychoanalysis than older ones. On the other hand, however, non-psychoanalytic therapies are better for psychotic patients in terms of improved capacity for adaptation, and successful psychoanalytic treatment of severe personality disorder very often requires a combination of supportive and expressive techniques.

Behavioural disorders also respond less well to psychoanalysis than to cognitive behavioural techniques. Furthermore, psychoanalytic therapy at a 'sub-clinical dose'—and, of course, unduly practised—may have negative outcomes and yatrogenic effects.

Medication Compliance

Even when formal psychotherapy is not part of the treatment, dynamic principles are very useful in prescribing psychotropic agents, especially when facing non-compliance, a major factor in the failure of pharmacotherapy. Reluctance to take medication can arise as a consequence of negative attitudes resulting from side effects which are, unfortunately, frequent and sometimes very disturbing. However, it has been shown that 'placebo side effects' are also common, in the form of adverse symptoms that cannot be explained pharmacologically (Gutheil, 1982). These negative placebo effects derive frequently from characterological resistance in the patients. Van Putten et al. (1976) showed that an ego-syntonic sense of psychotic grandiosity was the most powerful discriminating factor that distinguished schizophrenic patients who did not comply from those who did. An excessive tendency to deny the illness is the cause of many other patients having strong resistance to pharmacotherapy. Some other patients do not conform with pharmacotherapy due to the existence of secondary gains that make them prefer illness to health. These patients may even 'cling to their symptoms' when treated, thus making medication fruitless. Still others reject medication so as not to admit that they are really mentally ill.

The prescribing of medication by a psychiatrist can activate unconscious parental transferences, which may lead the patient to poor compliance (Beitman et al, 1984; Busch et al., 1993). This is particularly true in the case of the so-called 'manipulative help-rejecters'. The psychiatrists then frequently insists, in an authoritarian way, thus increasing the patient's opposition. Some psychiatrists may even threaten to discharge the patients from treatment if they do not comply, or induce guilt feelings so that patients obey in order to avoid offending their doctor. Some psychiatrists may accept the interruption of the treatment just to show reluctant patients how ill they will get (Book, 1987). On the contrary, some psychotherapists may fail to prescribe a much-needed medication because they narcissistically fear this would bring into question the efficacy of their technique.

Combined psychopharmacology and psychotherapy treatments are becoming commonplace with both many advantages but some difficulties (Balon, 1999).

Information is not always enough to improve medication compliance, so a certain number of interventions have been designed (Ciancetta, 1983;

Pakes, 1979). Thus, in a controlled study on the evolution of schizophrenic patients admitted to a day hospital, we were able to show that the patients following a group medication programme showed better attitudes (Eguiluz et al, 1999), compliance and clinical evolution than a control group, apparently due to the fact that both cognitive and affective elements of prejudice towards medication were confronted (Guimón et al., 1993).

PSYCHOANALYSIS IN PSYCHIATRIC INSTITUTIONS

The good results obtained with some patients by long-term psychoanalysis in the treatment of neurotic and personality disorders on a outpatient basis has not been paralleled with severe psychotic patients treated on an inpatient basis. However, psychoanalytic thinking and personnel training remains an essential tool in institutions, both for the maintenance of a therapeutic milieu and for understanding and improving the work of the therapeutic teams.

Indeed, in this kind of setting, it is assumed that the staff should play the role of an *alter familia* that would provide the clients with a 'corrective emotional experience'. However, various difficulties can arise in the team, coming from real problems and from projective identifications that clients put on the staff members. Therapists feel frequently compelled to act transferentially, as if they were moved by the patients' projections. Tensions arise in the team while its members try to become an adequate "container", a 'loving therapeutic team', able to take on the needs of the clients and avoid having to assume the difficulties of the staff members. Post groups and different kinds of supervision in therapeutic communities and in educational communities (Tsegos, 1995) are of great help in avoiding severe emotional difficulties arising in these professionals.

On the other hand, psychoanalytically oriented group psychotherapy is a basic therapeutic tool in short-term and long-term hospitalisation units for psychiatric patients. The well-known experiences of therapeutic communities, today unduly neglected, are an example of its efficacy. We have reported on our experience with several controlled group programmes which have been underway since 1975 in Bilbao, Barcelona, and Geneva for severe psychiatric patients in short-term and long-term in- and outpatient clinics (Guimón, 2001a; Guimón, 2001b; Guimón, 2001c; Guimón et al., 1992). The results of the establishment of such programmes were positive both from a clinical and organisational point of view. A special ward atmosphere develops which is unlike that of other units run using different approaches.

IMPLICATIONS FOR PSYCHIATRIC TRAINING

The role of psychoanalysis in the future of psychiatry will depend largely on the training programmes available, due to the resident's identification with his or her teachers and with their ideology during this period (Guimón et al., 1998). Certain personality traits affecting the way an individual approaches life play an important role in the choice of specialisation in psychiatry. The personality profile of physicians choosing psychiatry is changing, and becoming more technically than humanistically oriented. If this trend continues, there will be, in the future, a host of competent psychoneuroendocrinologists but a dearth of good psychiatrists (Guimón, 1990; Guimón, 1998).

On the one hand, specialists have a marked tendency of identifying with those who trained them during their internships and to adopt their ideology. It is true that when the future psychiatrist begins his training, a great part of his identity—in which his professional definition as physician plays a not-so-negligible role—is already in place. However, the prolongation of his period of dependence with regard to his trainers maintains him in a sort of prolonged adolescence. In what Erikson (1960) calls 'psychosocial moratorium', he has to question his identity as a physician, to adapt to his new identity as psychiatrist. In this process, the cognitive information received and the construction of his personality through the contact with his role models and mentors, thanks to a more or less unconscious process of identification, play a fundamental role. Indeed, the therapeutic orientation and, in general, the ideology of the psychiatrist are built in part throughout his training, and become increasingly similar to those of his teachers.

The type of activities that take place during his training and practice, modify his ideology. The human being has a tendency to invent beliefs to explain his acts. This tendency would explain the adoption of different ideological attitudes according to the psychiatrist's type of activity. Thus, it is entirely normal that the usual electroshock practice in a closed institution does not have the same influence on the one who implements it as the use of psychoanalytical therapy in a private practice.

It is necessary, therefore, to consider that the institutional path and expected activities in the training programme of postgraduates is particularly important for shaping their identity as psychiatrists. Along these lines, Beitman has stressed the need to begin training with similar activities to those of the other physicians (e.g., liaison psychiatry), and then to put residents in contact with a great number of seriously ill mental patients in a short-stay unit (Beitman et al., 1984).

A 'Brief Intensive Group Analytic Programme', which we established in 1994, is running in two short-stay units of the Department of Psychiatry at Bilbao University Hospital (Guimón et al., 1985; Guimón et al., 1988). A parallel programme of 'Group Analytic Training in Blocks' was developed in Barcelona during this same periods, and in Geneva since 1994 (Guimón, 2001e; Guimón, 2001c; Guimón et al., 1995). More than 1000 professionals working in these units have undergone this kind of training. The effects of this 'didactic community' kind of training on personnel and on the units where they work has been explored through different questionnaires.

REFERENCES

Adams, S., and Pitre, N. (2000). Who uses bibliotherapy and why? *Canadian Journal of Psychiatry*, 45 (7), 645–649.

Alexander, F., & French, T. M. (1946). *Psychoanalytic therapy: Principles and application*. Lincoln, NE: University of Nebraska Press.

Azcúnaga, D., Sacanell, E., & Guimon, G. (1986). Perfil sociolaboral y actividades clinicas de los psiquiatras españoles: implicaciones para la formacion de los residentes en psiquiatria. *Psiquis*, *242*(86), 21–32.

Balint, M., Omstein, P., & Balint, E. (1972). *Focal psychotherapy*. London: Tavistock.

Balon, R. (1999) Positive aspects of collaborative treatment, 1–31, In M.B. Riba and R. Balon (Eds). *Psychopharmacology and psychotherapy. A collaborative approach*. Washington DC, London: American Psychiatric Press, Inc.

Beitman, B. B., Chiles, J., and Carlin, A. The pharmacotherapy-psychotherapy triangles: psychiatrist, nonmedical psychotherapist, and patient. *Journal of Clinical Psychiatry* 45: 458–459, 1984.

Beitman, B. D., and Maxim, P. (1984). A survey of psychiatric practice: Implications for psychiatric training. *Journal of Psychiatric Education*, 8, 149–153

Book, H. E. (1987). Some psychodynamics of non-compliance. *Canadian Journal Of Psychiatry. Revue Canadienne De Psychiatrie*, 32, 115–117.

Busch, F. N., and Gould, E. Treatment by a psychotherapist and a psychopharmacologist: transference and countertransference issues. *Hospital Community Psychiatry* 44: 772–774, 1993.

Ciancetta, M. D. (1983). Individual vs group medication review programs for chronic Psychiatry patients. *Dissertation Abstracts*, B-44(2).

Davanloo, H. (Ed.). (1980). *Short-term dynamic psychotherapy*. New York: Aronson.

Durkin, H. E. (1975). The development of systems theory and its implications for the theory and practice. In L.R. Wolberg and M.L. Aronson (Eds.), *Group therapy* (pp. 8–20). New York: Stratton International.

Eguiluz, I., González Torres, M. A., and Guimón, J. (1999). Psychoeducational groups in schizophrenic patients. In J. Guimón, W. Fischer, and N. Sartorius (Eds.): *The image of madness* (pp. 208–215). Basel: Karger.

Erikson, E. H. (1960). The problem of Ego identity. In M. Stein, A. H. Vidich, and D. M. White (Eds.), *Identity and anxiety*. New York: The Free Press.

Ferenczi, S. (1967). *Teoría y técnica del psicoanálisis*. Buenos Aires: Paidós.

Fonagy, P. (2000). An open door review of outcome studies in psychoanalysis (www.ipa.org.uk/research/complete.htm). London: IPA.

Freud, S. (1918). Los caminos de la terapia analítica. In S. Freud (Ed.), *Obras Completas* (Vol. 2., pp. 449–453). Madrid: Biblioteca Nueva.

Greenberg, J., & Mitchell, S. (1983). *Object Relations i Psychoanalytic Theory*. Cambridge: Harvard University Press
Guimón, J., Ayerra, J. M., Sunyer, M., Ylla, L., et al. (1985). La formación en psicoterapia de grupo en Bilbao: descripción de una experiencia de 11 años. *Revista de Psicología General y Aplicada*, 40 (4), 811–820.
Guimón, J., Azcunaga, D., & Sacanell, E. (1987). Orientacion teórica de los psiquiatras espanoles. *Actas Luso-Espanolas de Neurologia, Psiquiatria y Ciencias Afines, XV*(2), 173–183.
Guimón, J., Gonzalez-Pinto, A., Sanz, C., and Gonzalez-Ceinos, M. (1988). Efectos terapéuticos en un programa de sensibilizacion grupal. *Psiquis*, 1, 11–28.
Guimón, J. (1990). *Psiquiatras: De brujos a burócratas*. Barcelona: Salvat Editores.
Guimón, J., Sunyer, M., Sanchez de Vega, J., and Trojaola, B. (1992). Group analysis and ward atmosphere. In F. P. Ferrero, A. E. Haynal, and N. Sartorius (Eds.), *Schizophrenia and affective psychoses*. Nosology in contemporary psychiatry (pp. 157–166). John Libbey CIC.
Guimón, J., Eguiluz, I., Bulbena, A. (1993). Group pharmacotherapy in schizophrenics: Attitudinal and clinical changes. *European Journal of Psychiatry* 7: 147–154.
Guimón, J. (1995). The use of group programs to improve medication compliance in patients with chronic diseases. *Patient Educ. Couns.* 26: 189–193.
Guimón, J., Fischer, W., Zbinden, E., Steiner-Konig, U., et al. (1995). Postgraduate psychiatric education in Switzerland: Elements for the building of a new programme. Paper presented at a symposium of the Assemblée Européenne de Psychiatrie, Strasbourg.
Guimón, J., Fischer, W., Goerg, D., Zbinden, E. (1997a). Orientations théoriques des psychiatres suisses. *Ann. Méd. Psychol.* 155, 3: 184–201.
Guimón, J., Fischer, W., Zbinden, E., and Goerg, D. (1997b). Consequences of recent changes in research and practice for the identity of psychiatrist. *European Psychiatry*, 12 (suppl. 2), 92s–98s.
Guimón, J., Fischer, W., Zbinden, E., and Goerg, D. (1998a). Therapeutic practice profiles, work settings and activities of Swiss psychiatrists. *Schweiz Arch. Neurol. Psychiatr.* 149.1: 29–39.
Guimón, J., Fischer, W., Zbinden, E., and Goerg, D. (1998b). Therapeutic practice profiles, theoretical models and representations of the psychiatry of Swiss psychiatrists. *Schweiz Arch. Neurol. Psychiatr.* 149.1: 41–50.
Guimón, J. (1998). *La profession de psychiatre. Evolution et devenir*. Paris: Masson.
Guimón, J., Fischer, W., Goerg, D., Zbinden, E. (1999). Use and misuse of pharmacological substances: The question of noncompliance. In J. Guimón, W. Fischer, and N. Sartorius (Eds.): *The image of madness* (pp. 143–151). Basel: Karger.
Guimón, J. (2001a). *Introduction aux thérapies de groupe*. Paris: Masson.
Guimón, J. (2001b). *Psiquiatría comunitaria*. Madrid: Core Academic.
Guimón, J. (2001c). *Salud mental relacional. Concepto, etiología y diagnóstico* (Vol. 1). Madrid: Core Academic.
Guimón, J. (2001d). Scope and limitations of psychonalysis in clinical psychiatry. In J. Guimón, J. (2001e). Training general practitioners in the psychoanalytical aspects of mental health. In J. Guimón and S. Zac de Filc (Eds *Challenges of psychoanalysis in the 21st century* (pp. 101–111). New York: Kluwer Academic.
Gutheil, T. (1982). The psychology of psychopharmacology. *Bulletin Of The Menninger Clinic, 46*, 321–330.
Malan, D. H. (1975). *La psychothérapie brève*. Paris: Payot.
Kohut, H., & Wolf, E. S. (1978). The disorders of the self and their treatment: an outline. *International Journal Of Psycho-Analysis, 59*, 413–425.
Milton, J. (2001). Psychoanalysis and cognitive behaviour therapy—rival paradigms or common ground? *International Journal of Psychoanalis*, 82(3), 431–447.

Pakes, G. E. (1979). Group medication counseling conducted by a pharmacist for severely disturbed clients. *Hospital Community Psychiatry*, 30 (4), 237–238.

Sifneos, P. (1977). *Psychothérapie brève et crise émotionnelle*. Bruxelles: Mardaga.

Tsegos, I. K. (1995). Further thoughts on group-analytic training. *Group Analysis*, 28 (3), 313–326.

Van Putten, T., and May, P. R. A. (1976). Milieu therapies of the schizophrenias. In L. J. Wets and D. E. Flinn (Eds.), *Treatment of schizophrenia: Progress and prospect* (pp. 217–243). New York: Grune and Stratton.

20

Group Therapy

FROM THE COUCH TO THE CIRCLE: HISTORICAL ASPECTS OF GROUP DYNAMIC PSYCHOTHERAPY

Techniques for use in groups have modified the traditional dyad relationship of psychiatric treatment. In recent decades, psychotherapists have had to take an interest not only in intrapsychic phenomena, but also in the phenomena arising out of groups and their interaction.

Freudian Concepts Regarding Groups and Institutions

Freud mainly expressed his concepts on the group in his books *Totem and Taboo* (Freud, 1913) and *Group Psychology and Analysis of the Ego* (1922). The ideas that he presented therein are clearly related to those of several of his contemporaries. Thus, Le Bon (1896) described certain precise phenomena arising in crowds: decrease in conscious states and outburst of unconscious phenomena, and massive contagion of affect among individual members of the crowd. McDougall (1920) referred to 'disorganised' and 'organised' masses of people, the latter being characterised by the existence of a common goal and convergent affects. Crocter (1921) pointed out the existence, in the individual, of a 'gregarious instinct' that he defined as a natural tendency to join groups. These are ideas that were taken up later by authors related to the British school of psychoanalysis, also known as the 'object relations' approach school.

Freud established psychoanalytical technique as a verbal process to resolve unconscious conflicts through the analysis of transference created between two persons. Psychoanalysis carefully distanced itself from methods of suggestion (Freud, 1918) but by the 1950s they had been forced to recognise that other specific techniques, such as those derived from behaviourism, had a place in psychotherapy. On the other hand, psychoanalysis had to make room for the many new categories of psychoanalytical psychotherapy, practised individually or in groups.

It became obvious that the group does not offer the ideal setting for analysis because of multiple cases of transference, the impossibility of practising free association, and a number of other factors. However, since the early 1930s a strong analytical group psychotherapy has developed, based on different theoretical approaches (object relations, the psychology of the ego, and self psychology) and techniques (e.g., Tavistock groups and group analysis).

The Group Context in the Development of Psychoanalytically Oriented Psychotherapy

It was only at the end of the 1920s that Tringant Burrow (Burrow, 1927) became interested in the application of individual psychoanalysis to small groups (Campos, 1998). During the same period, group psychotherapy benefited from the support of distinguished psychiatrists, such as Paul Schilder (Schilder, 1936). Impressed by the effects of unstructured discussion on the conflicts of seriously ill patients at Bellevue Hospital in New York, Schilder decided to start up a similar programme with small groups of patients suffering from neuroses. He favoured the interaction among the groups' members, who were considered to be the elements of one sole 'body', a concept similar to that which would be developed by Foulkes, under the influence (just as Schilder was) of the 'holistic' outlook of Kurt Goldstein (Goldstein, 1939) regarding brain function. He maintained a strict attitude of neutrality, and analysed transference and resistance according to classical psychoanalytical methods.

Wender (1940) noticed that, during his hospital visits, patients' replies were more often appropriate when he had an open and frank discussion with them about their psychodynamic problems. Encouraged by this observation, he began to organise therapeutic groups. Adler, for his part, stressed the importance of a social atmosphere of equality and mutual support that should reign in groups and insisted on the fundamental importance of these aspects in the therapeutic process.

Several experiences during the period between the World Wars showed that certain group techniques, as well as more global intervention in certain institutions, could be very effective, as we shall discuss further in chapter 21.

THEORETICAL CONSTRUCTS ON WHICH GROUP PSYCHOTHERAPY IS BASED

Bion and Foulkes

Bion (1959), who had been analysed by Melanie Klein, proposed some very original ideas based on his experiences in the recruitment units of the British army. Bion established an analogy between the relationship of the child with the mother and that of the 'group as a whole' with the leader. He considered that the emotional situation of the group showed a regression to the first steps in development of the ego (schizo-paranoid and depressive positions—Klein, 1946—), with a reactivation of psychotic anxiety and of primitive defences (projective identification and splitting) against them, characteristic of childhood development in accordance with Kleinian theories. He identified what he called 'the group mind' (functional unit of members of a group arriving at a determined goal, whether consciously or unconsciously) of the 'group culture' (the sum of the group's mind and the individual feelings of each of its members).

Bion distinguished between two different phases in the evolution of groups. In the first stage, the group functions according to the 'basic assumptions', that is to say, the primitive emotions that are always present in each individual and in each group: 'dependency', especially with regard to the therapist, considered as the provider and nurturer of all that is good; paranoid tendencies of 'fight/flight' towards internal or external enemies; and 'pairing' tendencies directed at the therapist or another member of the group. In the fantasy, the fruit of this union can give birth to a 'Messiah' who resolves all difficulties. A second stage is that of 'group work': in this stage, the attainment of an outcome or a goal dominates the group mentality and, in the case of therapeutic groups, it is finding a cure. Conscious co-operation among group members favours its realisation and 'valence', an instinctive process that is opposed to it and complicates it.

Bion called this interpretation the 'new idea'. He believed that the interpretation may then lead the 'basic assumptions group' to evolve into a 'work group'. Faced with the new idea, the group reacts by particular movements (changing the leader, changing its basic position, 'aberrant' reactions, and 'catastrophic' reactions). It considers the person who brings the new idea (or Messiah) to be a 'genius' or 'mystic'.

With regard to the techniques of the group itself, it must be noted that Bion only treated groups from 1947 to 1949. He did not write systematically on group therapy, and his approach was only implemented, after major modifications. It was Henry Ezriel (Ezriel, 1966) who, at the

Tavistock Clinic, contributed the most to the development of the method of 'group psychoanalysis'. However, Malan et al. (1976) only obtained meagre clinical results for such groups, and even if these methods are still in use at the Tavistock Clinic and the Scottish Institutes of Human Relations, it is mainly to train organisation administrators who must frequently face primitive group processes.

During the Second World War, Bion and Foulkes at Northfield Military Hospital and Maswell Jones (Jones, 1952) at the Mill Neurosis Centre organised some experiences that were eventually dubbed 'therapeutic communities', and which we shall discuss in chapter 21.

Foulkes described 'group analysis' as the self-analysis of the group by its members and its leader (Foulkes, 1946a, 1946b, 1948, 1963, 1964). His theoretical foundations (based on neurophysiology, psychoanalysis, medicine, neurology, psychiatry, gestalt psychology, and sociology) have not yet been well developed (Roberts, 1995), even if significant work has been accomplished by authors such as Malcolm Pines (Pines, 1976) and Brown and Zimnkins (Brown et al., 1994). Foulkes' most original theory was that of the 'group matrix': it presupposes that an individual mind might not exist and is in fact an illusory consequence derived from the dialogue between two or more members of a group. In the case of a person alone, the participants in the dialogue would have been interiorised. For Foulkes, mental illness comes from a perturbation in communication and an excessive attachment to the family; these difficulties are further reinforced in the different groups the subject belongs to during his or her life; the result is that therapy for adults is better undertaken in a group ('reticular theory of neurosis'). In interpreting group phenomena, all kinds of communication (whether a word or a gesture) must be taken into account, and any kind of communication coming from a single individual represents, in a certain manner, communication with the group as a whole. Although mainly used for neurotic patients, his techniques were also employed at the Institute of Psychiatry, and later throughout Europe, with psychotic patients.

After the Second World War, we witnessed a veritable explosion in group psychotherapy. Indeed, some psychiatrists in the United Kingdom–e.g., the Tavistock Clinic (Rees et al., 1955), the Cassel Hospital (Main, 1946), and he resettlement units–and in the United States–including the Menninger Clinic (Menninger, 1939) and the Group for the Development of Psychiatry (Menninger, 1939)—felt the need to break out of their traditional isolation from the public, by adapting the group experiences acquired during the war to the needs of daily practice (see chapter 21).

Dorothy Stock-Whitaker (Stock-Whitaker, 1992) and Morton Lieberman (Lieberman et al., 1968; Lieberman et al., 1996) proposed that the group process be viewed as a collection of foreseeable phenomena which could form the basis of a rigorous therapeutic method. This description of group phenomena, and the technique emerging from it, present a great resemblance to those developed by Ezriel (Roberts, 1995).

Bion's theories on the regressive phenomena in small groups were extended to the study of group processes, to the definition of the role of a leader, and to the authority and structure of major social organisations. A 'systemic' approach to analysing organisations was developed. Kernberg (1978b, 1979) applied these contributions by integrating object relations into the understanding of hospitals' organisational problems.

In Italy, Franco Basaglia, at Gorizia Hospital, criticised the concept of community therapy by proposing a programme of treatment based on large groups ('community meetings') with all patients in the hospital followed by meetings of personnel and leaders, with the objective of exchanging ideas about the preceding session. His experience led him to radically contest the role of the psychiatrist and psychiatric hospitals in mental health (Basaglia, 1970).

In France (Chanoit, 1995), the Centre for Treatment and Social Readaptation of the City of Evrard (Sivadon et al., 1963), the 13th Arrondissement of Paris (Diatkine, 1958; Lebovici, 1953; Racamier, 1979), and the Delaborde Clinic (Jeanoury, 1976) developed new therapeutic approaches with an orientation that was both sociological and psychoanalytical, which was called 'institutional psychotherapy' (Tosquelles, 1995).

On the psychoanalytical side, the movement towards institutional psychotherapy was enriched by the contributions of different authors, falling into three basic tendencies (Chanoit, 1995): psychoanalysts, who tried to apply analysis to the group situation (Di Nardo et al., 1983; Lebovici, 1953; Diatkine, 1958), such as Danon and Boileau (Kestemberg et al., 1964); psychiatrists, who tried to understand psychoses through psychoanalysis (Chaigneau et al., 1997), including Garabé and Racamier; and psychotherapists, who tried to define mental illness and social alienation (e.g., Tosquelles and Orury). These authors were interested in the analysis and interpretation of transference to the whole of the personnel in the hospital, which develops in a way differentiated from dual transference.

A law based on the general population rather than on institutions was enacted in France in 1985 concerning sectorisation, in order to ensure the continuity of care in various settings over different periods of time. This strategy for the continuity of care enables the same team to follow up the patient at the hospital and also in outpatient care, and favours a better and more dynamic care programme.

Over the past 30 years, whether using the more social approach of the British or the more dynamic one of the French and Americans, many traditional psychiatric hospitals and halfway structures (e.g., day hospitals, protected housing, and workshops) more or less adopted this philosophy, although they modified it, taking out the 'punch'—especially insofar as psychoanalytical elements were concerned. The idea of a therapeutic community was adopted by residential and day units, assisted by social services and volunteers who, as they did not have the necessary training, contributed to the model's loss of credibility (Roberts, 1995).

With the dramatic shortening of hospitalisations of mental patients (schizophrenics included) in the last decades, the usefulness of milieu therapy has been contested. However, in the United States and some other Western countries, therapeutic communities ideas have inspired the organisation of many day hospitals and some short-stay units.

For our part, as we said, over the past 20 years we have developed a number of group programmes involving many psychiatric units with an orientation towards community therapy, in a dozen different care units (short-stay units in general hospitals, rehabilitation units, and day hospitals) in Spain and in Switzerland (Guimón, 1998). The programmes include, as a minimum, a daily group of 'medium size', bringing together patients and staff, and a 'small' group of patients, with a dynamic orientation, but with occasional cognitive-behavioural tendencies, as well as group activities ('group work', in Foulkes's sense). From a clinical point of view, these programmes' results have been very positive. The patients' setting/group is the key element, from the standpoint of its creation of a 'home' in the consulting room and through the information it provides to patients. The other groups also give the patient orientation and emotional support. All this has enabled us to decrease the dosages of medication required and to create an agreeable atmosphere in the sessions, as well as lowered the number of incidents (e.g., aggression, suicide attempts, runaways). The tensions in the therapeutic team have eased. These different groups constitute a network for group analysis, which is favourable to the harmonious communication between the different services. This systemic vision of the institution is conducive to easier, quicker detection of problems and conflicts inside the institution. All of these elements furnish the input which feeds 'healthy precursor paranoia' (Kernberg, 1978a), which is so indispensable to managing these organisations.

GROUPS WITH PATIENTS IN ACUTE EPISODES

In most Western countries today, schizophrenic patients tend to be admitted to the psychiatric units of general hospitals. The trend towards shorter stays has encouraged the use of biological rather than psychodynamic treatments in these units. In order to minimise this bias, group-analytical programmes have been established at some short-stay units. In one of our studies, the results of the programme organised at Bilbao University Hospital over the last 17 years were viewed as positive from a clinical standpoint (Guimón et al., 1983). We believe that these positive effects were the result of the atmosphere created in the wards.

Staff Group

This group meets for half an hour early in the morning, from Monday to Friday, with all available personnel attending. The goals are to gather and share information on the evolution of the patients and problems arising in the ward since the last meeting. Interpersonal problems among the members of the staff are also occasionally taken up. This makes for a better understanding of the ward atmosphere, and a more comprehensive approach to the patient. Interpersonal difficulties and interprofessional competitiveness are often dealt with under the guise of theoretical disagreement, and become manifest at times in the form of lateness, absence or rationalisations.

Staff-Patient Group

This group's meetings are held early in the morning during the week, for periods of 45 minutes. All patients are urged to attend, and do so unless exceptional circumstances intervene. The sessions are conducted by a skilled group analyst. Approximately 40 chairs are arranged in a circle with the conductor seated always in the same position. Most of the personnel attend, and usually sit close to the more disturbed patients. The goals of this 'quick medium-size open group' are to facilitate the integration of the incoming patients to this new environment, the discussion of the situation of the outgoing patients, and to encourage the patients' active involvement in their therapeutic plans. Although a psychoanalytic reading of the communication is, of course, undertaken later by the staff, the interventions are carried out in a psycho-educational vein.

The conductor actively encourages each patient to participate in an open discussion. Patients are asked to talk about the tensions and conflicts arising among themselves and with the staff. Attempts are also made to show them how these reactions are often distorted by the psychopathology itself. They are invited to talk about their general condition, contrasting their assertions with those of the other patients. They share objective and subjective feelings about their symptoms. The therapist in charge conducts the group bearing in mind some ubiquitous topics: reluctance to take medication, side effects, unawareness of the illness, fears of being discharged, and so on.

Suggestions, protests and the patient's initiatives are worked out through structuring the group by giving the members responsibilities. Thus, once a week, the meeting takes the form of an administrative session, in which a president and a secretary of the assembly is elected by the patients from among themselves, and in which a plan of activities (plays, mural work, etc.) is organised. All of this contributes to the development of the healthy and creative aspects of the patient that otherwise would go unnoticed.

With this group, we try to guide the patient all along from the abstract to the actual, from the delusional to the real. We foster communication and interpersonal relationships. We try to integrate patients into an atmosphere that provides information concerning the many aspects of their lives, family, and friends. The presence of staff members in these groups enables the patients to have a closer relationship with them. This dispels persecutory feelings and resolves conflict that would otherwise persist. This environment fosters the transparency and directness of both patients and the therapeutic team. Resistance arising in the patients, such as fears of criticising others or being punished, tends to disappear soon. Irregular attendance on the part of the doctors arises during certain periods, under the pretext of overwork, but in reality reflecting a devaluation of the group approach, which can spread to the test of the team. This generally depends on the attitude of the ward leader towards group or milieu therapy. On the other hand, excessive nursing staff rotation results in sporadic attendance and a lack of commitment to the group. This is often fomented by the institution itself, which is reluctant to have its auxiliary personnel involved in these kinds of 'specialised' activities.

These problems are best worked out through the participation of the staff in the postgroup meeting created for this purpose. This meeting is, besides, a valuable means of sharing information about the patients.

Short-term Group Psychotherapy

In units for short-term hospitalisation, where the goal is to improve communication, patients who have kept their verbal ability and who are neither too regressive nor too agitated are integrated into a small group that meets five times a week, for one hour. This is called a 'verbal' session, and the leaders are very active. Certain leaders, in accordance with Yalom's precepts, put 'game' or 'go-around' techniques into play.

The leader encourages patients to take advantage of these sessions to voice their preoccupations and vent their frustrations and complaints, constantly stimulating verbal communication. This type of intervention commonly suits the state and characteristics of the personality type that, most often, is dominant in this kind of patient: oral gratification (often devouring and destructive), hostility (either passively self-directed and/or destructive to others), having major deficits insofar as defence of the ego is concerned, as well as problems in adaptation, refusal and/or flight when faced with reality.

We give patients a psychopedagogical understanding of the meaning of symptoms and their relationship to situations in real life. One of the principal objectives is to render the patient sensitive to the possibility of change, so that he might decide to engage in psychotherapeutic treatment after discharge.

Others (such as those in Bilbao), even if initially implementing this type of approach, have evolved towards more open meetings, by instigating conversations whose focus tends toward the usual, recurring themes in these groups (circumstances that resulted in destabilisation, problems caused by hospitalisation, the effects of medication, etc.).

Short-term Group Work

In short-term hospitalisation units, a type of group is organised that is informal in its atmosphere, intended to keep up psychomotor activities in patients, and promoting the possibilities of improving orientation and interaction with different members of the group. Patients suffering from severe mental disorganisation, incapable of maintaining a sufficient attention span, for which the 'verbal' groups described above are not suitable, take part five times a week, for one hour, in what Yalom (1983) termed a 'low group' and which we call a 'focus' or 'structuring' group. In this group are to be found patients who are not co-operative, hallucinating psychotics, patients suffering from delirium and in severe regressive states, or patients who, while not being psychotic, are too anxious or phobic to take part in groups at a higher level.

The session is organised, according to Yalom's method, into four stages: 1) orientation, lasting 2–5 minutes, during which the therapists introduce themselves, explain what the group is, its utility to patients, and so on; 2) a 5–10 minute warm-up, including several structured exercises, such as simple games and comments on participants (physical and mental states, feelings), in accordance with the group's situation in each session; 3) a 20–30 minute session of one or two structured activities, chosen in accordance with the group's daily needs, including sentences to complete, lists of values, and exercises intended to increase empathy; and 4) a review of the session with a quick conclusion covering the activities carried out.

We allow patients who take part in these groups to leave them when they wish, as the atmosphere of the session must be reassuring and show empathy for the patient. The therapist must focus his or her activities on helping patients, and help them to identify their problems, promoting relationships among them, and decreasing levels of anxiety, centring all the activity on the 'here and now'.

Patients who take part in this group sometimes perceive negatively the differences between it and the 'verbal' group. In our unit, we prefer to introduce patients into the different groups, not based on any diagnostic criterion, but with regard to their ability to communicate at the moment of their arrival. This explains the existence of heterogeneous groups at diagnosis level, but relatively homogenous ones insofar as the possibility of establishing relationships with others is concerned. Obviously, as we have already said, interventions do not address unconscious conflicts, but problems in daily life (Guimón, 2001).

Medication Information Group

There are three major factors that influence negative attitudes towards psychotropics, especially neuroleptics: the cognitive element, the affective element, and the behavioural element. It is obvious that public awareness campaigns on the indications of these products, and the precautions to take against possible drug interaction and side effects, could help decrease bias, which is especially important for persons coming from more modest cultural and educational backgrounds. However we are more pessimistic regarding the possibility of influencing the other aspects, based on affective elements, which are often unconscious and very difficult to change. It is useful, in this context, to recall that a campaign aimed at the general public in an American city, waged through various media, failed after several months to improve the population's attitudes in any appreciable manner. Rather, it wound up annoying the very people it was meant to influence. Attempts at modifying attitudes with regard to psychopharmacological substances require, in addition to public educational programmes, campaigns directed at specific target populations, for instance the physicians who prescribe these drugs and the patients who take them, and their families.

A programme intended to modify the negative attitudes of schizophrenic patients and their families towards medication has been ongoing since 1987 at the Bilbao City Hospital (Eguiluz et al., 1999). Patients took part in eight groups and families in two groups, lasting 90 minutes each. The first 45 minutes are given over to a theoretical explanation of schizophrenia as an illness, as well as information about neuroleptics and their collateral effects. The second part of the session is focused on an open discussion. Participating patients have shown better compliance and fewer hospitalisations than others who did not take part in this programme. These kinds of groups are also employed, with some modifications, in the management of chronic schizophrenic patients.

Multifamily Groups

Experiences in extended groups (more than 40 members and sometimes up to several hundred members) are not easy to manage (Roberts, 1995), but can constitute a strong incentive for personal and social change. The extended group, as described and implemented by Kreeger (1975), De Mare (1983, 1992) or Ayerra (1997), provides what initially would seem to be a disagreeable experience, allowing participants to experiment with 'psychotic' symptoms, primal defence mechanisms, and insight into the political process (Roberts, 1995) through which a veritable microcosm of life outside the family circle can be created. For more than 20 years, we have included groups of this type in our seminars on block group training, and Ayerra periodically organises, with the OMIE Foundation, specific seminars on extended groups, which are remarkably useful for those working with schizophrenics to have a first-hand experience of 'psychotic' feelings.

The objective of these groups is to provide support to families, by offering a 'disagreement' and a differentiated interpretation of the phenomena experienced in the family circle. They began as 'psychopedagogical groups' and were transformed little by little into groups that are 'evolving through open discussion'. The multifamily group tries to overcome resistance arising not only from the patient, but from the families themselves, who can find common ground with other families going through the same difficulties and identify with their ongoing struggle.

In the experiences of Garcia Badaracco (1990) and Ayerra, families take part with patients and professionals in groups made up of 30 to 35 people. The sessions last 90 minutes, and are held on a weekly basis. The therapeutic attitude is based on the idea of a 'disagreement' which explains the presence of several members of the team who sit at strategic locations, next to those patients or their families who are undergoing the most delicate situations. In the same way, as usual, patients choose to sit in 'protected' locations, according to their state, very often next to the group's therapists. In this group, hallucinations arising from the subconscious or from transference are not interpreted although, in contrast, anxieties, subconscious desires and defence mechanisms are mentioned. Behaviours and interpersonal relationships are analysed in an attempt to highlight the positive aspects, the affective compulsions, and deep-seated needs which are often hidden beneath each conflict. It is a question of helping patients to find the path that lies between the rational and the irrational and to go beyond it, to the emotional stage. Confronted with the most primal anxieties, the response takes the form of a more intensive investment and greater self-control. Prolonged silence is counter-productive. One characteristic of the therapeutic team of the group is the spontaneity of its intervention, its renunciation of omnipotence and absolute knowledge by preferring to appear simply as fellow beings, furnishing daily examples intended to promote trust. The members of the group become co-therapists, treating aspects that they have slowly succeeded in resolving. The presence of families who have had positive experiences of this process is invaluable: they can guide others, giving them hope.

The multifamily group is also useful when important decisions must be made (hospitalisation, a possibly ill-considered and premature choice to leave the hospital too early, changes in therapeutic projects), and to help to prevent legal difficulties. Little by little, the group becomes more homogeneous, and we progressively leave behind the dissociated pedagogical group (families/patients, the sick and the healthy, people who are knowledgeable and those who are uninformed). We start to recognise that the same problems can be encountered for children and for families. In couples, conflictual situations start to appear. With the understanding that all the members are in the same predicament, have similar experiences, and that no one can manage to save themselves without help, acceptance crystallises around the fact that this principle also applies to institutions and to society.

Garcia Badaracco (1990) developed these groups to act as an exceptionally useful instrument in treating patients with schizophrenia and other serious illnesses within the context of their 'multifamily, psychoanalytical therapeutic community'. He also, additionally, records on videotape multiple therapy sessions of this type, which have a great value not only for teaching but also for research.

REFERENCES

Ayerra, J. M. (1997). Grupo grande. *Boleíin*, 7 (28–46).
Basaglia, F. (1970). *L'institution en négation*. Paris: Edition du Seuil.
Bion, W. (1959). *Experiences in groups and other papers*. New York: Basic Books.
Brown, D., and Zinkin, L. (1994). *The psyche and the social world*. London: Routledge.
Burrow, T. (1927). The group method of analysis. *Psychoanalytic Review*, 10, 268–280.
Campos, J. (1998). *Una historia de la AIPG: hechos y hallazgos*. Barcelone: Gràfiques MAES.
Chaigneau, H., Chanoit, P., and Garrabe, J. (1997). *Les thérapies institutionnelles*. Paris: Masson.
Chanoit, P. S. (1995). *La psychothérapie institutionnelle*. Paris: Presses Universitaires de France.

De Mare, P. (1983). Michael Foulkes and the Northfield Experiment. In M. Pines (Ed.), *The Evolution of Group Analysis*. London: Routledge.
Di Nardo, P. A., O'Brien, G. T., Barlow, D. H., Waddell, M. T., et al. (1983). Reliability of DMS-III anxiety disorder categories using a new structured interview. *Archives of General Psychiatry*, 40 (10), 1070–1074.
Diatkine, R. (1958). Activité de psychothérapie de groupe et de psychodrame. *Group psychotherapy, psychodrama and sociotherapy*, 11, 187–188.
Eguiluz, I., González Torres, M. A., and Guimón, J. (1999). Psychoeducational groups in schizophrenic patients. In J. Guimón, W. Fischer, and N. Sartorius (Eds.), *The image of madness*. Basel: Karger.
Ezriel, H. (1966). Le rôle du transfert dans le traitement psychanalytique de groupe, *Pratique de la psychothérapie de groupe*. Paris.
Foulkes, S. H. (1946a). On group-analysis. *International Journal of Psycho-Analysis*, 27 (46–51).
Foulkes, S. H. (1946b). Principles and practice of group therapy. *Bulletin of the Menninger Clinic*, 10, 85–89.
Foulkes, S. H. (1948). *Introduction to group-analytic psychotherapy*. London: W. Heinemann.
Foulkes, S. H. (1963). Psychotherapy and group psychotherapy. In A. L. Kadis, J. D. Krasner, C. Winick and S. H. Foulkes (Eds.), *A practicum of group psychotherapy*. New York: Harper and Row.
Foulkes, S. H. (1964). *Therapeutic group analysis*. Wheaton and Co.
Freud, S. (1913). *Totem und Tabu* (G-W IX, translated into French, 1947 ed.). Paris: Payot.
Freud, S. (1918). Los caminos de la terapia analítica. In S. Freud (Ed.), *Obras Completas* (Vol. 2, pp. 449–453). Madrid: Biblioteca Nueva.
Freud, S. (1922). *Group Psychology and Analysis of the Ego*. London: International Psychoanalytic Press.
García Badaracco, J. E. (1990). *Comunidad terapeutica psicoanalítica de estructura multifamiliar*. Madrid: Tecnipublicaciones.
Goldstein, K. (1939). *The organism: A holistic approach to biology*. New York: American Book Company.
Guimón, J., Sunyer, M., Sanchez de Vega, J., & Trojaola, B. (1992). Group analysis and ward atmosphere. In F. P. Ferrero & A. E. Haynal & N. Sartorius (Eds.), *Schizophrenia and affective psychoses. Nosology in contemporary psychiatry*: John Libbey CIC.
Guimón, J. (1998). Thérapie groupale dynamique intensive et brève. *Psychothérapies*, 18 (1), 15–21.
Guimón, J., Luna, D., Totorika, K., Diez, L., et al. (1983). Group psychotherapy as a basic therapeutic resource in psychiatric community care from the general hospital. In J. J. López Ibor and J. M. López Ibor (Eds.), *General hospital psychiatry*. Amsterdam: Excerpta Medica.
Guimón, J. (2001). *Introduction à la psychothérapie de groupe*. Paris: Mason.
Jones, M. S. (1952). *Social psychiatry: A study of therapeutic communities*. London: Tavistock Publications.
Kernberg, O. (1978a). Leadership and organizational functioning: Organizational regression. *International Journal of Group Psychotherapy*, 27, 3–25.
Kernberg, O. (1978b). Leadership and organizational functioning: organizational regression. *International Journal of Group psychotherapy*, 28, 3–25.
Kernberg, O. (1979). Regression in organizational leadership. *Psychiatry*, 42, 24–39.
Kestemberg, J., and Decobert, S. (1964). Approche psychanalytique pour la compréhension de la dynamique des groupes thérapeutiques. *Revue Française de Psychanalyse*, 28, 393–418.
Klein, M. (1946). Notes on some schizoid mechanisms. *The writings of Melanie Klein* (Vol. 1). London: Hogarth Press.

Kreeger, L. (Ed.). (1975). *The large group. Dynamics and therapy*. London: Constable and Company Limited.
Le Bon, G. (1896). *Psychologie des foules*. Paris: PUF 1990.
Lebovici, S. (1953). A propos de la psychanalyse de groupe. *Revue Française de Psychanalyse*, 17, 266–268.
Lieberman, M. A., Lakin, M. E., and Whitaker, D. S. (1968). The group as a unique context for therapy. *Psychotherapy: Theory, Research and Practice*, 5, 29–36.
Lieberman, M. A., and Yalom, I. (1996). Brief group psychotherapy for the spousally bereaved: A controlled study. *International Journal of Group Psychotherapy*, 42 (1), 117–133.
Main, T. F. (1946). The hospital as a therapeutic institution. *Bulletin of the Menninger Clinic*, 10 (66–70).
Malan, D. (1976). Group psychotherapy: A long-term follow-up study. *Archives of General Psychiatry*, 33, 1303–1315.
McDougall, W. (1920). *The group mind*. New York: G.P. Putnam.
Menninger, W. (1939). Psychoanalytic principles in psychiatric hospital therapy. *Southern Medical Journal*, 32, 354–384.
Menninger, W. C. (1942). Experiments and educational treatment in a psychiatric institution. *Bulletin of the Menninger Clinic*, 6, 38–45.
Oury, J. (1976). *Psychiatrie et psychothérapie institutionnelle*. Paris: Payot.
Pines, M. (1976). *The evolution of group analysis*.
Racamier, P. C. (1979). *De psychanalyse en psychiatrie*. Paris: Payot.
Rees, T. P., and Glatt, M. M. (1955). The organization of a mental hospital on the basis of group participation. *International Journal of Group Psychotherapy*, 5, 157–161.
Roberts, J. P. (1995). Group psychotherapy. *British Journal of Psychiatry*, 166 (1), 124–129.
Schilder, P. (1936). The analysis of ideologies as a psychotherapeutic method, especially in group treatment. *American Journal of Psychiatry*, 93, 6601–6617.
Sivadon, P., Davies, R. L., and Baker, A. (1963). *L'hôpital psychiatrique public*, 1. Geneva: World Health Organization.
Stock-Whitaker, D. (1992). Transposing learnings from group psychotherapy to work groups. *Group Analysis*, 25, 131–150.
Tosquelles, F. (1995). *De la personne au groupe: à propos des équipes de soins*. Ramonville Saint Agne: Erès.
Wender, L. (1940). Group psychotherapy: a study of its application. *Psychiatric Quarterly*, 14, 708–718.
Yalom, I. D. (1983). *Inpatient Group Psychotherapy*. New York: Basic Books Publishers.

21

Milieu Therapy

FROM THE CIRCLE TO THE INSTITUTION

During the period between the World Wars, a series of experimental treatment programmes showed that some group techniques, as well as more global interventions in certain institutions, could be very effective. For instance, in the early 1930s, the Spanish psychiatrist Mira y Lopez (quoted in Campos, 1998) began to form groups and, at the beginning of the Spanish Civil War, he took steps to ensure that the 1300 patients in Barcelona's San Baudilio Hospital could learn to manage to some extent their own therapy, which made him a forefather of therapeutic communities.

As we have seen in the previous chapter, during the Second World War the sudden increase in stress-related psychiatric illnesses led to the utilisation of therapeutic group techniques and to the employment of non-medical personnel, which meant important savings in time and money. Similarly, the treatment in group settings (both inpatient and outpatient) of veterans presenting mental disorders became necessary. This led to the creation of halfway houses, clubs, and other o to promote their re-adaptation into society.

In 1942, at the height of World War II, Bion was sent as a psychiatrist to the Northfield Military Hospital. There he promoted with Rickman a very interesting programme (known as 'the first Northfield experiment') to try to modify the functioning of the institution by means of groups, considering the institution 'as a whole'. However, conflicts arising with the military administrators of the hospital led to a premature end of the experiment after six weeks.

The second experience was more the result of a team effort, and lasted till the end of the war. One month after Bion's departure, Foulkes arrived, and he was able to continue and enlarge the movement over four years in what has been called the 'second Northfield experiment'. The account of the first trial, published in the *Bulletin of the Menninger Clinic* (Menninger, 1942) and the ensuing comments by Foulkes (Foulkes, 1946, 1948) and by other participants (De Mare, 1983; Main, 1946, 1977; Anthony, 1983) are of great interest in helping to understand the genesis of therapeutic communities. Foulkes was the only psychoanalyst at Northfield, and brought his experience as a leader of small therapy groups, which he had previously developed at a psychiatric service in Exeter.

Meanwhile, Maxwell Jones (Jones, 1952) initiated at the Mill Neurosis Centre a programme that was based on the same principles as Northfield (with whose leaders he was in contact) although his had a more sociotherapeutic than psychoanalytical orientation. His therapeutic approach became very popular, and the term 'therapeutic community' is commonly associated with this author, who later specialised in the treatment of delinquents presenting what today would be diagnosed as 'personality disorders' (especially borderline personality disorder).

Therapeutic communities were thus originally used for the treatment of neurosis and personality disorders, and only later, principally after Main's experiences at Cassel Hospital, were they used for schizophrenics (Main, 1946).

After these first experiences in Britain, therapeutic communities were created in several countries. In Latin America, this occurred mainly in the private sector, for example at Garcia Badaracco's Buenos Aires clinic (Garcia Badaracco, 1990). In France, Tosquelles (1995), in an 'institutional psychotherapy' context (see chapter 20), developed techniques that underline the singularity of illness, teamwork, the system of meetings, and active therapies. Meetings were planned to facilitate the transmission of information, while reducing the intensity of the "corridor noise" generated by various meetings of the profesionnals, the patients, the management, etc. The active therapies were based on methods of eliciting participation, such as occupational therapy and social therapy, through the use of groups. The therapeutic groups were used to promote autonomy in occupational therapy (Tosquelles) and directed by patients.

These ideas also inspired the work of others in several countries (Rees et al., 1955; Rickman, 1935; Sivadon et al., 1963), since they showed the usefulness in psychiatric hospitals of open rooms and more open communication links between patients and those responsible for their treatment. In the United States, the liberalisation of the hospital environment was already active in the 1950s. The therapeutic team of Woodbury started a study in a ward, Chestnut Lodge at St. Elizabeth's Hospital of Washington, which became the first experience of community therapy carried out in that country. However, the most complete example of community therapy was given by the Menninger Clinic in Topeka, Kansas.

Other authors extended Bion's theories on regressive phenomena in small groups to the study of group processes, to the definition of the role of a leader, to the authority and structure of great social organisations. They developed a 'systemic' approach in order to analyse organisations. Later, Kernberg (1978, 1979) applied these ideas by integrating object relationships into the understanding of hospital organisational problems.

However, the concepts of 'individual institutional transference' and counter-transference have been questioned widely. A number of psychoanalytical authors have urged that they be used with caution. In any case, thanks to these approaches, progress has been made regarding knowledge of the therapeutic function of the institution, and that of the modification of institutional settings necessary to put into action psychoanalytical treatments for seriously ill patients and, through certain modifications in psychoanalytical theory, for psychoses, as well. For instance, since the patient is only connected to the institution for the duration of hospitalisation, a differentiation was made between psychoanalytical interpretation, which must rarely be formulated, and the psychoanalytical understanding that the therapist acquires of the phenomena of the group and the institutional relationship (Racolt, 1970). Therefore, for psychotic patients, Racamier (1983) proposed a 'bifocal' treatment, combining a psychiatrist, who takes charge of the aspects centred on reality, and a psychoanalyst, who works at the level of unconscious fantasy.

THERAPEUTIC MECHANISMS

As Gunderson (1983) said, in the treatment programmes proposed by Menninger (1939) and Bettelheim (1950), two factors present in the course of treatment in certain psychiatric hospitals were recognised: 'containment' (in Bion's sense), which furnishes a feeling of security in the face of the infantile pain, rage and despair that are frequently re-experienced in the therapeutic community; and 'structuring the environment' to make it less uncertain and to facilitate modifications in ill-adapted behaviour in the patient. The activities designed to furnish this structure ranged from the organisation of hierarchical systems of reward and privilege to the use of contracts, setting up meetings and issuing guidelines for patients' daily routine and hygiene. These authors (Menninger, 1939; Bettelheim, 1950) set up programmes that offered a structure through the organisation of space, activities, certain privileges and contracts, and the planning of daily activities.

Other factors with an impact on the efficacy of a therapeutic milieu have been described, notably, the 'support' of whatever can foster patients' personal investment in the treatment plan, to fight against passiveness and to promote acceptance of the expression of their pathology ('validation'), which enables patients to assume their individuality. In these programmes, it is stipulated that the patient's desire for solitude must also be respected—including the patient's need to keep secrets—as well as his or her disability and symptoms. 'Implication' is the mechanism through which patients are encouraged to interact with their environment, to escape from passiveness, and encourage them to collaborate.

These different mechanisms act in a specific fashion for different kinds of patients. Thus, containment can be necessary for a schizophrenic in an acute phase, confused and impulsive, but can have a negative effect on chronic patients. Support can be very useful for depressed or frightened patients, but may be harmful for paranoid or borderline patients. "Providing structure" can also be useful for chronic schizophrenics, as implication is for paranoid schizophrenics, whereas an active psychotic can be overwhelmed by the demands of community inclusion. Validation can be very useful for paranoid and borderline patients, but can be dangerous for suicidal patients and can lead to the neglect of certain passive or verbose patients.

In addition, from a psychoanalytical point of view, certain ingredients derived from theories of object relations, of the psychology of the ego, and group analysis represent the quintessence of therapeutic communities and explain their therapeutic effect. In following a developmental sequence (Haigh, 1999; Hinshelwood, 1999; Hinshelwood et al., 1998), several therapeutic ingredients have been described, of which the first was *attachment*. The theory of attachment shows that if the link with the mother has not been reassuring, the adult will lack confidence in him- or herself, which is notably the case of certain patients suffering from personality disorders. The therapeutic community creates a culture in which belonging is highly prized, and where the members themselves are validated, which is reassuring for the patient. However, for an individual to develop, he or she must be able to confront other complex experiences—such as love, hate, anger, frustration, sadness, attack, defence, and comfort—that facilitate disillusion regarding the phantasy of symbiotic fusion and early attachment, thus rendering the patient capable of 'growing up and leaving home'. In this sense, the therapeutic community offers experiences of inclusion (a process of derivation and evaluation) and of departure (such as farewell rituals).

Another fundamental therapeutic factor of development (Haigh, 1999; Hinshelwood, 1999) is, of course, the already mentioned concept of *containment*, which relates to the 'mothering element' of these institutions. But there also exists a 'paternal element', which consists of establishing limits and rules and reinforcing boundaries, which contradicts to a certain extent the notion of 'permissiveness' demanded in a therapeutic community.

Once the therapeutic community has mastered primitive preverbal work with a patient, a fundamental challenge is to establish *communication,* in the form of contacts with other patients and caregivers, which allows them to build mutual understanding through the use of 'symbolic representations' and the process of 'identification'. For this to occur, there must exist a 'communal identity' (Rapaport, 1974), which comprises a set of intimate experiences that are forged through the participation of all the members in therapeutic, social, and informal activities in a 'culture of enquiry'. Stable, protected groups with well-defined boundaries enhance this process.

Another factor specific to therapeutic communities is the compromise obliging patients to accept that all interpersonal interaction belongs to all the members of the community. Effectively, everything that goes on in the community can be utilised from a therapeutic point of view, leading then to an inseparable union between 'living and learning' (Jones, 1972).

On the other hand, therapeutic communities hold to a basic belief according to which the patient's unconscious is a better judge than the analyst's of the direction therapy should take, thereby bringing into play the idea that the most important therapeutic effect is brought into being by the patient, not by the therapist. The lack of symmetry between the therapist and the patient is accepted, but the automatic assumption of the therapist's superiority is rejected. This attitude fosters accountability in patients, who assume responsibility for their own therapeutic process, which, while facilitating its improvement, can also be a source of ambivalence, for example engendering feelings of guilt.

The majority of severely affected patients have a fragmented internal world, with a disorganisation of their identity and of their mental processes. Disorganised institutions threaten to increase disorganisation in their members who, in turn, will disturb the institution. Effectively, patients project their difficulties onto the community that surrounds them and introject elements of organisation into that community. The concepts of 'internalisation of object relations' have been used in most therapeutic communities.

The life of a community is in constant evolution, due to the curiosity of its members (*'epistemophilic'* drive), which is evident from the process of the search for self which constitutes a 'culture of enquiry' (Main, 1977). Bion coined a term for relations of curious enquiry in psychoanalysis, which he called K (i.e., 'knowing') *relations* (Bion, 1959). This 'K approach' is the equivalent of the attitude of "community enquiry" which, at each step, seeks to know why certain things are done. If things are not called into question, memories disappear, and are replaced by a moralist tone: 'We do this like that'. The result is that rules are made by the superego rather than the ego (Main, 1977). It is, however, true that even this culture of enquiry can become ritualised, and that it is necessary to have a sort of 'metavigilance' to avoid it (Levinson, 1996).

EXAMPLES OF CLINICAL PROGRAMMES

True Therapeutic Communities

Therapeutic communities have had difficulties in surviving in the medicalised atmosphere wrought by the managed-care strategies that are now prevalent in most Western countries (Schimmel, 1997). However, this type of approach should be an antidote to the biases of managed care. Indeed, patients with serious psychiatric illnesses (incompetence, suicidal tendencies, dependency) who suffer from a feeling of profound insecurity will continue to need long-term, intensive therapy, and we should show some reticence when faced with attempts to reduce or dilute the services we offer (Campling and Dixon Lodge, 1999a, 1999b; Campling and Haigh, 1999). A training process that adheres to therapeutic community principles should encourage the growth and differentiation of patients and, as Campling and Haigh warn, avoid the indoctrination and infantilisation that are typical not only of medical training, but also of psychoanalytical training. As noted above, although the philosophy of therapeutic communities has become especially widespread over the last few years in half-way institutions, the hospital-based therapeutic community will remain valid. In fact, the latter combines sociotherapeutic treatment and psychotherapeutic treatment with the advantages of a hospital context (Schimmel, 1997); moreover, such an approach has shown itself to be useful in the treatment of borderline personality disorder and the rehabilitation of certain delinquents. More research is needed in order to evaluate its efficacy for other diagnostic groups, but it seems that the intensive approach, permitting therapeutic regression while diminishing anti-therapeutic behavioural regression, can be very appropriate for psychotic patients, who have shown themselves to be resistant to treatment by other means (Nieminen et al. , 1994). Over the course of the last 20 years, Ciompi (1997) has developed the concept of 'psychosociobiological integration of logic to affect' in therapy for schizophrenia—an innovative therapeutic approach that is particularly useful for these patients, in which the style of the environment and the assistance given lend themselves to a relaxation of the emotions.

Access to *quality* therapeutic community treatment will represent, therefore, an important element in furnishing a complete psychiatric service. But it must be noted that there is a need for quality: as shown in several studies (Isohanni et al., 1992), the lack of participation or the passiveness of patients is principally linked to certain aspects of the programme, such as ward policy; consequently, we have noted that when the programme is good, participation and commitment progress. Thus, it is important to improve therapeutic programmes, and the skills of their leaders. A study by Nieminen et al. (1994) found that patients who obtained better immediate results, generally stayed 10 to 20 days longer in the hospital than those who did not. For our part (Guimón, 1998) as we said earlier, over the past 20 years we have developed a certain number of group programmes, dubbed 'decaffeinated therapeutic communities' (Guimón 1999) in many psychiatric units, with an orientation towards community therapy in a dozen different care units (short-stay units in general hospitals, rehabilitation units, day hospitals) in Spain and in Switzerland (Guimón, 2001). The programmes (see chapter 20) of these units include, as a minimum, a daily medium-sized group bringing together patients and staff and a 'small' group of patients, with a dynamic orientation but with occasional cognitive-behavioural tendencies as well as group activities ('group work' in Foulkes's sense). We shall look at some of these units below.

Short-Stay Units

It used to be generally accepted that short-stay units constituted a totally inadequate setting to undertake psychotherapy and to organise the systems of assistance oriented around the therapeutic community model. Indeed, the patients' serious symptomatology, the heterogeneity of diagnoses, and the typically short stays result in an extremely fluctuating, variable setting which undermines and can even render impossible the usual psychotherapeutic approaches. In addition, the care required by patients placed in these facilities through a court order, who pose a threat to themselves and to others, necessitates the establishment of a closed system and compels staff to act in a sometimes overly authoritarian manner. Obviously, such conditions represent a major obstacle to the establishment of a therapeutic community.

In spite of all this, within the framework of different short-stay units for patients with acute illness, it has been possible to show the efficacy of psychotherapy and the value of the introduction of certain characteristic elements of the community therapy philosophy into the organisation itself. At Bilbao University Hospital (Guimón et al., 1983), a standard group analytic programme has been functioning since 1980 in a closed unit with 20 beds receiving between 350–450 patients annually. Stays last, on average, 20 days and the most frequently encountered disorders are schizophrenia and schizophreniform, neurotic and personality disorders, as well as affective and other psychoses. The clinical state of these patients is characterised by poor functioning insofar as reality testing is concerned, presenting varying degrees of mental regression, and a predominance in the thought processes of primal defence mechanisms. The environment becomes, in these circumstances, an essential support for the mental process, and the therapy atmosphere constitutes therefore an important therapeutic tool.

We introduced in 1984 a group therapy programme (see chapter 20) including the participation of all the patients with staff, preceded and followed by two short staff meetings. Two types of small groups are organised, as described in the previous chapter, in accordance with the patients' level of mental disorganisation. Once or twice a week we organise group art therapy on a voluntary basis. Occupational therapeutic groups are also conducted several times a week. From a clinical point of view, the programme's results have been very positive, enabling us to decrease the dosages of medication required and to create a pleasant atmosphere in the sessions, as well as leading to a drop in the number of incidents (e. g. , aggression, suicide attempts, escapees) and level of tension on the part of the therapeutic team.

Rehabilitation Units for Psychotic Patients

A certain number of psychotic patients, mostly schizophrenic, need long-term hospitalisation, either because of a lack of response to treatment, or for social or even legal reasons. An appropriate ward atmosphere, obtained through a *milieu therapy* approach, is essential if a rehabilitation programme is to be successful.

A rehabilitation unit for 12 psychotic patients has been set up in the psychiatric hospital of Belle-Idée, which depends of the University of Geneva's Department of Psychiatry (Guimón, 2001). The average stay is 51. 61 days; the mean is 20 days; the average patient age is 38, and the median, 35. The care programme for patients includes individual and group activities, each professional category taking part in both aspects of treatment. The multidisciplinary team includes psychiatrists, psychologists, nurses, social workers and psychomotor therapists. The patients generally have a low functioning level, resulting in social and family problems, and difficulties and resistance to a care programme in an outpatient setting. For younger patients and those with a more recent onset of illness, the work is centred on integration and acceptance of the illness itself, on the meaning that the illness may have for each patient, and on maintenance and the possibility of improvement of skills.

Day Hospitals and Day Centres

Over the past 30 years, whether with the more social approach of the British or the more dynamic one of the Americans and the French, many traditional psychiatric hospitals and halfway structures (day hospitals, protected living quarters, workshops, etc.) have adopted this philosophy to varying degrees. However, by modifying it, they have taken away much of its effective force, especially insofar as psychoanalytical elements are concerned. The idea of a therapeutic community was adopted by residential and day units, assisted by social services and volunteers who, since they lacked the necessary training, contributed to its loss of credibility (Roberts, 1995).

With the dramatic shortening of hospitalisations of mental patients over the last decades, the usefulness of milieu therapy has been contested. However, in the United States and in some other Western countries, therapeutic community ideas have inspired the organisation of many day hospitals and some short-stay units. Now that the optimism born 30 years ago from the efficacy of neuroleptics has diminished, much of the general public considers the deinstitutionalisation of schizophrenic patients as a threat to the security and the well-being of the population, and this increases opposition to their departure from hospitals even further. Nevertheless, rigorous studies have found that the costs—at the clinical, social and economic levels—of deinstitutionalision efforts are financially viable for a great number of schizophrenic patients, as long as an appropriate outpatient structure exists to lend assistance.

The day hospital and other halfway houses are indispensable structures for maintaining schizophrenics in the community. In a day hospital, group psychotherapy is the basic therapeutic instrument. Some day centres treat patients from the very first manifestations of their disorder through to complete remission, whereas others focus on rehabilitation of patients following treatment in hospital. We shall describe here a day hospital in Geneva where both types of patients are accepted, in different but complementary programmes. The first therapeutic function of this day hospital is to offer the patient a setting, which allows him or her to shore up internal checks and balances, and to receive psychiatric attention. A second function is to furnish emotional support, so that the patient's self-esteem is reinforced. The group dynamic seeks to create an atmosphere in which 'pathogens and pathogenic ties' can surface, and then be addressed and modified.

The day programme at Geneva University Hospitals (Guimón, 2001) is planned for a maximum of 20 patients, five days a week, seven hours a day. On average, it handles around 15 patients at the same time, with an average age of 26.5 years ±7.8 years and an average hospital stay of 9.9 months ±7. The most common diagnosis is schizophrenic disorder. This unit offers a range of corrective group experiences that make it possible to modify the patient's clinical symptomatology, social adaptation and, ideally, relationship structures.

The programme includes the prescription and control of medication, the organisation of psychotherapeutic activities based on the comprehension of the dynamic factors that intervened in triggering the illness, and the techniques which aim to combat the symptoms characteristic of schizophrenic deterioration: difficulties of an intellectual type, apathy and libidinal objectal withdrawal, isolation in the patient's introverted world. The days begin with a coffee break and include lunch and three small groups a day, which comprise verbal psychotherapy (dynamic and cognitive) twice a week as well as group activities in the form of discussion (free, on medication, on social information, on daily life) and various activities (artistic expression, theatre and video, body movement, cooking, games). In addition, there are two median groups: general assembly (which unites all caregivers and patients once a week) and the multifamily group (which unites all patients, their families and caregivers) once a month.

On the therapeutic team, in varying percentages, can be found psychiatrists, psychologists, social workers, occupational therapists, and psychomotor therapists. Professionals have in general received training in individual and group psychoanalysis, and possess a certain amount of knowledge regarding family therapy and social networks. Communication between therapists is in the form of meetings of working groups.

GROUP PSYCHOTHERAPY AND INTERACTION

While most authors agree on the benefits of group psychotherapy for a large proportion–80%, according to Kanas (1986)–of schizophrenics on an outpatient basis, studies analysing its global effectiveness with hospitalised schizophrenics are inconclusive. However, in thorough evaluation of the literature, Kanas (1991) found that group therapy was effective in two-thirds of the inpatient studies. Our previous study on two wards (Guimon, 1998, 2001) showed that the group-analytic programme resulted in the use of lower doses of medication and fewer serious disturbances (e.g., aggressions, attempts at suicide, and escapees) in the ward. Moreover, patients tended to seek psychotherapeutic help more frequently when discharged.

Mosher and Gunderson (Mosher et al., 1980) found that the outcome with group psychotherapy was favourable in studies where the aims to be achieved (for example 'interaction' in Corder et al., 1971) and the specific activities designed to achieve those aims were well defined. May and Simpson (May et al., 1990) emphasised that good results are obtained when therapy concentrates on daily life, difficulties in social relationships, compliance in taking medicine and recreational activities. In the same way, two studies have shown the positive effect of group treatment in the variables socialisation and 'interpersonal skills' (Levine, 1980; O'Brien et al., 1972) in schizophrenic patients. Interaction-oriented groups were more effective than those using an insight orientation (Kanas, 1991), which could even be harmful for schizophrenics. In the same way, in our study, those items that were rated higher in our wards referred to the aspects that could be enhanced by interaction.

This favourable effect of groups on patient interaction is probably more evident in the case of prolonged treatments. In the inpatient literature, therapy groups lasting longer than three months were more likely to be successful than those conducted for shorter periods of time. Only five of the studies favoured the use of short-term group programmes with schizophrenics. However, recently there has been an upsurge of interest in time-limited therapy groups with these patients. Kanas has developed a model of nine sessions of discussion-oriented inpatient groups and 12 sessions of closed outpatient groups which has shown empirical evidence of efficacy when used in conjunction with antipsychotic medication.

Kanas favours homogeneous groups for schizophrenics, since these enhances cohesiveness and protect them from the anxiety-provoking uncovering techniques (long silences, emphasis on past conflictual events), frequently used in groups where other kinds of patients (borderline, neurotic, etc) are present. In our units, we preferred to assign the patients to one of the two small groups, not in accord with their diagnosis but to the severity of the impairment of their overall cognitive fonctionning. This gives rise to groups heterogeneous in diagnosis but relatively homogeneous in their ability to relate with others. Of course, interventions, as noted previously, do not address unconscious conflicts, but questions from every day life, in a supportive vein.

The good results obtained by long-term psychoanalytically-oriented group psychotherapy in the treatment of neurotic and personality disorder patients on an outpatient basis has not been paralleled with severe psychotic patients treated on an inpatient basis, although Kanas (1986, 1991) found that group therapy was effective in two-thirds of the inpatient studies in his review. In any case, group work remains an essential tool in institutions both for the maintenance of a therapeutic milieu (Guimón et al., 1998) and for understanding and improving the work of therapeutic teams (Guimón et al., 2001).

REFERENCES

Basaglia, F. (1970). *L'institution en négation*. Paris: Edition du Seuil.

Bettelheim, B. (1950). *Love is not enough*. New York: Free Press.

Bion, W. (1959). *Experiences in groups and other papers*. New York: Basic Books.

Campling, P., and Dixon Lodge, F. (1999a). Boundaries: Discussion of a difficult transition. In P. Campling and R. Haigh (Eds.), *Therapeutic communities. Past, present and future*. London: Jessica Kingsley Publishers.

Campling, P., and Dixon Lodge, F. (1999b). Chaotic personalities: Maintaining the therapeutic alliance. In P. Campling and R. Haigh (Eds.), *Therapeutic communities. past, present and future*. London: Jessica Kingsley Publishers.

Campling, P., and Haigh, P. (1999). Introduction. In P. Capling and R. Haigh (Eds.), *Therapeutic communities. past, present and future*. London: Jessica Kingsley Publishers.

Campos, J. (1998). *Una historia de la AIPG: hechos y hallazgos*. Barcelona: Gràfiques MAES.

Ciompi, L. (1997). The concept of affect logic: an integrative psycho-socio-biological approach to understanding and treatment of schizophrenia. *Psychiatry*, 60(2), 158–170.

Corder, B. F., Corder, R. F. , and Hendricks, A. (1971). An experimental study of the effect of paired-patient meetings on the group therapy process. *International Journal of Group Psychotherapy*, 21(3), 310–318.

Foulkes, S. H. (1946). Principles and practice of group therapy. *Bulletin of the Menninger Clinic*, 10, 85–89.

Foulkes, S. H. (1948). *Introduction to group-analytic psychotherapy*. London: W. Heinemann.

Garcia Badaracco, J. E. (1990). *Comunidad terapeutica psicoanalitica de estructura multifamiliar*. Madrid: Tecnipublicaciones.

Guimón, J. (1998). Thérapie groupale dynamique intensive et brève. *Psychothérapies*, 18(1), 15–21.

Guimón, J. (2001). *Introduction à la psychothérapie de groupe*. Paris: Mason.

Guimón, J., Luna, D., Totorika, K., et al. (1983). Group psychotherapy as a basic therapeutic resource in psychiatric community care from the General Hospital. In J. J. L. -Ibor and J. M. L. -Ibor (Eds.), *General hospital psychiatry*. Amsterdam: Excerpta Medica.

Gunderson, J. G. (1983). An overview of modern milieu therapy. In J. G. Gunderson (Ed.), *Principles and practice of milieu therapy*. London: Jason Aronson.

Haigh, R. (1999). Psychotherapy for severe personality disorder. Evolution is part of the therapeutic process of therapeutic communities [letter]. *British Medical Journal*, 319 (7211), 709–711.

Hinshelwood, R. D. (1999). Psychoanalytic origins and today's work. The Cassel heritage. In P. Campling and R. Haigh (Eds.), *Therapeutic communities. Past, present and future*. London: Jessica Kingsley Publishers Ltd.

Hinshelwood, R. D. , and Skogstad, W. (1998). The hospital in the mind: the setting and the internal world. In J. Pestalozzi, S. Frisch, R. D. Hinshelwood, and D. Houzel (Eds.), *Psychoanalytic psychotherapy in institutional settings*. London: Karnac.

Isohanni, M. , and Nieminen, P. (1992). Participation in group psychotherapy in a therapeutic community for acute patients. *Acta Psychiatrica Scandinavica. Supplementum*, 86(6), 495–501.

Jones, M. (1972). *Au-delà de la communauté thérapeutique*. Villeurbanne: Simep Editions.

Jones, M. S. (1952). *Social psychiatry: A study of therapeutic communities*. London: Tavistock Publications.
Kanas, N. (1986). Group therapy with schizophrenics: A review of controlled studies. *International Journal of Group Psychotherapy*, 36, 339–351.
Kanas, N. (1991). Group Therapy with schizophrenic patients: A short-term, homogeneous approach. *International Journal of Group Psychotherapy*, 41, 33–48.
Kernberg, O. (1978). Leadership and organizational functioning: Organizational regression. *International Journal of Group Psychotherapy*, 1978(27), 3–25.
Kernberg, O. (1979). Regression in organizational leadership. *Psychiatry*, 42, 24–39.
Levine, H. B. (1980). Milieu biopsy: the place of the therapy group on the inpatient ward. *International Journal of Group Psychotherapy*, 30(1), 77–93.
Levinson, A. (1996). The struggle to keep a culture of enquiry alive at the Cassel Hospital. *Therapeutic Communities*, 17, 47–57.
Main, T. F. (1946). The hospital as a therapeutic institution. *Bulletin of the Meninger Clinic*, 10(66–70).
Main, T. F. (1977). The concept of the therapeutic community: variations and vicissitudes. *Group Analysis*, 10 (Suppl.), 2–16.
May, P. R. , and Simpson, G. M. (1990). Schizophrenia: Evaluation of treatment methods. In H. I. Kaplan and A. M. Freedman and S. B. J. (Eds.), *Comprehensive textbook of psychiatry* (Vol. 2, pp. 1240–1275). Baltimore: Williams and Wilkins.
Menninger, W. C. (1939). Psychoanalytic principles in psychiatric hospital therapy. *Southern Medical Journal*, 32, 354–384.
Menninger, W. C. (1942). Experiments and educational treatment in a psychiatric institution. *Bulletin of the Menninger Clinic*, 6, 38–45.
Mosher, L. R. , and Gunderson, J. G. (1980). Group, family, milieu, and community support systems treatment for schizophrenia. In L. Bellak (Ed.), *The disorders of the schizophrenic syndrome*. New York: Basic Books.
Nieminen, P., Isohanni, M. , and Winblad, I. (1994). Length of hospitalization in an acute patients' therapeutic community ward. *Acta Psychiatrica Scandinavica*, 90(6), 466–472.
O'Brien, C. P. , Hamm, K. B. , Ray, B. A. , et al. (1972). Group vs. individual psychotherapy with schizophrenics. A controlled outcome study. *Archives of General Psychiatry*, 27(4), 474–478.
Racamier, P. C. (1983). *Le psychanalyste sans divan-la psychanalyse et les institutions de soins psychiatriques*. Paris: Payot.
Racolt, M. (1970). Psychanalyse et psychothérapie institutionnelles: bases théoriques et collaboration entre psychanalystes. *Information Psychiatrique*, 46(8), 775–783.
Rapaport, R. N. (1974). *La communauté thérapeutique*. Paris: François Maspéro.
Rees, T. P. , and Glatt, M. M. (1955). The organization of a mental hospital on the basis of group participation. *International Journal of Group Psychotherapy*, 5, 157–161.
Rickman, J. R. (1935). A study of Quaker beliefs: The Lister Memorial Lecture given to the Quaker Medical Society. *Unpublished*.
Roberts, J. P. (1995). Group psychotherapy. *British Journal of Psychiatry*, 166(1), 124–129.
Schimmel, P. (1997). Swimming against the tide? A review of the therapeutic community. *Australian and New Zealand Journal of Psychiatry*, 31(1), 120–127.
Sivadon, P., Davies, R. L. , and Baker, A. (1963). *L'hôpital psychiatrique public*, n° 1. Geneva: WHO.
Tosquelles, F. (1995). *De la personne au groupe: à propos des équipes de soins*. Ramonville Saint Agne: Erès.

22

Combined Treatments

For many years, the combination of psychotherapy and pharmacotherapy was considered a difficult undertaking, and even inadvisable. Indeed, psychotherapy alone was deemed sufficient treatment, if well conducted. Medication, it was believed, could facilitate resistance, since by diminishing anxiety and symptoms intensity, the motivation for psychotherapy was then less apparent.

With the great development of psychopharmacology in the last decades, it became apparent that pharmacotherapy was a useful treatment for many psychiatric disorders; that psychotherapy could be more effective in conjunction with psychopharmacological treatment, in many cases; and that the combined use of pharmacology and psychotherapy gave frequently better results than the use of one of these procedures alone (Lam et al., 2003). Although the combined use of pharmacotherapy and psychotherapy has become a widespread practice all around the world, efforts to include the teaching of this procedure in resident programmes have yet to see parallel development.

In this chapter, we shall first comment on the different possible combinations of pharmacotherapy and psychotherapy. We shall then present the results of a survey on the extent to, and the conditions under which, combined treatment is used in the clinical practice of Swiss psychiatrists, the advantages and disadvantages of combined psychotherapy, and the problems arising in collaborative psychotherapy. We shall finally give some recommendations on how to overcome these difficulties.

THE DIFFERENT POSSIBLE COMBINATIONS OF PHARMACOTHERAPY AND PSYCHOTHERAPY

Combined treatment is neither a unique nor a simple treatment method: a very wide variety of combinations exist.

Pharmacotherapy and individual or group psychotherapy can be carried out by a single psychiatrist, a procedure which is frequently called 'combined pharmacological and psychotherapeutic treatment'. But the term 'combined' is also used for the so-called collaborative treatments, so these terms will be used here interchangeably. Individual psychotherapy and pharmacotherapy can be implemented by different therapists and, in this case, pharmacotherapy can be administered by a psychiatrist or a non-psychiatric physician, and psychotherapy can be carried out by a psychiatrist (or a psychotherapist who is not a physician), a procedure which is frequently referred to as 'collaborative pharmacological and psychotherapeutic treatment'. The same could be said when pharmacology is undertaken in parallel with group psychotherapy. Pharmacotherapy can thus be combined with individual or group psychotherapy, using a treatment team of two or three clinicians, either psychiatrists, non-psychiatric physicians, or non-physician psychotherapists. Finally, under inpatient and 'half-way' conditions, a 'multiple treatment setting' is the rule, featuring a wide variety of professionals involved in different activities. Clearly, these multiple combinations give rise to different technical problems, which should be addressed with particular strategies.

THE EXTENT OF THE PRACTICE

A survey of all psychiatrists in Switzerland was carried out by Geneva University's Department of Psychiatry in collaboration with the Swiss Psychiatric Association and the Swiss Society for Child and Adolescent Psychiatry (Guimón et al., 1998a). A questionnaire was mailed, in 1994, to about 2300 psychiatrists, established either in private practice or working in the public sector. The response rate was 44%. Out of 1,000 questionnaires returned, 964, which came from psychiatrists giving information on the different types of treatment they utilised, were included in this analysis.

The questionnaire was mainly concerned with psychiatrists' professional activities (including work setting, time spent on different activities, and clinical practice) and their theoretical orientations, areas of interest, and representations of psychiatry.

The overall results of this survey have been published elsewhere (Guimón et al., 1997, 1998a, 1998b), where we have analysed in more detail

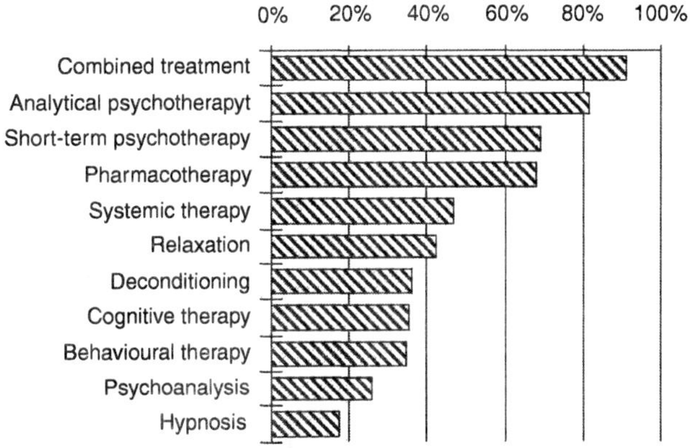

Figure 22.1. Percentage of psychiatrists employing different therapies

the data concerned with the combination of pharmacotherapy and psychotherapy, summarised here.

When asked about the different therapies they used, 94% of Swiss psychiatrists indicated that they practised combined pharmacological and psychotherapy treatment. Combined treatments thus ranked first among individual therapies, before analytically inspired psychotherapies (84%), short-term psychotherapy (72%) or pharmacotherapy alone (70%) (Figure 22.1). These figures are higher than those obtained in a similar survey made among Spanish psychiatrists (Table 22.1).

When respondents who stated that they used combined treatment frequently or very frequently (68%) were differentiated from those who used

Table 22.1. Activities at the individual level in percentages (several answers possible)

	Switzerland	Spain
Analytically inspired psychotherapy	81.3%	28.2%
Psychoanalysis	25.8%	9.1%
Short or focal psychotherapy	69.2%	18.2%
Relaxation	42.6%	49.0%
Hypnosis	17.7%	
Behavioural therapies	34.3%	
Cognitive therapies	35.4%	
Systemic therapies	46.8 %	
Deconditioning	35.9%	33.0%
Psychotherapy + medication	91.2%	71.2%
Principally medication	68.1%	27.3%

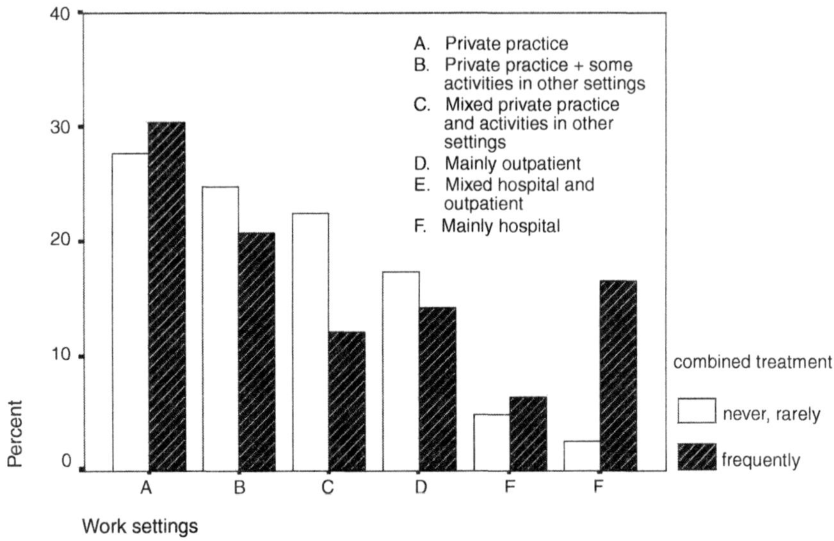

Figure 22.2. Distribution of work settings according to the frequency of combined treatment

it rarely or never (32%), we found that this procedure was mainly carried out in institutional practice. Frequent users worked more often in the public sector than non- or infrequent users (37% vs. 25%, $p < 0.001$). They were more often men (73% among frequent users vs. 61%, $p < 0.001$), who, in any case, worked more often in this setting overall than did women psychiatrists. Combined treatment was particularly favoured by psychiatrists working in hospitals, and less often by psychiatrists in private practice who also had activities in other settings.

A typology of therapeutic practice profiles was constructed according to two criteria: 'frequency' (therapy with the orientation concerned must be carried out fairly often or very often) and 'dominance' (the orientation concerned must apply to at least a third of all of a psychiatrist's therapeutic activities) (Guimón et al. 1998a). Psychiatrists with a biological practice profile were much more liable to use combined treatment than were those with a psychoanalytical one.

The same was true of theoretical orientations: psychiatrists adhering to the so-called eclectic model of treatment were more frequent users of mixed treatment than psychiatrists ascribing to the psychological model.

Women psychiatrists, psychiatrists in private practice, and those working in a psychoanalytical practice profile and adhering to a psychological model of psychiatry appeared more reluctant to use combined treatment.

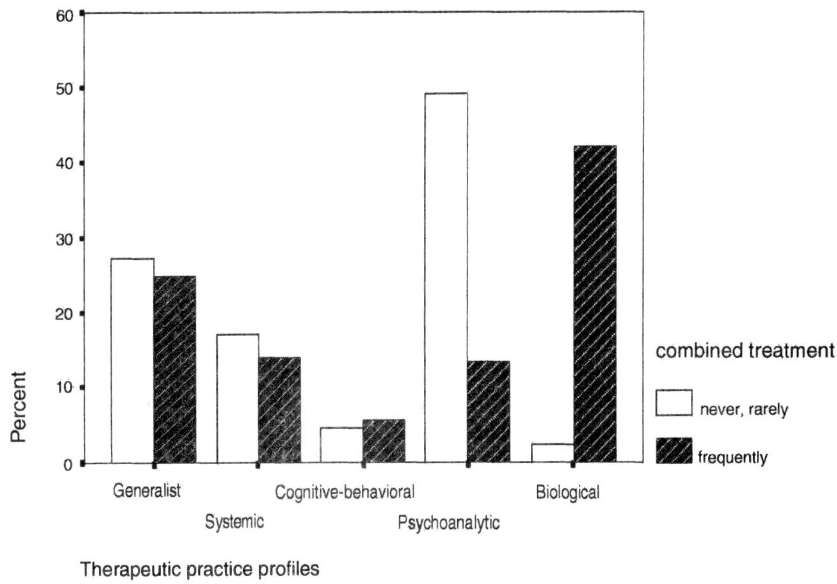

Figure 22.3. Distribution of therapeutic practice profiles according to the frequency of combined treatment

THE ADVANTAGES AND DISADVANTAGES OF COMBINING PSYCHOTHERAPY AND PHARMACOTHERAPY

In our survey, we found that combined psychotherapy is very frequently carried out by the same clinician, especially in the case of psychiatrists working in public services and those with a biological orientation. This kind of practice has, of course, the advantage saving time and concentrating the information emanating from the resulting effects of both treatments in the person of the same clinician. However, transferential issues arising in psychotherapeutic treatment can produce a negative effect on the pharmacological treatment, leading to non-compliance or to negative placebo effects. Furthermore, when the treatment involves psychotic, borderline, or substance-abuse patients, or others with severe disorders, primitive defence manoeuvres and acting-out frequently burn out the therapist.

To avoid this, an alternative strategy consists of collaborative treatment among two or three different clinicians (Beitman et al., 1984). Among the advantages of this approach, there is a sense of relief for the therapist based on sharing the burden of difficult patients (Balon, 1999). In fact, such a triangle is a well-known approach to containing conflict and anxiety, as has been shown by couple and family therapists. Patients, for their part, usually report a greater sense of containment and better tolerate the occasional absences of one of the clinicians.

It is, however, well known that transference and counter-transference issues can seriously deteriorate collaborative treatment (Busch and Gould, 1993). A great number of coalitions can form among the three sides of the triangle, with the resultant partiality, competition, envy and jealousy (Kahn, 1991). Problems arise mainly when communication among therapists fails and when each of them wants to be the 'favourite parent,' which leads to therapeutically destructive power struggles. For example, some psychiatrists are accustomed to being the primary therapist and feel narcissistically injured by having to share power, believing that their approach is the superior one. Apart from the type of profession, intergenerational differences can add to the difficulties. Under these circumstances, patients can be transformed into narcissistic objects.

A particular risk for the therapist resides in the temptation to collude with the patient's negative transference due to projective identifications and splitting. Because of this last mechanism, a polarisation of good and bad feelings results in some members of the treatment team being perceived as 'totally good' (the longed-for, idealised parent) and others as 'totally bad' (the authoritarian parent, an intruder in a previously harmonious relationship).

If triangular relations are usually difficult, the collaborative group psychotherapy and pharmacological treatment creates additional problems because they tend to elicit rivalry among some members, stigmatisation of others, and other group phenomena.

'Multiple treatment settings' (in hospitals or day centres) have many advantages because the therapeutic relationship between staff and patients with a severe pathology makes for a potentially very positive environment where re-enactments of internal object relations can be interpreted. The therapeutic team offers itself as an alternative family able to provide a corrective emotional experience, which can help the patient, as was conceptualised by Adshead (1998) in terms of attachment theory. However, therapeutic teams do not always behave as an ideal family. Certain manifestations signal negative counter-transference reactions, such as inappropriate restrictions applied to the patients, some pejorative terms applied to certain patients and so on. On the other hand, as we said earlier, external demands of the system such as the pressure of insurance companies, poor leadership, boundary violations and so on, can deteriorate the therapeutic milieu.

A PARTICULAR CASE: NON-COMPLIANCE

Cramer and Rosenheck (1998), in a review of the literature, found that the mean compliance rate for patients with physical disorders was 76% (ranging from 60% to 92%), whereas psychiatric patients receiving antipsychotics had an average compliance rate of 58% (ranging from 24% to 90%). In fact, other studies have shown that up to 40% of schizophrenic patients abandon medication during the first year, and that 24–63% of outpatients take less antipsychotic medication than prescribed. According to a review of the literature by Jamison (1984) concerning tricyclic antidepressant drugs, the non-compliance rates reported ranged from 32% to 76%. However, they decreased appreciably when medicinal treatment was accompanied by psychotherapy, in which case non-compliance dropped to 10–32%.

Reluctance to take medication can be linked to numerous factors (Guimón et al., 1999). It might be a consequence of both real side effects and negative attitudes, giving rise to a 'placebo side effect' in the form of adverse symptoms that cannot be explained pharmacologically. These manifestations frequently derive from a particular meaning the patient attaches to the drug, from characterological resistances, and from transferential responses of the patients.

As Goin (1999) points out, patients who are not psychotic are especially likely to provoke uncomfortable reactions in psychiatrists, because their psychological pain is often more disguised and their psychopathology is more obscure. On the other hand, an ego-syntonic sense of grandiosity and denial of the illness (anosognosia) are frequent in non-compliant psychotics. It is easy, in the case of such patients, for the clinician to see that there is nothing 'personal' in the resistance or reluctance to take medication, although it is not uncommon to feel a surge of anger when they sabotage the psychiatrist's recommendations. But as Goin observes, when we move up the diagnostic ladder to neurotic or borderline patients, we are more likely to personalise patients' reactions.

Secondary gains are a frequent cause of resistance, making patients 'cling to their symptoms' when treated. Some patients reject medication so as not to admit that they are really mentally ill. In many patients, unconscious parental transferences are activated by the prescribing psychiatrist.

In any case, clinicians' negative countertransference can affect medication decisions, such as the dose or the frequency of patients' visits, making the clinician either unnecessarily or excessively protective. Psychiatrists' reactions may frequently include insistence on authoritarian methods. Some even threaten to discharge patients from treatment, accepting its interruption just to show the patient how ill he or she may get.

SOME RECOMMENDATIONS ON HOW TO OVERCOME THESE DIFFICULTIES

Splitting, which is more frequent in borderline and psychotic patients, can be prevented by open communication among all parties and when therapists share a basic belief system—including an agreement regarding which treatment works for which aspects of the patient's psychopathology. However, communicátion is frequently difficult, especially when the therapists do not work in the same place. For private practitioners, communication is frequently hampered by the fact that it is not reimbursed by third-party payers. Some problems of confidentiality can also deteriorate communication, but in any case, a patient needs to be aware that communication exists between the different therapists and that even sensitive information must be shared there is a risk of putting the patient or others in danger (for instance, homicidal or suicidal desires).

Finally, in dealing with non-compliance, therapists have to remember that reluctance is especially conditioned by the affective aspects of attitudes. Public campaigns do not easily change attitudes, but some studies (Guimón et al., 1993; Guimón, 1995; Eguiluz et al., 1999) have shown the efficacy of group techniques in the modification of their cognitive, affective and psychomotor components, thus leading to better medication compliance and clinical evolution. In fact, the group format is optimal for facing transferential problems because transference in groups spreads horizontally. Masochistic attitudes are also best interpreted by the other members in a group setting, thus avoiding the resistance to accept therapists' (parental) interventions.

In conclusion, combined psychotherapy and pharmacotherapy is a common treatment strategy. We can even predict that with advances in both biological and psychological research, combined treatment will become universal. An effort should be made to prepare psychiatrists, general practitioners and non-medical psychotherapists to face the difficulties involved in this kind of approach—something that is currently sorely lacking.

REFERENCES

Adshead, G. (1998). Psychiatric staff as attachment figures. Understanding management problems in psychiatric services in the light of attachment theory. *British Journal of Psychiatry* 172: 64–69.

Balon, R. (1999). Positive aspects of collaborative treatment, 1–31. In M. B. Riba and R. Balon (Eds.). *Psychopharmacology and Psychotherapy. A Collaborative Approach*. Washington DC, London: American Psychiatric Press, Inc.

Beitman, B. B., Chiles, J., and Carlin, A. (1984). The pharmacotherapy-psychotherapy triangles: psychiatrist, nonmedical psychotherapist, and patient. *Journal of Clinical Psychiatry* 45: 458–459.

Busch, F. N., and Gould, E. (1993). Treatment by a psychotherapist and a psychopharmacologist: transference and countertransference issues. *Hosp. Community Psychiatry* 44: 772–774.

Cramer, J. A., Rosenheck, R. (1998). Compliance with medication regimens for mental and physical disorders. *Psychiatr.* Serv. 49: 196–201.

Eguiluz, I., González Torres, M. A., Guimón, J. (1999). Psychoeducational groups in schizophrenic patients. In J. Guimón, W. Fischer, and N. Sartorius (Eds.), *The image of madness*. Basel: Karger.

Goin, M. K. (1999). Countertransference in general psychiatry. In G. O. Gabbard (Ed.), *Countertransference issues in psychiatric treatment, Review of Psychiatry*, vol. 18. Washington, D.C. and London: American Psychiatric Press, Inc.

Guimón, J, Eguiluz, I, and Bulbena, A. (1993). Group pharmacotherapy in schizophrenics: Attitudinal and clinical changes. *European Journal of Psychiatry* 7: 147–154.

Guimón J. (1995). The use of group programs to improve medication compliance in patients with chronic diseases. *Patient Educ. Couns.* 26: 189–193.

Guimón, J., Fischer, W., Goerg, D., and Zbinden, E. (1997). Orientations théoriques des psychiatres suisses.*Ann. Méd. Psychol.* 155, 3: 184–201.

Guimón, J., Fischer, W., Zbinden, E, and Goerg, D. (1998a).Therapeutic practice profiles, work settings and activities of Swiss psychiatrists. *Schweiz Arch. Neurol. Psychiatr.* 149, 1: 29–39.

Guimón, J., Fischer, W., Zbinden, E., and Goerg, D. (1998b). Therapeutic practice profiles, theoretical models and representations of the psychiatry of Swiss psychiatrists. *Schweiz Arch. Neurol. Psychiatr.* 149, 1: 41–50.

Guimón, J., Fischer, W., Goerg, D., and Zbinden, E. (1999). Use and misuse of pharmacological substances: The question of noncompliance. In J. Guimón, W. Fischer, and N. Sartorius (Eds.), *The image of madness*. Basel: Karger.

Jamison, K. R. (1984). Psychological management of bipolar disorders. Pharmacologic prevention of recurrence. Consensus Development Conference of Mood Disorders, Washington, D.C.

Kahn, D. A. (1991). Medication consultation and split treatment during psychotherapy. *J. Am. Acad. Psychoanal.* 19: 84–98.

Lam, D., Watkins, E., Hayward, P., Bright, J., Wright, K., Kerr, N., Park Davis, G., & Sham, P. (2003). A randomized controlled study of cognitive therapy for relapse prevention for bipolar affective disorders. *Arch Gen Psychiatry, 60*(2), 145–152.

23

Community Mental Health Interventions

The Present and the Future of Psychiatric Care

Over recent decades, mental health services in the West have developed in three phases (Talbott, 1983): the *institutional* period, the era of *alternatives* to hospital, and the *management* period. Looking at these phases, which came to be more or less successively superimposed, enables us to understand the development of care which was, in turn, influenced by technical evolutions in medicine, socio-economic phenomena (as well as changes in management technique), and ideology (Guimón, 2001).

Regarding the latter, it must be stressed that mental health care is confronted by highly sensitive human rights issues, and that psychiatry is a discipline with low technological input. Consequently, it is more frequently subjected to political influences than are other branches of medicine. In concrete terms, questions such as patients rights, the potential danger of patients, the restriction of their liberties, the very existence of psychiatric hospitals, the power conferred by society on psychiatrists, administrators and jurists, and the treatment of psychologically disturbed children and delinquents are issues which have arisen throughout the world over the centuries whenever decisions have had to be made concerning mental health treatment (Guimón, 1998).

THE PHASES OF EVOLUTION OF MENTAL HEALTH SERVICES

During the *institutional* period, psychiatric hospitals were the only institutions in existence, and as many patients as necessary were hospitalised for excessive, often indefinite lengths of time. Because of the isolation of users, there was a tendency to hospitalise and marginalise underprivileged minorities.

The era of *alternatives* to the hospital phase, with emphasis on the so-called *preventive* phase, inspired by progressive ideologies orientated toward the positive acquisition of mental health, led to *community psychiatry* and *deinstitutionalisation* in the 1970s.

The *management* period essentially began in the 1980s, as a result of the need to contain costs, and is ongoing.

THE FUTURE OF MENTAL HEALTH CARE

The phenomenon of globalisation no doubt carries considerable advantages, which have contributed to the success of psychiatry today, but it also carries risks, which may jeopardise the future of psychiatry if corrective measures are not taken.

The Evolution of Psychiatric Practice

Diagnosis

The remedicalisation of the psychiatric profession has provided new specialists with solid training in neurobiology, and given them access to the new medications developed. While this diagnostic approach has led to considerable advances in psychiatry over the last 20 years, it has also given rise to highly debatable theoretical concepts regarding the very idea of mental illness and a distorted view of the reliability and validity of the diagnoses proposed. Meanwhile, it has substantially weakened the relational approaches, particularly the psychoanalytical, regarding patients' diagnosis and treatment.

Therapeutic Guidelines

Evidence-based psychiatry is increasingly used, employing the various guidelines that have been developed in this speciality. It is important that treatment be increasingly based on the most appropriate diagnosis and therapeutic procedures, rather than on practices inspired by ideological prejudice. But, as we said earlier, even if the new therapeutic guidelines have introduced rationality and discipline into determining and ranking treatment measures, they should not be overestimated. Indeed, they are based more on a consensus of experts than on specific markers to ensure proper aetiological treatment.

The Future of Psychoanalysis as Therapy

Science, like any of man's other domains, is subject to the influence of fashion and economic factors. In line with cost containment procedures, the trend in the West has been to use psychiatric hospital units not to treat the patient as a whole, but merely to stabilise his or her symptoms and arrange for discharge. Following this, in outpatient treatment, 'low cost' therapies are sought (behavioural, cognitive), dispensed by staff with little training, assisted by occasional supervision.

Although the theoretical orientation of psychiatrists has changed over the last 20 years as a result of the remarkable progression of the biological model, most psychiatrists, around the world (Guimón et al., 1997), adopt an eclectic approach, one called *dynamic psychiatry*.

As we said above (see chapter 4), dynamic psychiatry adopts a 'generic' model based on universal data from all psychotherapies, regardless of their theoretical orientation. Indeed, it has been noted that most of the benefits of psychotherapy are attributed to common factors, and that conversely, the theoretical orientation of clinicians only partially accounts for what they do in their work, given that, very often, effective therapists use a mixture of common therapeutic ingredients which they later justify by using the jargon of their theoretical models. Be this as it may, studies on the effectiveness of psychoanalysis (Fonagy, 2000) demonstrate the undeniable efficacy of psychoanalysis for certain disorders.

Our view is that mental health should continue to be based on this dynamic approach; it may be quite a distance from neurobiology, but not from psychiatry, which will continue to form the scientific basis of this field of health.

Managed Care

With the changes that have taken place in psychiatric practice in terms of cost containment, psychiatrists are in the process of losing a large degree of their autonomy. Simultaneously, the doctor-patient relationship is being challenged as psychiatrists are faced with ethical constraints in the conflict of interests between patients, hospitals and managed care organisations (Guimón et al., 1999).

Under managed care, emergency psychiatry, consultation-liaison psychiatry, and crisis intervention take on added importance. Psychiatrists have to provide brief, symptom-centred psychotherapeutic support, co-ordinate treatment with non-medical therapists and primary care doctors, and offer supervision and consultation. Managed care organisations would find the combined use of psychotherapy and pharmacology of inestimable value, given that a single professional (the psychiatrist) is in a position to offer both a therapeutic relationship and specific biological intervention. Moreover, private psychiatrists would be motivated to develop multidisciplinary team practices, based on networks. This type of practice requires assigning different tasks to different professionals, as well as offering a comprehensive response to demand.

If the goal is greater co-operation between the providers and financiers of mental health services, and if psychiatrists are expected to actively promote the practice of managed care, they must be given a voice in its management and take part in developing national policies. Partly as a result of managed care policies, and thanks to global communications through the Internet, the care provision systems in all Western countries have witnessed a change in recent decades: patients have become clients, well-informed on technological developments and treatment choices, compelling psychiatrists to provide more information and to be able to assess the chances of success and the risks involved in the treatments they propose—with the possible threat of legal action. This will unfortunately lead to a defensive attitude among professionals in the future, which may undermine the doctor-patient relationship.

The Organisation of Care

The Quality of Care: Optimal Versus Maximal Positions

The recent cost containment system operating in certain Western countries imposes restrictions on treatment, which may conflict with providing quality psychiatry (Thornicroft et al., 2001). Even if it is acceptable to propose an 'optimalist' medical attitude (i.e., the best quality at a reasonable cost) rather than the 'maximalist' attitude (only optimal treatment is acceptable, regardless of cost), psychiatrists must at least make sure that the same effort is made in psychiatry as in the other medical specialities in terms of the quality of care. The reimbursement of psychiatric treatment (hospital and outpatient) for patients in this speciality is confronted with more restrictions than in the case of patients suffering from somatic illnesses, both in terms of length of stay and in the number and type of outpatient consultations. Moreover, financial compensation for a mental handicap is lower than that granted for a physical handicap.

Overall, psychiatric patients have more difficulty than the rest of the population in obtaining care, particularly in the case of elderly patients or those suffering from mental retardation. This has led some structures to create the position of 'case manager': these professionals are responsible both for detecting the problems of those who have not yet had access to psychiatric care, but who are in need of it, and for assisting chronic patients in the complicated process of transferral from one service to another.

The Place of Psychiatry within the Health System

While it is important to avoid 'psychiatrifying' life and 'psychologising' health to excess, some attempt must be made to mark out the frontiers between psychiatry and neighbouring specialities, as a sense of competition sometimes reigns regarding territorial limits.

Difficulties also arise in clearly distinguishing the frontiers of activities that are the traditional domain of the psychiatrist. Moreover, the community psychiatry movement has blurred the distinctions between training in the various mental health specialities; the result is a mixture, with confusion over domains of activity. Indeed, in recent decades, psychiatry has increasingly tended to hand over the practice of psychotherapy to psychologists; the latter have furthered their knowledge of biology and now vindicate their right to prescribe certain medications. On the other hand, general practitioners increasingly undergo psychiatric training, which is all to the good.

WHAT PROGRAMMES FOR THE FUTURE?

Reinforcing the Practice of Psychiatry in Primary Care

It is common knowledge that most people presenting mild or moderate psychiatric disorders are seen by general practitioners who, while they fulfil a fundamental role, often fail to recognise these problems. They may even make an incorrect diagnosis and thus prescribe unsuitable treatment. In countries where state health services are highly developed, psychiatry is practised in health centres alongside general medicine and paediatrics, thereby improving provision for those with psychological problems. Generalists and internists are increasingly demanding admission to certain advanced psychiatric training modules. A major effort should be made to make this training available.

Emergencies and Crises

Home emergency services are on the increase in big cities, and have already proved to be successful. Alternatives to hospitalisation have been successfully developed in some countries. In Geneva, there are two crisis centres, not in hospitals, referred to as 'short therapy centres' (*Centres de*

Thérapie brève), which also have eight beds each. This could be a highly effective, although costly solution.

A Cochrane Review on the effect of crisis intervention for people with severe mental illnesses (Joy et al., 2002) concludes that home care crisis treatment, coupled with an ongoing home care package, 'is a viable and acceptable way of treating people with serious mental illnesses'.

Sectorisation

Sectorisation, which emerged from the French post-war policy and American psychiatry in the 1960s, has rendered a valuable service to psychiatric care by allowing the deinstitutionalisation of many psychiatric patients, and by avoiding hospitalisation for many new cases. Sectorisation has made possible the continuity of care between the hospital and non-hospital services, particularly in catchment areas of under 200,000 inhabitants, where there are smaller-sized teams and more fluid communication.

In recent years certain limitations have been detected in sectorisation:

1. The dispersion of populations in the city suburbs. Other features of urbanisation mean that for certain groups of the population, there is no advantage in seeking care near home. There are even indications that, as the Internet develops, some people's social networks may be very far from where they actually live.
2. In areas where the sector is too small, there are a number of specialised programmes (substance abuse, detection of certain early psychoses, specific treatment for rare pathologies) which should be inter-sectorial.
3. The irregular distribution of hospitals in cities often means that patients in a sector are admitted to hospitals at a considerable distance from their homes.

Psychiatric Admission to the General Hospital

Over the past 30 years, and in keeping with recommendations such as those issued by the WHO, most Western countries have set up small, short-stay psychiatric hospital units within general hospitals. In some countries, such as Italy, there is even a stipulation that psychiatric patients be sent to a general hospital for first admissions. Admissions to general hospitals have contributed to reducing the stigmatisation of psychiatric patients and mental health professionals, and to the development of biological psychiatry. Finally, these patients present a far better course of evolution than those who are admitted to specifically psychiatric hospitals.

On the other hand, it has been argued that this type of procedure weighs excessively in favour of the biological approach, to the detriment of the psychosocial model of intervention. Moreover, professionals who work in general hospitals tend to develop a certain all-powerful attitude, with the impression that short-term biological treatment is highly effective, whereas they lack any feedback on the chronic evolution of these patients outside hospital. Finally, depending on where the patient is admitted, whether to a general hospital or to a psychiatric hospital, according to sector or to the stage of the course of illness, there is a risk of creating psychiatry with a fast track and a slow track.

The Role of the Psychiatric Hospital

The transformation of the dominant role traditionally played by the psychiatric hospital is one of the fundamental features of new trends in psychiatric care in Western countries. A large number of beds in psychiatric hospitals throughout the world remains permanently occupied by patients with social handicaps rather than psychiatric illnesses. The majority should in the future be able to live in establishments that are state funded and suitably equipped, rather than in health care organisations.

Nevertheless, there will always be a number of patients who, for the most part, suffer from chronic functional psychoses and dementia syndromes, for whom long-stay will continue to be necessary. It will be difficult to modify psychiatric hospitals due to the particularities inherent to their organisation, and we have come to question the justification for maintaining them. However, some kind of psychiatric hospitalisation will continue to be necessary, to fulfil certain functions. The first of these is the role of protecting the patients themselves (asylum), in a case where their survival mechanisms prove insufficient in an increasingly conflict-ridden world. Then there is a therapeutic role for particular patients whose condition demands a series of treatment in a specific 'milieu', which can only be found in certain specialised psychiatric centres, difficult to create in a general hospital. Major efforts have been made in many hospitals to improve the functioning of long-stay units. Although its historical background is often unrecognised, the spirit of the therapeutic community has been reintroduced into the range of psychiatric care, albeit often in a 'decaffeinated' form (Guimón, 2001a, 2001b).

In recent years the philosophy of the therapeutic community has tended to spread to interim institutions (short therapy centres, day hospitals, hostels). A number of programmes based on therapeutic communities in the wider sense have also been initiated in the last twenty years, in different care units (e.g., short-stay units, rehabilitation units in psychiatric hospitals). These different programmes and their therapeutic orientation have been described elsewhere (Guimón, 2001a, 2001b).

A more intensive approach, allowing for therapeutic regression while alleviating anti-therapeutic behavioural aggression, has proven to be appropriate for patients suffering from chronic psychosis, for certain drug addicts, for borderline personality disorders, and for rehabilitating certain delinquents (Hinshelwood, 1999). In effect, it combines socio-therapeutic and psychotherapeutic treatment with the advantages of the hospital context.

General or Specialised Hospital Units?

A great deal of controversy has been created in many countries between those professionals favouring the creation of many specialised units, and those opposed to this approach. Psychiatric beds are usually ranked in the literature, according to length of stay, as short-stay beds (less than 1 month), medium-stay beds (1–3 months) and long-stay beds (more than 3 months). Short-stay beds are sometimes referred to as 'acute patient beds' and medium-stay beds as 'rehabilitation beds'. As a rule, short-stay beds have gradually been placed in general hospitals, and this tends to be true throughout the world, but some short-stay units remain within psychiatric hospitals. However, it is in psychiatric hospitals where one finds more long- and medium-stay beds (Jenkin and Glover, 1997).

There are also 'general' psychiatric units, which admit patients of all types, and units that are 'specialised' according to age (geriatrics, adolescents, children) or diagnosis (e.g., double diagnosis of substance abuse/psychiatric disorder, mentally retarded patients, eating disorders and physical/psychiatric comorbidity). Regarding long-stay beds, these are chiefly aimed at patients subjected to legal restrictions, patients with resistant depression, and for the rehabilitation of schizophrenic patients.

Highly specialised programmes, designed for specific pathologies, now exist that are mainly for outpatients, mainly in the United States. In some countries, geriatric psychiatry, child psychiatry, and adult psychiatry have obtained recognition as subspecialties with academic prerogatives and related funding (specificities for reimbursement). In other countries, criteria have been applied to maintaining a single speciality.

At a time when the role of the general practitioner is being reappraised after decades of an excessive tendency towards specialisation, a cogent argument can also be put forward for maintaining and reinforcing the role of the general psychiatrist. Clearly, as a corollary to the preceding remarks, training is becoming very long, but it is true that the six years currently required for psychiatric training should be adequate to cover this. It is also clear that the domain is spreading, and the merging of the different theoretical models often creates a sense of insecurity, resulting from the feeling of being incapable of understanding everything in depth. This is precisely why the ability to synthesise and the capacity to accept frustration are among the characteristics that the future psychiatrist needs to possess.

Outpatient Care

Treatment of severe psychiatric patients in community-oriented settings has been the most important contemporary development in mental health planning. A recent Cochrane Review (Marshall et al., 2002) compared day hospital versus outpatient care for psychiatric disorders, and found that there was evidence from one trial suggesting that day treatment programmes were superior to continuing outpatient care in terms of improving psychiatric symptoms. However, there was no evidence that day treatment programmes were better or worse than outpatient care for any other clinical or social outcome variable, or regarding costs. Another Cochrane review (Catty et al., 2002) did not find any randomised trial evaluating the effects of non-medical day centre care for people with severe mental illness.

REFERENCES

Alanen, Y. O., Lethtinen, V., Aaltonen, J., and Rakkolainen, V. (2000). The Finnish integrated model for early treatment of schizophrenia and related psychoses. In B. Martindale, A. Bateman, M. Crowe, and F. Margison (Eds.), *Psycosis: Psychological approaches and their effectiveness*. London: Gaskell.

Catty, J., Burns, T., and Comas, A. (2002). *Day centres for severe mental illness (Cochrane Review)* (Vol. 1). Oxford: Update Software.

Fonagy, P. (2000). *An Open Door Review of outcome studies in psychoanalysis* (www.ipa.org.uk/research/complete.htm). London: IPA.

Guimón, J. (1990). *Psiquiatras: De brujos a burócratas*. Barcelona: Salvat Editores.

Guimón, J. (1998). *La profession de psychiatre*. Evolution et devenir. Paris: Masson.

Guimón, J. (2001a). *Intervenciones en Psiquiatría comunitaria* (Vol. 3). Madrid: Core Academic.

Guimón, J. (2001b). *Introduction aux thérapies de groupe*. Paris: Masson.

Guimón, J. (2001). *Psiquiatría comunitaria*. Madrid: Core Academic.

Guimón, J., Fischer, W., Zbinden, E., and Goerg, D. (1997). Consequences of recent changes in research and practice for the identity of psychiatrist. *European Psychiatry*, 12 (supp. 2), 92s–98s.

Guimón, J., and Sartorius, N. (Eds.). (1999). *Manage or perish? The challenges of managed mental health care in Europe*. New York: Kluwer Academic/Plenum Publishers.

Hinshelwood, R. D. (1999). Psychoanalytic origins and today's work: The Cassel heritage. In P. Campling and R. Haigh (Eds.), *Therapeutic communities. Past, present and future*. London: Jessica Kingsley Publishers Ltd.

Jenkin, R., and Glover, G. (1997).The importance of service level measures for mental health policy. In M. Tansella (Ed.), *Making rational mental health services*. Rome: Il Pensiero Scientifico Editore.

Joy, C., Adams, C., and Rice, K. (2002). *Crisis intervention for people with severe mental illnesses (Cochrane Review)* (Vol. 1). Oxford: Update Software.

Marshall, M., Crowther, R., Almaraz-Serrano, A., and Tyrer, P. (2002). *Day hospital versus outpatient care for psychiatric disorders (Cochrane Review)* (Vol. 1). Oxford: Update Software.

Talbott, J. A. (1983). *Psychiatric administration*. New York: Grune and Stratton.

Thornicroft , G., and Tansella, M. (2001). The planning process for mental health services. In G. Szmukler (Ed.), *Textbook of community psychiatry*. New York: Oxford University Press.

24

Efficacy of Psychosocial Interventions

RESEARCH ON PSYCHOTHERAPY ASSESSMENT

A Historical Controversy

The controversy regarding the efficacy of psychotherapy does not end with the man in the street. Mental health professionals also have different ideas on this issue. If we hear a psychotherapist conversing with a researcher, we shall see that the former will state that the human personality and psychotherapy itself are so complex and multidimensional that they cannot be evaluated experimentally. The researcher will argue that if, indeed, such therapy can bring about some change in the personality, this change must be observable and measurable. The therapist, on the contrary, will insist that the really important things cannot be measured, and that feelings and emotions cannot be translated into abstract mathematical figures. The researcher will hold that the therapist's conviction concerning the efficacy of his therapy is rather like the bloodletting practised in centuries past, and that the therapist's predecessors were like magicians. The therapist will then accuse the researcher of being a nihilist, saying that his resistance to therapy arises from his psychodynamic problems. Outside of jeopardising their interpersonal relations, little will be gained by such a dialogue.

Therefore, can psychotherapy be assessed scientifically? If that is the case, what studies have been done concerning the efficacy of different techniques, for different patients with different problems, and conducted by different therapists?

First, we must bear in mind that in psychotherapeutic assessment, the problems are even greater than they may seem, since in addition to the difficulty of evaluating the mental condition is the difficulty of defining the impact of therapists' personal characteristics, their level of technical knowledge, the aims that they pursue during the treatment, and the degree of compatibility existing between the therapist and the patient.

Studies on the efficacy of psychotherapy can be divided according to their degree of objectivity in the study of a particular case, or an outcome review using more objective criteria, and finally the controlled experiment, using adequate measures and a control group. However, the use of a control group creates many problems; prominent among these is the improvement of some untreated persons. This last issue was addressed in depth by Denker (1946), in a survey of 500 patients who were expecting compensation from an insurance company. He noticed that within a year. 44.6% were apparently cured, and within 1–2 years, 71.6% were cured, without any specific treatment from general practitioners. He compared his findings with the results of other psychoanalysts in Berlin, Chicago, and London, who had reported 0% improvement. This led him to conclude that there was really no difference between those who had progressed, thus proving, in his view, that psychoneurosis takes a self-limiting course. However, it is evident that the data he handled were not at all comparable, since the studies had used different recovery criteria, and had reported on different kinds of patients, with different assessment measures. Moreover, these studies did not compare their data with those of patients who had not received any kind of treatment.

In a well-known paper, Eysenk (1952), stated that providing psychotherapeutic treatment to neurotics was no more efficacious than not giving it, a view shared by many other authors at the time. In his paper he compared the 72% of neurotics who had improved without psychotherapy with another set who had received "eclectic" treatment, 66% whom improved, and a third group receiving psychoanalysis, of whom 44% improved. Several authors soon criticised these findings. In 1960, Eysenk stated that another survey carried out with a control group confirmed that psychotherapy was not efficacious.

By 1964, there were more than 70 controlled surveys that Eysenk neglected to cite. Meltzoff and Kornreich (Meltzoff et al., 1970) reviewed them and found that 80% of the patients had improved with the psychotherapy employed, and that only 20% had negative or no results, particularly regarding delinquents, chronic schizophrenics, drug addicts and eneuretics. They concluded that psychotherapy was clearly useful, although that did not imply that any kind of psychotherapy practised by anyone on anybody was going to be successful. The criticisms of Eysenk, Truax (Truax et al., 1965), and others were based on incomplete reviews of existent research, which did not evaluate the data adequately. The better the quality of research, the more positive were the results observed.

In the last few years, surveys have multiplied concerning the efficacy of psychotherapy, using sophisticated and valid and reliable instruments of evaluation. Their results leave no doubt about the efficacy of psychotherapy. But is there evidence concerning the superiority of some technical and theoretical approaches over others?.

Some Uncontrolled Studies on the Problem of Indication

On the basis of serious but uncontrolled studies, during the last decades of the last century it was proposed that neurotic patients respond well to psychoanalytically orientated verbal psychotherapy. A smaller group of them would be good candidates for short dynamic psychotherapy. Among these patients, relaxation techniques and behavioural procedures would be beneficial for syndromes of generalised anxiety. Phobics and some obsessive patients could achieve good results using behavioural techniques.

By the 1980s, there was a general consensus that some personality disturbances, for example borderline and narcissistic patients, could be treated successfully with modifications in the psychoanalytic technique in line with the ideas of Kohut (1984) and Kernberg (1986). Cognitive therapies could be remarkably useful with depressive patients. However, except for successful results obtained in the treatment of schizophrenic patients by certain very skilled psychoanalysts, there was general agreement that psychoanalysis has little effect on these patients, and can even on occasions be harmful, although some behavioural techniques could be successful in the modification of some symptoms of psychotics, and in the rehabilitation of their social skills.

Around this time, Toseland (1987), in a review, compared some published studies on the results of individual and group psychotherapy. He evaluated 74 studies, which were reduced to 32 when only those with a classical experimental design were selected. In 24 of them, no significant differences were found between the two therapeutic categories; in the remaining eight, group treatment was found to be significantly more effective when compared with individual treatment. Ten studies, moreover, concluded that it was more efficient economically, and that there were fewer dropouts in the groups than in the individual context. These authors, however, drew attention to the fact that with these data, the superiority of group treatment cannot be stated categorically. They pointed out, on the other hand, that of the studies carried out, there was no clear pattern regarding what kind of problems of what kind of patients evolves better in group treatment, and maintained that the clinical point of view continues to be important.

Variables of the Therapist

It would seem easy to determine what kind of things make it possible for one therapy to be useful and another not. Unfortunately, there is too much information, too many details in which one kind of therapy differs from another. Many authors have assumed that the most important factor in psychotherapy is how the patient perceives the therapist and the relationship between the two.

In fact, the patient and the therapist do not see therapy in the same light. Board (1959) proposed that, according to the patient, success was related to his feelings towards the therapist, particularly in those cases where the doctor felt that the therapy had not been successful. To the question 'Do you feel that your therapist appreciates you?', the patients answered 'Yes' Feifel and Eells (Feifel et al., 1963) showed that the therapist's estimation of the success of psychotherapy is related to the disappearance of certain symptoms and an increase in social adaptation. The patients, for their part, emphasise the changes in their subjective, internal feelings. While the therapist thinks that the results depend on the techniques, the patients relate them more to personal qualities: being able to talk to someone about their difficulties in a warm, tolerant, and sympathetic atmosphere. In another study, what most impressed the patients was the personality and attitude of the therapist, especially the conviction of having his respect.

For psychotherapy to be successful, it is necessary for the psychotherapist to be seen as loyal and honest. He should give priority to the emotional needs of the patient during the session. The patient needs the assurance that the psychotherapist understands him and respects his right to be the final judge of his own feelings and experiences. No matter what its theoretical orientation may be, one of the therapist's functions seems essential for the success of psychotherapy: providing adequate space for the patient to put his worries, desires, and anguishes on the therapist himself. The therapist thus becomes a container in which all those affections can be processed and, once modified, taken in again by the patient. As a container, the therapist meets the patient's need for emotional contact, and the cognitive information that leads to a passive learning. From that moment, the patient is ready to accept the conceptual framework of the therapist concerning his view of the world, man, the causes of his disturbances, and the means of curing them. At this point, we are dealing with an active learning process in which there is an attempt at modifying the patient's perceptions, feelings, cognition, and behaviour. All of the above involve existential, philosophic, and educational connotations.

CONTROLLED STUDIES

Scope and Limits

Psychotherapists as a whole, but mainly psychoanalysts, have long overestimated the potential damage of research constraints on psychoanalytic process and outcome (Busch et al., 2001). However, in recent years, there has been a strong movement toward 'evidence-based medicine,' which has significantly affected approaches to the delivery of mental health care through the emphasis on randomised controlled trials (RCTs). According to the criteria of the American Psychological Association Task Force, to be considered 'well-established', treatments for specific disorders must be shown to be efficacious in at least two independent randomised clinical trials (Buchkremer et al., 2001). Some excellent journals, such as *Clinical Evidence* (BMJ, 2002), periodically inform practitioners on the results of such evaluative reviews on the efficacy of different interventions, including psychosocial ones.

However, there are many ethical difficulties for controlled research in psychotherapy (Quitkin, 1999), mainly issues concerning the use of placebo. To overcome some of these limitations, Kendall (Kendall et al., 1999) proposed 'normative comparisons', a procedure consisting of comparing data on treated individuals with that of normative individuals.

Other relevant forms of review, not using the Cochrane methodology, have also been published, such as the Patient Outcomes Research Team programme in Baltimore, using a structured expert review method that includes RCT and non-RCT data for the evaluation of psychotherapeutic treatment that might be delivered by community mental health teams (Thornicroft et al., 2001). However, other authors recommend adding naturalistic outcome studies to complete the limitations of RCTs.

On the other hand therapy research has only a vague resemblance to what goes on in actual clinical practice (Goldfried et al., 1999), and most practising therapists continue to work on the basis of their clinical experience, not the available research findings. Thus, Margison et al. (2000) support 'practice-based evidence', a complementary paradigm, to improve clinical effectiveness in routine practice via the infrastructure of Practice Research Networks (PRNs). In addition to scientific criteria, those deriving from mental health policy and economics are also important (Buchkremer and Klingberg, 2001).

Some Results

It is essential to note that evidence-based assessment is no more (but no less) than a tool to detect which treatments are most likely to help. Finding no good evidence does not mean that the intervention does not work. Thornicroft et al. (2001) contend that mental health teams have produced improved patient outcomes in several domains, although notably not in symptom reduction. Psycho-educational methods and cognitive-behavioural treatments (less well established) are efficacious for patients with schizophrenia under experimental conditions; however, there is little evidence that dynamic psychotherapy has any beneficial effects (Lehman and Steinwachs, 1998).

On the overall results of different techniques, Hager et al. (2000) reviewed 22 studies comparing behaviour therapies and short-term psychodynamic therapies, and concluded that there is no evidence of a 'highly significant' superiority of behaviour therapies over short-term psychodynamic therapies.

For Alzheimer's disease, a systematic review of controlled trials compared reality orientation with no treatment and found improvement in cognitive functions (Spector et al., 2000). Regarding other interventions, such as reminiscence therapy and music therapy, evidence is still insufficient. Cognitive-behavioural therapy reduces symptoms in anorexia nervosa (Jacobi et al., 1997; Loeb et al., 2000; Treasure et al., 1999), and cognitive therapy has been found useful for depression (Gloaguen et al., 1998). Interpersonal therapy, problem-solving therapy, and non-directive counselling may be as effective as medication in mild-to-moderate syndromes. There seems to be little evidence in severe depression, but the addition of drugs to interpersonal or cognitive psychotherapy is more effective than either psychological therapy alone (Thase et al., 1997).

Craighead (Craighead et al., 2001) contends that short-term and maintenance empirical data support the effectiveness of using behavioural therapy and cognitive-behavioural therapy as adjunctive interventions with medications for bipolar I disorder and schizophrenia. The combination of psychotherapy and psychotropic medications is not always additive for acute treatment effects, and especially for the maintenance of treatment effects, so that the combination of psychotherapy and medications is not the most effective treatment for all psychiatric disorders.

Cognitive therapy has been found superior to no treatment (Fisher et al., 1999) and to relaxation (Ost et al., 2000) for generalised anxiety disorders, and behavioural therapy is as useful as cognitive therapy and better than relaxation (Abramowitz, 1997) for obsessive-compulsive disorders.

Lutz et al. (2001) combined a dose-response model with growth curve modelling to determine dose-response relations for wellbeing, symptoms, and functioning. Their results provide further empirical support for the dose-response model and the "two phases model" of psychotherapy, as well as for the usefulness of patient treatment response profiling for individual treatment management.

Psycho-education (Pekkala et al., 2002), as well as family interventions (McFarlane, 2000; Pharoah et al., 2002), significantly reduce relapse in schizophrenic patients and improve treatment compliance.

THE EFFICACY OF MILIEU THERAPY

An Increasing Interest

As discussed previously, the therapeutic community approach has been used for a multiplicity of patients having different diagnoses, with variable results. For some authors, such as Van Putten (1976), the usefulness of creating such environments in psychiatric hospitals has not been clearly established. In fact, some research projects that attempted to show the efficacy of therapeutic communities failed to come up with conclusive results because of differences between patients and in the length of hospitalisation, as well as due to differing techniques. However, more recently, an important body of work has shown the therapeutic value of programmes especially based on group techniques.

The best early studies are those of Rapoport (1974) and Whiteley (Whiteley et al., 1987), both conducted at the Henderson Hospital, and that of The Association of Therapeutic Communities Research Group. More recently, other studies have been carried out in Britain. The methodologies used to carry out these studies were descriptive or evaluative, ideographic or nomothetic, sociological vs. psychological, or a combination of the above.

A controlled experimental study at Kingswood House concluded that it was almost impossible to link effect to cause when discussing multidimensional treatments such as those being offered in a therapeutic community. An alternative method to experimental design is represented by the 'cross-institutional design', which can be completed by several quantitative methods. An example of this methodology is that proposed by Moos, using the 'ward atmosphere scale' in therapeutic communities (Moos, 1987, 1997; Guimón, 2001) to evaluate the social and physical atmospheres in some treatment units.

Several studies have been centred on a single therapeutic community (Clark et al., 1969; Clark, 1999). Some of them utilised simple measures, such as re-hospitalisation, or penal relapses (Whiteley et al., 1987); other studies have a psychological orientation (De Leon et al., 1997; Dolan et al.,

1997); and finally, studies have recently been published on the relationship between cost and efficiency (Dauwalder et al., 1995).

Variables Associated with Efficacy

Insofar as variables associated with therapeutic results (Guimón, 2001) are concerned, Holmqvist did not find important differences in any comparison when analysing the relationships between psychiatric diagnoses of patients, their self-image, and the feelings of personnel towards patients in 17 treatment units for psychiatric patients presenting severe disorders (Holmqvist et al., 1996). Werbart studied exploratory and support factors in insight-oriented milieu therapy at three Swedish therapeutic communities for psychotic patients, using the scales of the Community-Oriented Programmes Environment Scales (COPES), and found that a beneficial psychotherapeutic environment requires organisation and a setting that corresponds to a well-defined treatment philosophy. The several structured studies that have been carried out indicate that community meetings had the effect of reducing unfavourable ward incidents, in particular those of an aggressive nature (Ng, 1992).

Regarding the value of specific techniques used in these programmes, Winer and Klamen (Winer et al., 1997) presented a model of community relations for hospitalised patients which was led as a large-group interpretative psychotherapy centred on the examination of relationships between patients and personnel in the here-and-now. This model is useful even in short-term hospital units and with severe patients, because it can provide a gauge of milieu, throwing light on the undesirable conduct of both staff and patients, discovering anti-therapeutic attitudes in personnel, helping to improve compliance with treatment in patients, and reducing tension within the unit.

Several studies have indicated the fundamental value of group therapy in these programmes. Kahn et al. (1992), in a short-term hospital unit, made a comparison between the dynamics of groups that met there and the atmosphere in the unit, finding very clear parallels between the processes of group therapy and those of the ward. Isohanni et al. (1992) studied the degree of participation in group psychotherapies in a therapeutic community for severe patients and observed, for example, that lack of participation (4% in all episodes) or passiveness (14%) were associated with an inferior therapeutic result and depended principally on programme characteristics (ward policy, short treatment times) and on diagnoses of personality disorder. The results suggested that participation in the group, the therapeutic programme, the patient's characteristics, and the success of treatment are inter-related.

Concerning the efficacy of different therapeutic mechanisms, Holmqvist et al. (1994, 1996) proposed a method to follow up the development of relations and to study those that are useful and useless, through a recapitulative list of words given to nurses, which makes it possible to reliably measure the quantity of emotional arousal. In another study, Holmqvist and Fogelstam (1996) studied, in 21 small treatment houses, the feelings of countertransference of therapists in the milieu towards patients and their influence on the psychological climate in the unit .

The Evaluation of Psychiatric Wards

Several instruments have been designed to measure different ward aspects. They allow a certain 'taxonomy of wards' that can be related to the differences in the therapeutic response. Kellam et al. (1966) developed a 'Ward Information Form' that aims to measure visible aspects of the atmosphere in psychiatric wards. Elsworth et al. (1971) designed a 'Perception of Ward' scale to measure the perceptions of patients and hospital personnel as well as attitudes towards the therapeutic programme, and there is another instrument that tries to measure different aspects of the ward climate (Spiegel et al., 1972). Nevertheless the most used scales are those developed by Paul et al. (1977), the 'Chronography of Interaction between Hospital Personnel and Patients', and that of Moos (1987), called the 'Psychiatric Ward Atmosphere Scale' (WAS). Moos assumed that the scale would enable patients and staff to describe the atmosphere as they see it. The behaviour of the subjects in an environment is determined by certain aspects of their perception. Thus, the scale would describe, to a certain extent, the climate of the ward, even when the perceptions of patients and personnel vary considerably.

Moos developed his scale after noting that three dimensions could be described in an environment: the relational dimension (including such factors as involvement, support, and spontaneity); therapeutic or human growth dimension (including autonomy, orientation towards practice, orientation towards personal problems, expression of anger, and aggressiveness) and system maintenance dimension (including order and organisation, programme clarity, and staff control).

THE EVALUATION OF MENTAL HEALTH SYSTEMS

The World Health Organization is frequently asked for advice concerning new policies in mental health. The Mental Health Programme at the WHO Regional Office for Europe in Copenhagen established a task force on mental health assessment to work on such policy decisions. Its members are European experts in psychiatry who, along with the WHO collaborating centres, assist a European network on mental health made up of 47 state-nominated national *counterparts* for mental health. The task force collaborates closely with other international panels active in mental health. During its two years of existence, several mental health care audits have been carried out. In a recent paper (Guimón et al., 2002) we described the audits and the experiences in mental health care assessment gathered by the task force in seven eastern and southeastern European countries, as well as techniques to create assessments and gather information from different sources.

The Model for Mental Health

The WHO subscribes to a precise model of mental health promotion and mental health care. Moreover, the European region has identified some of the central features that should guide development as per international recommendations regarding human rights of persons with mental health problems:

a) mental health care should be provided in a participatory approach, involving clients and their families in decision-making;
b) the size of large mental hospitals should be reduced and inpatient treatment minimalised;
c) whenever possible, inpatient treatment should be provided in general hospitals;
d) in- and outpatient care should be provided as close as possible to the population served, and offered in community-based mental health facilities;
e) outpatient facilities and day care should be widely available and involve primary health care;
f) non-medical extramural care by social workers, nurses, etc. should be developed;
g) the principle of multidisciplinary teamwork should be followed in mental health care;
h) mental health concerns all areas of society and all these areas of society are responsible for it.

The goals of the Task Force for Mental Health Assessment is to evaluate the degree of accordance of a given system to these criteria.

In line with this WHO policy, the task force was assigned the following goals:

a) to collect evidence-based knowledge on the topics;
b) to produce a position paper on the state-of-the-art in Europe;
c) to co-ordinate research to be carried out;
d) to develop evidence-based strategies, and to implement these strategies in one or two places as 'good examples';
e) to prepare and hold a meeting on the topic in the year 2002;
f) to develop an action plan on the topic to be presented and adopted at this meeting;
g) to integrate work done by the task force in the preparation of the WHO ministerial conference on mental health proposed to be held in 2004.

The task force agreed throughout the discussion and approval of a position paper, that in order to assist member states in the process of implementation of adequate services in mental health a certain number of steps should be taken:

a) establish the *model of service;*
b) set the *boundary* conditions;
c) assess population *needs;*
d) assess current *provision;*
e) formulate a *strategic plan* for a local system of mental health services;
f) implement *service* components at local level;
g) establish a *monitoring* and review cycle.

Methodology

The task force has responded to assessment requests via evaluative visits to countries and establishment of reports and recommendations. However, before taking any engagement, the *instances* requesting an evaluation and the extent and limits of the assessment that could be offered have had to be clarified. An assessment could in fact be requested by *supranational* organizations—such as the United Nations or the WHO itself—wishing to obtain information regarding the state of mental health planning and services offered in their respective countries. The evaluation could be also requested by *private instances,* such as private associations, e.g., the World Psychiatric Association and national or international non-governmental organisations, whose purpose is to improve the present situation. However, to date consultancies have been requested (directly or indirectly) by member states themselves, who wish to change policies via the WHO, which has the required knowledge and objectivity. Obviously, the kind of assessment to be carried out depends on the source of and reason for the request.

In order to accomplish its mission, the task force has sought the following information:

a) a panorama of the mental health situation of services in the country;
b) needs evaluation of the patient population;
c) mental health promotion plans;
d) investment in mental health;
e) inter-relationship of mental and physical components of health;
f) evaluation of mental health services;
g) evaluation of management quality;
h) evaluation of equity and human rights legislation.

However, the extent and methodology of interventions depend largely on precise definition of demand. Thus, assessments can be carried out via audits, accreditation visits, quality assurance screening procedures, or fact-finding missions; they can focus on a given target patient population or a complete health organisation; and existing or newly created instruments for evaluation of needs can be used, as well as operational manuals and indicators of stigma, discrimination and equity issues. A particular model proposed by a consulting member of this task force (the *Matrix Model*, Thornicroft , 1999) brings critical issues for mental health service planning and provision into focus, and was considered a good set of guidelines to be followed by the task force.

Time and budget limits are proportional to the task, and strategy varies from simple consultation of data provided by the client to in-depth and costly epidemiological studies. Thus, the origin of funding is a critical issue in terms of impartiality and task efficiency.

To date, the task force has made (or is in process of making) several visits to Poland, Kyrgyzstan, Romania, Lithuania, Slovenia and Switzerland and fact-finding missions were made in Russia and Georgia, all countries within the European region, in order to re-establish contacts and to introduce the re-emerged mental health programme and its policy, explore the present situation of mental health, and create interest in fundraising for different projects of the programme. More countries have applied, and should be evaluated soon.

In Romania, a relatively full evaluation has been made, providing an insight into the scope of mental health issues there. For other assesments, one or several members—in the case of Russia, the whole task force itself—visited the countries on fact-finding missions looking at some specific areas. They met with political and health officials, mental health professionals and representatives of organisations active in mental health. Furthermore, they visited educational and research institutions and mental health facilities, mostly hospitals.

Conclusion

Since the re-opening of the European Mental Health Programme, the Task Force for Assessment of the WHO's Regional Office for Europe has undertaken a series of activities. The task force followed the recommendations of the policy paper of the Regional Office, HEALTH21, which stressed the need for inter-sectorial co-operation within societies on different programmes covered by the Regional Office. During a 30-month working period, the task force was able to collect evidence-based knowledge on health assessment, and to produce a position paper on the state-of-the-art in Europe in order to develop strategies to be able to carry out a number of audits and fact-finding missions in seven east European countries.

Evaluations made in the east European countries involved in the project showed the existence of important inequities between these and other more developed nations regarding socio-economic determinants of health, lifestyles, mental health resources, and access to health services.

The task force discussed many instruments for the evaluation of population needs, resources and efficiency of the systems, and some of these instruments were used during the visits. However, most of the instruments are proposed for individuals in target populations, and this requires costly and lengthy field studies, which will rarely be possible in the context of this kind of evaluation. Therefore, in the future a great effort should be made in order to agree on simple and reliable procedures for assessing these parameters and monitoring evolution.

Time and budget limits greatly conditioned the task permitted, but an overall appraisal of models of the system, its boundary conditions, population needs, and current provision could often be made. In some cases, recommendations could be set forth for a strategic plan for a local system of mental health services. On the whole, an increasing interest in and sensitivity to mental health issues has put mental health issues into the limelight of policy in most countries. Some have requested an in-depth mental health evaluation, which could lead to implementing the service components at local level and eventually to establishing a monitoring and review cycle.

However, most politicians and administrators remain reticent regarding mental health issues, and they argue that no clear relationship exists between diagnosis and needs, and that it is difficult to evaluate results. To improve the situation, we need to give simple, relevant, information to the general population, employers, groups at risk, patients and families, primary care professionals, educators, mental health professionals, and administrators. However, these are evidently costly and long-term interventions.

Partially due to the activities of this task force, co-operation with the EU is at a stage of bilateral development. The wish for synergistic activities, co-ordination of work and exchange of experience as well as mutual technical assistance, has been pointed out by both sides. A joint conference and brainstorming session on mental health promotion and a European conference on mental health promotion has been presented as a joint effort. On the other hand, the Regional Office has strengthened links with WHO headquarters, other networks of the Regional Office, WHO advocacy groups, the World Federation of Mental Health (WFMH) and the World Psychiatric Association (WPA).

REFERENCES

Abramowitz, J. (1997). Effectiveness of psychological an pharmacological treatment for obsessive-compulsive disorders. *J. Consult. Clin Psychol.* 65, 44–52.

BMJ. (2002). *Clinical Evidence Mental Health.* London: BMJ Publishing Group.

Board, F. A. (1959). Patients' and physicians' judgements of outcome of psychotherapy in an outpatient clinic: a questionnaire investigation. *Archives of General Psychiatry*, 1, 185–196.

Buchkremer, G., and Klingberg, S. (2001). What is science-based psychotherapy? On the discussion of guidelines for psychotherapy research. *Nervenarzt*, 72(1), 20–30.

Busch, F., et al. (2001). How treating psychoanalysts respond to psychotherapy research constraints. *J. Am. Psychoanal. Assoc.*, 49(3), 961–984.

Clark, D. H. (1999). Social therapy, the therapeutic community approach. In P. Campling and R. Haigh (Eds.), *Therapeutic communities. Past, present and future.* London: Jessica Kingsley Publications.

Craighead, W., and Craighead, L. (2001). The role of psychotherapy in treating psychiatric disorders. *Med. Clin. North Am.*, 85(3), 617–629.

Dauwalder, J. P., and Ciompi, L. (1995). Cost-effectiveness over 10 years. A study of community-based social psychiatric care in the 1980s. *Social Psychiatry and Psychiatric Epidemiology*, 30(4), 171–184.

De Leon, G., Melnick, G., and Kressel, D. (1997). Motivation and readiness for therapeutic community treatment among cocaine and other drug abusers. *Am. J. Drug Alcohol Abuse*, 23(2), 169–189.

Denker, P. G. (1946). Results of treatment of psychoneuroses by the general practitioner—a follow-up of 500 cases. *New York State Journal of Medicine*, 46, 2164–2166.

Dolan, B., Warren, F., and Norton, K. (1997). Change in borderline symptoms one year after therapeutic community treatment for severe personality disorder. *British Journal of Psychiatry*, 171, 274–279.

Ellsworth, R., Maroney, R., Klett, W., Gordon, H., and Gunn, R. (1971). Milieu characteristics of successful psychiatric treatment programs. *American Journal of Orthopsychiatry*, 42(3), 427–441.

Eysenck, H. J. (1952). The effects of psychotherapy: an evaluation. *Journal of Consulting and Clinical Psychology*, 16, 319–324.
Feifel, H., and Eells, J. (1963). Patients and therapists assess the same psychotherapy. *Journal of Consulting Psychology*, 27, 310–318.
Fisher, P., and Durham, R. (1999). Recover rates in generalized anxiety disorders following psychological therapy. *Psychol. Med.* 29, 1425–1434.
Gloaguen, V., et al. (1998). A meta-analysis of the effect of cognitive therapy in depressed people. *J. Affect. Disord.* 49, 59–72.
Goldfried, M., Borkovec, T., Clarkin, J., et al. (1999). Toward the development of a clinically useful approach to psychotherapy research. *J. Clin. Psychol.*, 55(11), 1385–1405.
Guimón, J. (2001). Introduction à la Psychothérapie de Groupe. Paris: Mason.
Hager, W., Leichsenring, F., and Schiffler, A. (2000). When does a study of different therapies allow comparisons of their relative efficacy? *Psychother. Psychosom. Med. Psychol.*, 50(2), 51–62.
Guimón, J., Baro, F. C. J., Becker, T., Breier, P., Czabala, J. C., Dilling, H., Henderson, J. H., Meulenberg, L., Tudorache, B., Yastrebov, V. S., Rutz, W., & Bramesfeldt, A. (2002). WHO Tak Force on Mental Health Assesment: A reflection on an experience of three years. *The European Journal of Psychiatry*, *16*(4), 233–239.
Holmqvist, R., and Armelius, B. A. (1994). Emotional reactions to psychiatric patients. Analysis of a feeling checklist. *Acta Psychiatrica Scandinavica*, 90(3), 204–209.
Holmqvist, R., and Fogelstam, H. (1996). Psychological climate and countertransference in psychiatric treatment homes. *Acta Psychiatrica Scandinavica*, 93(4), 288–295.
Isohanni, M., and Nieminen, P. (1992). Participation in group psychotherapy in a therapeutic community for acute patients. *Acta Psychiatrica Scandinavica. Supplementum*, 86(6), 495–501.
Jacobi, C., Dahme, B., and Rustembach, S. (1997). Comparaison of controlle psycho and pharmacotherpy studies in bulimia anorexia nervosa (in German). *Psycother Psychosom Med Psychol* (47), 346–364.
Kahn, E. M., Sturke, I. T., and Schaeffer, J. (1992). Inpatient group processes parallel unit dynamics. *International Journal of Group Psychotherapy*, 42(3), 407–418.
Kellam, S. G., Shmelzer, J. L., and Beman, A. (1966). Variation in the atmospheres of psychiatric wards. *Archives of General Psychiatry*, 20(1), 169–183.
Kendall, P., Marrs-Garcia, A., Nath, S., and Sheldrick, R. (1999). Normative comparisons for the evaluation of clinical significance. *J. Consult. Clin. Psychol.*, 67(3), 285–299.
Kernberg, O. (1986). *Internal world and external reality. Object relations theory applied.* New York: Jason Aronson.
Kohut, H. (1984). *How does analysis cure?* In A. Goldberg and P. Stepansky (Eds.). Chicago: University of Chicago Press.
Lehman, A. F., & Steinwachs, D. M. (1998). Patterns of usual care for schizophrenia: initial results from the Schizophrenia Patient Outcomes Research Team (PORT) Client Survey. *Schizophr Bull*, *24*(1), p11–20; discussion 20–32.
Loeb, K., Wilson, G., Gilbert, J., and Labouvie, E. (2000). Guided and unguided self-help for binge eating. *Behav. Res.* Ther. 38, 259–272.
Lutz, W., Lowry, J., Kopta, S., et al. (2001). Prediction of dose-response relations based on patient characteristics. *J Clin. Psychol.*, 57(7), 889–900.
Margison, F., Barkham, M., Evans, C., et al. (2000). Measurement and psychotherapy. Evidence-based practice and practice-based evidence. *Br. J. Psychiatry*, 177, 123–130.
McFarlane, W. R. (2000). Psychoeducation multi-family groups: adaptations and outcomes. In B. Martindale and A. Bateman and M. Crowe and F. Margison (Eds.), *Psychosis. Psychological Approaches and their Effectiveness* (pp. 68–95). London: Gaskell.

Meltzoff, J., and Kornreich, M. (1970). *Research in psychotherapy*. New York: Atherton Press, Inc.
Moos, R. H. (1987). *The social climate scales. A user's guide*: Consulting Psychologists Press.
Moos, R. H. (1997). *Evaluating treatment environments. The quality of psychiatric and substance abuse programs* (2nd ed.). New Brunswick: Transaction.
Ng, M. L. (1992). The community meeting: a review. *International Journal of Social Psychiatry*, 38(3), 179–188.
Ost, L., and Breitholts, E. (2000). Applied relaxation versus cognitive therapy in the treatment of generalized anxiety disorder.
Paul, G. L., and Lentz, R. J. (1977). *Psychosocial treatment of chronic mental patients: Milieu vs. social learning programs*. Cambridge. Mass.: Harvard University Press.
Pekkala, E., and Merinder, L. (2002). *Psychoeducation for schizophrenia (Cochrane Review)*. Oxford: Update Software.
Pharoah, F., Mari, J., and Streiner, D. (2002). *Family intervention for schizophrenia (Cochrane Review)* (Vol. 1). Oxford: Update Software.
Quitkin, F. (1999). Placebos, drug effects, and study design: a clinician's guide. *Am. J. Psychiatry*, 156(6), 829–836.
Rapaport, R. N. (1974). *La communauté thérapeutique*. Paris: François Maspéro.
Spector, A., Orell, M., and Davies, S. (2000). *Reality orientation for dementia. The Cochrane Library* (3).
Spiegel, D., and Younguer, J. B. (1972). Ward climate and community stay of psychiatric patients. *Journal of Consulting and Clinical Psychology*, 39(1), 62–69.
Thase, M. E., Reynolds III, C. F., and Houck, P. R. et al. (1997). Treatment of major depression with psychotehrapy or psychotherapy-pharmacotherapy combinations. *Archives of General Psychiatry*, 54, 1009–1015.
Thornicroft , G. (1999). *The Mental Health Matrix. A manual to improve services*. Cambridge: Cambridge University Press.
Thornicroft , G., and Susser, E. (2001). Evidence-based psychotherapeutic interventions in the community care of schizophrenia. *Br. J. Psychiatry*, 178(1), 2–4.
Toseland. (1987). The results of group psychotherapy. *International Journal of Group Psychotherapy*, 21, 406–428.
Treasure, J., Katzman, M., Schmidt, U., et al. (1999). Engagement and outcome in the treatment of bulimia nervosa. *Behav. Res. Ther*. 37, 405–418.
Truax, C. B., and Carkhuff, R. R. (1965). Experimental manipulation of therapeutic conditions. *Journal of Consulting and Clinical Psychology*, 29, 119–124.
Van Putten, T. (1976). Milieu therapy of schizophrenia. In W. Flinn (Ed.), *Treatment of schizophrenia, progress on prospect*. New York.
Whiteley, J. S., and Collis, M. (1987). The therapeutic factors in group psychotherapy applied to the therapeutic community. *International Journal of Therapeutic Communities*, 8, 21–32.
Winer, J. A., and Klamen, D. L. (1997). Interpretive psychotherapy in the inpatient community meeting on a short-term unit. *Psychiatric Services*, 48(1), 91–92.

25

Mental Health Professionals

The community mental health movement stressed the importance of sectorisation, teamwork, involving the general population in service management responsibilities, prevention, crisis intervention, deinstitutionalisation, and the development of *therapeutic communities*. As a result, from the 1960s on, the old professional roles were redefined, and a large number of workers coming from new fields entered the different psychiatric services.

The need to contain health care costs has led, over the last two decades, to the so-called *managed care psychiatry* movement in mental health, which has produced fresh transformations in how services are offered, as well as more major changes in the activities of the professionals involved. This chapter aims to provide an overview of the range of activities that they carry out, and give an idea of the numbers of individuals from different specialities working in this field today.

WHO ARE THEY?

As Goode pointed out (cited by Gracia, 1996), in order to speak of a *profession*, it is necessary for those who exercise it to undergo prolonged specialised training in 'a body of abstract knowledge', and perform services oriented towards a collective. Traditionally, a differentiation has been made between *professionals* (e.g., physicians, lawyers, and the clergy) and other occupations (whether mercantile or industrial), in which the first group acted 'altruistically', since their role in society was so important that it could not be paid for with money, so that they not receive a formal 'salary' for their services, but rather symbolic amounts to 'honour' them, *honorariums*.

However, many sociologists believe that altruism cannot be considered a defining characteristic of these professions, and that in the case of medicine, it became accepted as a profession when it obtained official recognition, with its own course of university study, and the physician was guaranteed the exclusive right to determine the adequacy of his knowledge and most effective methods for treating a patients. Later, medical practitioners became a 'legally privileged' group, a kind of monopoly (Berlant, cited by Gracia, 1996), which has had a series of exclusive functions, including: strict control of the market in order to rule out competition from other groups, using a specialised language not directly understandable by non-initiates; a body of transmittable theoretical doctrine; an educational system; control of professional practice; monopoly on that practice; and autonomy in fixing its own regulations.

For their part, the rest of the health care 'occupations', sometimes called medical 'paraprofessionals', have tried to gain the rank of true professions without complete success, as is the case of nurses, who have created institutions similar to those of physicians. As Freidson put it (cited by Gracia, 1996), they have developed standardised curricula, as much of it as possible on a university level. They have created or described abstract theoretical concepts to transmit to their students, written ethical codes, sought support to create licensing or special registration procedures in order to exercise some control over who is allowed to work in their field. 'But,' he added, 'they inevitably fail when they try to gain complete autonomy in the formulation of their education and licensing norms, and also in the real execution of their work. Their autonomy is somewhat partial, second-hand, and limited by a dominant profession. These are the uncompromising criteria that maintain these occupations on the paraprofessional level, in spite of their success in attaining many of the institutional attributes associated with the professions'. Therefore, according to this view, the basic criterion for defining an occupational group as a *profession* cannot be found in its education, nor in its licensing procedures, nor even in the existence of particular ethical codes, but rather in its autonomy. All of these considerations are important to gaining a better understanding of the evolution that we have seen over the past few decades in the health care occupations, and the tensions that have arisen among those who work in these areas.

In fact, in the 1970s, within the context of the community psychiatry movement, the different mental health occupations did indeed acquire a certain autonomy, which created a certain amount of confusion in the field's different areas. Consequently, over the course of the last two decades, and all over the world (with few exceptions, such as Switzerland), psychiatrists have been increasingly delegating the practice of psychotherapy to other professionals, such as psychologists, social workers, and nursing school graduates.

Meanwhile, in some countries, psychologists have worked to gain more biological knowledge, and even lobbied to acquire the right to prescribe medication. Likewise, a new clinical psychology speciality called *health psychology* is invading the field of psychophysiological medicine, which has traditionally been the domain of liaison psychiatrists. By the same token, nurses, social workers, occupational therapists, and others have been raising their own profile within the area of mental health care, and have been honing the theoretical and practical content of their respective disciplines.

Therefore, although Gracia's comments regarding who, strictly speaking, should be called professionals are worth bearing in mind (Gracia, 1996), the use of this term has been expanding so much in every language that we are using it here to designate all of the categories of workers in the mental health field, excluding administrative and general services personnel.

The professionals represented in the different health care systems of different parts of the world are not the same, but, if we consider only Western countries, we can find, at least, the following varieties (Table 25.1):

Table 25.1. Professional categories

CATEGORIES
1. PSYCHIATRIST PHYSICIANS
Interns and Residents
2. NON-PSYCHIATRIST PHYSICIANS
Dentists
Gynaecologists
Radiologists
3. PSYCHOLOGISTS
Clinical psychologists
Research psychologists
Speech therapists
4. SOCIAL WORKERS
5. NURSES
6. NURSES' AIDS
7. OCCUPATIONAL THERAPISTS
Occupational therapist's aids
8. PHYSIOTHERAPISTS
9. SOCIOTHERAPISTS
10. REHABILITATION SPECIALISTS
11. ART THERAPISTS
Musical therapists
Ceramics teachers
12. EDUCATORS
Orientators (counsellors and therapists)
Socio-professional teachers (workshops)

In some countries, *professionals* are considered those included in the first five categories, and the rest are called *paraprofessionals*.

HOW MANY ARE THERE?

According to the latest data from the World Health Organization (WHO, 2001a) (Table 25.2), there is a worldwide average of 3.96 psychiatrists per 100,000 inhabitants (with a median of 1/100,000); however, this rises to 9 psychiatrists per 100,000 in the rich countries. Regarding nurses, the worldwide average per 100,000 inhabitants is 9 (with a median of 2), but in rich countries, the average is 33.5.

The contrasts are also huge in other mental health professions. Worldwide, there is an average of 6.43 psychologists per 100,000 inhabitants (median of 0.4), although this average is 26.7 in the more developed countries. The average number of social workers is 8.64 per 100,000 (median of 0.3), although in rich countries it is 25.5. The numerical representation of these different categories varies a great deal from one country to another, regardless of whether we consider hospital or outpatient services, public or private.

If we look at the public hospital services of a certain number of Western countries, we can find the following averages. Physicians (psychiatrists and non-psychiatrists) represent 6.8% of the staff. Psychiatrists, specifically, are the best-trained professionals, continue to head most hospital psychiatric departments, and are relatively scarce.

The most striking aspect of this distribution is, naturally, the enormous preponderance of nurses, who account for 54% of the total personnel in hospital psychiatric departments (if we include administrative and service

Table 25.2. Professional categories per patient

Type of professional	Number
1. Psychiatrist and non-psychiatrist physicians	0.0635
2. Psychologists	0.0155
3. Social Workers	0.0260
4. Nurses	0.5080
5. Nurses' aids	0.2062
6. Occupational therapists	0.0177
7. Physiotherapists	0.0062
8. Sociotherapists	0.0105
9. Rehabilitation specialists	
10. Art therapists	0.0018
11. Educators	0.0635

personnel). Nurses' aids represent 22% of the personnel in clinical units, which means that, if we add them to the nurses, together they constitute 76% of the employees in these treatment units. However, it should be noted that the category of 'nurses' includes workers with very different levels of qualification. In any case, these professionals have become the key element in mental health care, not only due to their numbers, but also to the many hours that they spend with the patients.

Regarding the personnel in outpatient services, data are harder to come by, and vary a great deal more from one country to another, according to their respective sectorisation policies. In any case, it would not be an exaggeration to say that in outpatient public clinics, the number of professionals does not, on average, reach even one-fifth of those in hospitals, and that the nurses have a much less clout, except for in those few countries where there is a highly developed programme of home psychiatric care programme.

The number of professionals in the private sector also varies a great deal in different countries, according to whether the health care insurance system is public, private, or mixed.

We cannot end this section on human resources without mentioning the role played by family members and volunteer workers, which is extremely important in mental health, although not always recognised, and which almost never receives economic or educational support.

MOTIVATIONS FOR CHOOSING MENTAL HEALTH PROFESSIONS

Psychiatrists

If we judge the motivations that lead physicians to choose the speciality of psychiatry, as based on their personality traits, these have changed notably over the last decades. Rogow (1970) described those who were interested in psychiatry as being genuinely interested in alleviating psychological suffering, not very interested in economic compensations, holding advanced social and political ideas, progressive in their habits, nonconformists, agnostics, and with literary and artistic affinities. The type of activities that they carry out today have become much more technical and bureaucratic, and this professional profile, now that the field has been stripped of its former romantic aura, no longer interested those doctors with artistic, literary, or humanist tastes, and now attracts those with a more 'psycho-neuro-endocrinological' orientation, which has considerably altered the profile of future specialists.

New medical school graduates prefer other, more attractive specialities, seen as more effective and requiring less of a personal commitment. It does not seem, as some fear, that the profession is becoming extinct, but it is true that there is a tendency to limit its field of action to behavioural neurobiology, delegating to other specialists, who are not physicians, the more psychological aspects of mental suffering.

'Caring' Professions

It is true that a great deal of the conscious choices that psychiatrists and other mental health professionals make are based on certain aspects of our personalities, such as authoritarianism, altruism, or idealism. In any case, as Vega Zagier Roberts (1994) points out, the choices that we make regarding what profession to select, with which group of clients, and in which setting we would prefer to work, are all deeply influenced by our need to negotiate unresolved issues from the past. We are often inclined to work in a particular setting because it offers us the chance to manage our own unresolved problems. It is well known that many of those who choose professions within the field of health care have had serious conflicts due to the presence of sick relatives within their families. In principle, this can be considered an appropriate motivation, but it can lead to anomalous reactions if the motivation is not adequately explored and elaborated.

The attachment theory proposes that human beings are social animals and that, to survive, we need relationships, which are moulded by early attachment experiences with parental figures. Thus, internal models of the self and others are established as internal cognitive structures, which have a neuropsychological basis. In later life, when we feel threatened, we show attachment behaviours, especially with figures who are close to us (Weiss, 1994).

In children (Ainsworth, 1969) different attitudes of 'insecure attachment' (avoiding, ambivalent, and disorganised) have been observed, which when they interact with other vulnerability factors, predispose subjects to developing psychiatric disorders: depression, pathological mourning, and personality disorders. Many adults seek to help others because they themselves, in infancy, experienced inadequate attachment, leading them to have a need for compulsive caring, which is seen in some professionals. The problem is that some of these professionals are hesitant to accept that they have difficulties or to seek help, which leads them to suffer from substance abuse of 'burnout'.

From a psychoanalytical viewpoint, the reparation impulse, partly conscious, but mainly unconscious, is the fundamental impetus to all creative, productive, and caring activities. This drive has its roots in our own experiences with our first 'caretakers': the mother and maternal substitutes. When the child acquires a sufficient perception of his surroundings, he becomes conscious of the fact that his mother is the only person whom he both loves and hates at the same time. When he realises this, he feels remorse, worry, and guilt for the damage that this avidity and aggression may have caused her. Thus, the urge to repair (redeem, protect) arises, and also to express gratitude for the good care received. Normally, the child's reparation activities keep his anxieties at bay. However, when the guilt is too strong, this repairing activity is inhibited. In its place, the child – and the adult who is reliving these early conflicts – reverts to the more primitive mental attitude of splitting objects into good and bad ones, which can be loved and hated separately, without ambivalence.

Some mental health specialities, centres, or institutions can attract personnel with internal needs similar to those of their clients, and a similar propensity to use certain types of defences, which can contribute to the appearance of certain defensive institutional processes. Bion (1959) calls this phenomenon *valence*.

Normally, having discovered many times that the mother, and later, others survive his attacks, the child learns to have confidence that his love dominates his hate, and that his reparation activities are successful. This reduces his fears of persecution and retaliation by the bad mother whom he has attacked. But when external reality fails to refute the child's anxieties, for example, if the mother dies, or retires, or retaliates, then the depressive anxieties can be too heavy to be borne. The individual then abandons his failed reparation activities, and recurs instead to more primitive paranoid, manic, and obsessive defences.

Paranoid defences imply denial and the projection of aggression so that the patient experiences it as coming from the outside, in the form of persecution. Manic defences are directed at denying that the harm has occurred, and involve omnipotent phantasies of magical reparation. Contrary to genuine reparation, which requires the ability to accept that harm has been done and cannot be undone, manic reparation must be total, so that no anxiety, pain, or guilt is felt. When manic reparation fails, individuals may resort to obsessive defences, the ritual repetition of certain acts, as an added effort to control and dominate anxiety, especially when their aggressive drives are concerned (Klein, 1948; Segal, 1988). Those who work in the 'caring' professions often, and inevitably, fail in their work with damaged and needy clients. If this failure sparks intolerable guilt and anxiety, these professionals (like infants) may regress to these primitive defences with the aim of maintaining their precarious self-esteem, and defend themselves from the retaliation they feel is coming to them for failing to effect a cure.

The working situation in the caring professions is sometimes similar to that of situations in early life, with which the worker may still unconsciously be in conflict, and which led him to seek this particular line of work. There is an awareness that the caring professions require special technical skills, but it is often forgotten that the main instrument for producing a beneficial effect on the patient is the professional *himself*. Professionally, he perceives this potential, and tries to devote himself to serving as an instrument, hoping unconsciously to confirm that he has enough 'internal goodness' to repair harm in others. This is a source of enthusiasm and devotion, but simultaneously it causes a great deal of anxiety, and frequently leads to 'burnout'. Indeed, success in caring that is attained through using the love or goodness that one has within greatly strengthens the capacity to act constructively. But failure, or even limited success, is experienced as showing some inner deficiency, and is intolerable (Roberts, 1980).

Non-Psychiatric Professionals

During the 1970s, as part of the counterculture movement, the power of psychiatrists came under fire. Parallel to this phenomenon, in the previous decade, some other occupational groups in the mental health field had begun to transform themselves into professions.

Since the appearance of asylums, caring for the illnesses of the patients confined therein was assigned to physicians, who only later became interested in their mental problems, thus becoming the first 'psychiatrists'. The custody and 'care' of patients in these asylums was the charge of ill-paid guardians from the lower classes. In many of these institutions which were in the hands of the church, members of the clergy took care of the mental patients. Saint John of God decided to educate these carers in treating them humanely, so that he was a precursor of what would later come to be called 'moral treatment'.

It was, however, the experience of the two World Wars that made manifest the need to provide specific training in mental health principles to those who were in charge of caring for patients with these disorders, especially general practitioners and psychiatric nurses. Thus, the professional identify of nurses, social workers, occupational therapists, and others received social recognition, and they began to draw up training programmes for their activities and, in some places, acquire a certain degree of autonomy vis-à-vis physicians.

General Practitioners

Medicine has long had a particular power ('medical domination') similar to that of priests and politicians (Max Weber, cited by Gracia, 1996).

This power was based on 'corporate government': define what illness is; determine who should be subjected to examination to see if he is ill; control the therapeutic processes. As Gracia puts it (1996), 'the doctor has seen himself as a little king who acts with patients in an autonomous, unconditional fashion.... However, in today's society, where all of its individuals are autonomous moral agents, with different criteria regarding what is good and what is bad... the medical relationship, insofar as it is an interpersonal relationship... has become mechanical, plural, secularised, and conflictive'.

Indeed, the technification of medicine, with the demand for complex complementary explorations and teamwork, has made private practice increasingly difficult. Attempts at cost containment on the part of governments and insurance companies have led them to control the work of doctors (including psychiatrists), who have become anonymous cogs in a complex health care machine, with very little autonomy. They receive modest salaries, and find themselves subjected to abusive control of their prescription practices on the part of the administration, and to the influence of pharmaceutical companies, which sometimes leads them to make not very edifying concessions. Called into question by their clients, who are increasingly well informed and demanding, increasingly legally persecuted by malpractice suits, they have lost their former aura of prestige, which was the source of much of their therapeutic influence. All of this has led them to adopt excessively defensive attitudes, to the detriment of their relationship with patients and their families.

Be that as it may, doctors continue to be the professionals who are best prepared to detect and treat mental disorders, whether at the level of primary care (general practitioners, paediatricians) or a more specialised level (psychiatrists). In specialised services, neurologists have, for their part, developed a subspeciality, *behavioural neurology*, and they also treat dementia, as do geriatrists.

According to the Epidemiological Catchment Areas study, 19.1% of the population had suffered some DSM-III-R mental disorder in the previous 6 months. It is generally accepted that approximately one-third of the patients who consult a general practitioner present psychiatric symptoms, especially neurotic ones. Demand for mental health in a primary care area of a town like Barcelona was found to be nearly 10% of the population (Tizón, 1992).

However, general practitioners' ability to identify psychiatric patients is very low, gauged at approximately 60%. In a country like Spain, they refer an excessive number of patients to psychiatrists; if, on the other hand, they treat these patients themselves, they mainly prescribe psychopharmaceuticals and vitamins, which is not always the most appropriate approach.

The relationships between mental health and primary care staff (when they exist) are based on three models: *consultation*, *referral* and *liaison*. The consultation model involves discussing cases with the general practitioner, and proposing guidelines or recommendations. In the referral model, the general practitioner sends the patient with psychological problems to the mental health team, which sends him back once he has been treated, in order for the general practitioner to continue to handle the case. The liaison model (preferred by most professionals) involves a mental health team in the primary care system, together with the general practitioner.

The classic model of psychiatric practice has little value in a primary care setting (Guimón, 2001). However, a certain amount of dynamic training can be very helpful for general practitioners and paediatricians, in order to teach them to use simple psychotherapeutic techniques, and, above all, to acquire an ability to hold patients.

Other Non-Medical Practitioners

As we mentioned earlier, Gracia (1996) pointed out that medicine achieved the rank of a profession when it was able to autonomously fix its own norms of functioning. However, since the end of the 18th century, it is clear that the physician has had to share his power, to a certain extent, in order to continue to enjoy his privileges. 'This represented the step from a strictly monarchical phase to an oligarchic one. Paternalism and tyranny continued, or rather increased in intensity, since now not only the doctor was exercising them, but also the surgeon and the pharmacist'.

Psychiatric Nurses

A psychiatric nurse is, according to the WHO (WHO, 2001) a person who has graduated from a recognised, university-level nursing school, and who has undergone further training to specialise in psychiatry, in a programme recognised by the competent authorities, and who works in the psychiatric field.

Today, around the world there is major shortage of well-trained nursing personnel, and there is not a psychiatric nursing corps with universal standards. Indeed, there is a wide range of occupations that, in Spain for example, correspond to at least five functions of psychiatric nursing: carers, psychiatric nurses' aids, members of religious orders, non-specialist nurses, and nurses who are specialised in psychiatry.

Nurses are the most numerous professionals in the field of mental health. According to WHO statistics (WHO, 2001), there is an average of 12.3 nurses and a median of 2 nurses per 100,000 inhabitants. In Southeast Asia, 97% of the population has access to at least 1 psychiatric nurse per

100,000 inhabitants, but also in the eastern Mediterranean, more than 63% have access to the same proportion. In Southeast Asia the median is 0.16 per 100,000, whereas in Europe it is 27.5, and in the wealthier countries, 33.5.

The ratio of psychiatric nurses to psychiatrists is 3 to 1 in the Americas and Europe, whereas it is 8 to 1 in Africa and Southeast Asia. Nurses are especially important in providing home care, and their numbers need to grow, and their training improve.

The Birth of a Profession

The first true schools of psychiatric nursing arose in Germany in 1836, and the United States in 1870, but it was not until the 1950s that this sort of training became generalised, although such a school was founded in the Spain in 1930 (Franco, 2000).

Indeed, in clinical practice, there are hardly any specialised nurses holding positions in psychiatric centres. The vast majority work at inpatient hospital units, and there are practically no psychiatric nurses working in the community. Therefore, it is essential for future professional training to be more oriented towards working in the community.

The Activities of Psychiatric Nurses

General Activities

Nursing school graduates must be able to carry out a series of activities, which are described in a number of standard professional manuals.

In hospital psychiatric departments, nurses are in charge of admitting patients, filling out the necessary registration sheets for hospitalising the patient. Once this has been done, the nursing personnel must make sure that the patient is well received (e.g., showing him the physical space where he is going to move about, noting his reactions to being admitted). If the unit context allows it, and always respecting patients' need for privacy and confidentiality, the nurse may participate in some of the interviews that are carried out, in order to later collaborate in the teams decisions.

The nurse should then plan how care is to be given in order to satisfy the patient's basic needs, ensure security and risk prevention, and note any kind of incidents. In rehabilitation units, the nurse should collect data on the patient through his family, and collaborate in establishing the patient's needs before embarking on any rehabilitation and social reinsertion programme.

The Helping Relationship

The work of psychiatric nurses differs from work carried out in other clinical fields (Franco, 2000), due to the very special attention given to the interpersonal relations between the nurse and the patient based on a 'helping relationship'. This relationship has characteristics different from those of the social relationships that are usually established with other people, insofar as the objectives that they aim to accomplish are concerned, and the involvement of those who intervene, as well as in their precise limits regarding both time of duration and the phases that the process entails.

As many psychiatric patients present problems in relational areas, it is difficult to achieve efficient communication able to obtain the objectives proposed—but when it occurs, it enables the patient to acquire a different perspective regarding himself and his problems, which can have a therapeutic effect that cannot be produced outside of this professional framework.

Nurses interact with patients 24 hours a day, in all aspects of daily life—feeding, games, hygiene. The relationship established has to serve the patient as a model for acquiring different patterns of functioning, to increase his autonomy and adaptive capacity.

The interpersonal aspect, then, is an essential part of their work; but the nurse's participation should be less intense, on an emotional level, than in a personal relationship. Besides these more 'everyday' interactions, in which a helping relationship is produced, nurses should, in the context of patients' day-to-day experiences, set guidelines for behaving and programme a series of periodical interviews, where a more specifically therapeutic process is produced. In order to do this, nursing professionals should have training that enables them to respond to patients needs, which demands, in any case, having better knowledge of themselves.

Psychologists

According to the WHO atlas (2001), a psychologist in the mental health sector is a graduate of a recognised university-level psychology programme, who has had special training in clinical psychology. Psychologists should be licensed to practice by the competent authorities (according to the regulations of their respective countries) and work within a mental health framework. There is an average of 6.43 psychologists per 100,000 inhabitants, and a median of 0.4 (showing a very wide standard deviation).

In Africa and southern Asia, 90% of the population has access to less than 1 psychologist per 100,000 inhabitants, but even in Europe, nearly half of the population also has less than 1. The mean in economically disadvantaged countries is 0.4 psychologists per 100,000 inhabitants, compared with 26.7 in rich countries. In some countries, no data is available regarding the number of psychologists practising different activities, such as diagnosis or readaptation, which are the most important tasks that they carry out. In any case, their numbers are insufficient, and although many countries train a large number of psychologists, a great many of them do not then practise in the mental health field. Psychologists' activities centre on co-operating in establishing a diagnosis, and in psychotherapy. In most countries, these professionals play a leading role in research, since their programme of study at university prepares them better than others for this work.

Social Workers

The WHO atlas (2001a) defines social workers in the mental health field as being graduates of a recognised university-level social work programme, licensed to practice by the competent authorities (according to the regulations of their respective countries), and who work in the mental health field.

Their average number worldwide is 8.64 per 100,000 inhabitants (with a median of 0.3, a large standard deviation). More than 90% of the population in Africa and the eastern Mediterranean has access to less than 1 social worker per 100,000 inhabitants, and the same is true for 63% of the population in Europe, although the region's average is 2.35. In economically disadvantaged countries, the average is 0.03, whereas in rich countries it is 25.5 per 100,000. No data is available regarding their distribution in different professional settings, such as hospitals, outpatient clinics, and home treatment.

Social workers' activities, in most countries, focus on co-operating in patients' social and occupational concerns, helping them and their families through the intricate pathways to accessing medical and psychiatric services. In addition, today, psychotherapeutic functions are increasingly delegated to them, above all in rehabilitation and home-care programmes.

Community nurses and social workers also take pride of place in providing care to chronic psychiatric patients living in the community, whether in half-way houses, residences, outpatient clinics, or the patients' home. Usually, these patients are more or less dependent on their families, lacking in rehabilitating resources, and they represent a considerable burden on their environment, which increases discrimination against them. These professionals can provide them with a permanent means of contacting a therapeutic team, which contributes to their compliance with prescriptions. They are also in a position of provide information, and to educate the patients' family and others in his setting.

Occupational Therapists

Occupational therapy had its origins in the field of social work. Indeed, Eleanor Clarke Slangle, a social worker interested in the negative effects of inactivity on mental patients during their time in hospital, developed tasks to keep them occupied, the responsibility for which became a specific post in mental institutions. In the United States, the psychiatrist and psychoanalyst Adolf Meyer (Meyer, 1957) provided occupational therapy with its own theoretical basis, hypothesising that an adequate balance in vital rhythms (rest, work, play, and sleep) is basic for mental health. Another psychiatrist, William Rusch Dunton, introduced occupational therapy as a treatment for mental patients in Baltimore in 1895. In Britain, Henderson also used this approach during World War I.

Soon, psychoanalytical theorists advanced the view that these activities, besides keeping the patient busy and entertained, have a high communicative value: they make it possible to open up a space for dialogue, detect the patient's ego resources, and observe the difficulties that he finds in relation to his activities. In addition, since the activities are carried out in a group context, they facilitate patients' integration through a 'co-existence without demands', which favours the participants' spontaneous expression of their feelings. These programmes have integrated the findings from child psychotherapy regarding the therapeutic value of play.

PARTICIPATION IN PRIMARY PREVENTION

McGorry (2000) pointed out that until 1960, dynamic psychotherapy was the prevalent treatment for psychosis, but it later lost favour, and training of personnel in this field dropped off. Training was then more oriented towards a 'dehumanising and inefficient behaviouralism', and later cognitive aspects were added as a compromise. In recent years, there has been a rebirth in interest regarding dynamic treatments, because of findings regarding their efficacy in certain disorders. Although there were pioneers in early intervention for schizophrenia, such as Sullivan (1927), only in recent years has their optimism become consolidated, especially in the Scandinavian countries (Alanen et al., 2000).

Early Intervention Programmes

Indeed, it was in Scandinavia that Johannenssen et al. (2000), assessed an early intervention programme that they developed for reducing the duration of untreated psychoses (DUP), using public information campaigns regarding methods for recognising early warning symptoms, with positive results. In Finland, Alanen (Alanen et al., 2000) successfully introduced an integrated model (mainly following a dynamic-systemic psychotherapeutic approach) for early treatment of schizophrenia, working intensely with their families and carrying out house calls. The incidence of schizophrenia fell from 24.6 cases per 100,000 inhabitants during 1986–1989 to 10.4 in the 1990–1994 period of the programme. Of the schizophrenics who had previously been hospitalised, 40% were treated as outpatients.

Interest in these programmes has led to the creation of the International Society for the Psychological Treatment of the Schizohrenias and Other Psychoses (ISPS), and the Early Psychoses Prevention and Intervention Centre (EPPIC) Programme in Australia.

Psychotherapeutic Treatments in Primary Care

Formal treatments are very difficult to apply in primary health care (Goldberg et al., 2001), so they should be undertaken in 'secondary' units. In primary care, new strategies need to be applied (Coderch, 1991; Perez Sanchez, 1996), such as brief and focused psychotherapy, support therapy, specific brief interventions for working through mourning, psychological follow-up, psychotherapeutic flash processes, and so on. There are mixed techniques, with a psychoanalytical orientation, incorporating behavioural, cognitive-behavioural, or psychodynamic techniques, e.g., protocols for functional enuresis and relaxation techniques.

Tizón recommends using so-called 'flash techniques' in daily clinical practice, which were mentioned at the end of their lives by the husband-and-wife team of the Balints.

REFERENCES

Ainsworth, M. (1969). Object relations, dependency and attachment: a theoretical review of the mother–infant relationship. *Child Development*, 40, 969–1025.

Alanen, Y., Lehtinen, V., Lehtinen, K., et al. (2000). The Finnish integrated model for the early treatment of schizophrenia and related psychoses. In B. Martindale, A. Bateman, M. Crowe, and F. Margison (Eds.), *Psychosis. Psychological approaches and their effectiveness*. London: Gaskell.

Bion, W. (1959). *Experiences in groups, and other papers*. New York: Basic Books.

Coderch, J. (1991). *Psiquiatría dinámica* (5th ed.). Barcelona: Herder.

Franco, J. (2000). *Memoria*. Universidad del País Vasco, Bilbao.

Goldberg, D., Mann, A., and Tylee, A. (2001). Primary care. In G. Thornicroft and G. Szmukler (Eds.), *Textbook of community psychichiatry*. New York: Oxford University Press.

Gracia, D. (1996). El poder médico. In P. Ridruejo , A. Medina and J. L. Rubio (Eds.), *Psicologia médica*. Madrid: McGraw Hill Interamericana.

Guimón, J. (2001). Scope and Limitations of Psychonalysis in Clinical Psychiatry. In *Challenges of psychoanalysis in the 21st century*. New York: Kluwer Academic.

Johannessen, J. O., Larsen, T. K., McGlashan, T., and Vaglum, P. (2000). Early intervention in psychosis: the TIPS project, a multi-centre study in Scandinavia. In B. Martindale,

A. Bateman, M. Crowe, and F. Margison (Eds.), *Psychosis. Psychological approaches and their effectiveness*. London: Gaskell.
Klein, M. (1948). Mourning and its relation to manic-depressive states. In M. Klein (Ed.), *Contributions to Psychoanalysis* 1921–1945. London: Hogarth Press.
McGorry, P. (2000). Psychotherapy and recovery in early psycosis: a core clinical and research challenge. In B. Martindale & A. Bateman & M. Crowe & F. Margison (Eds.), *Psycosis. Psychological Approaches and their Effectiveness* (pp. 266–293). London: Gaskell.
Meyer, A. (1957). *Psychobiology: A science of man*. Springfield, Illinois: C.C. Thomas.
Perez Sanchez, A. (1996). *Prácticas psicoterapéuticas*. Barcelona: Paidos.
Roberts, J. P. (1980). Destructive processes in a therapeutical community. *International Journal of Therapeutical Communities*, 1 (3), 159–170.
Roberts, V. Z. (1994). The self-assigned impossible task. In A. Obholzer and V. Z. Roberts (Eds.), *The unconscious at work*. New York: Routledge.
Rogow, A. A. (1970). *The psychiatrists*. New York: Putnam's Sons.
Segal, H. (1988). *Introduction to the work of Melanie Klein*. London: Karnac and the Institute of Psycho-Analysis.
Sullivan, H. S. (1927). The onset of schizophrenia. *American Journal of Psychiatry*, 105, 135–139.
Tizón, J. L. (1992). *Atención primaria en Salud Mental*. Barcelona: Doyma.
Weiss, M. F. (1994). Children's attitudes toward the mentally ill: an eight-year longitudinal follow-up. *Psychol. Rep.*, 74 (1), 51–56.
WHO. (2001). *Atlas. Resources humaines consacrées à la santé mentale dans le monde*. Geneva: WHO.

26

Psychiatrists

From Sorcerers to Bureaucrats

WHAT IS A PSYCHIATRIST?

People with little direct knowledge often have a highly confused image of the psychiatrist, confusing him with other medical specialists, such as neurologists, or even members of other professions, such as psychologists. The enormous range of tasks that the psychiatrist has to carry out today adds to this confusion. Indeed, in accordance with the different theoretical orientations discussed in previous chapters, psychiatrists fulfil tasks that are highly varied. Some turn their attentions to the ultramicroscopic study of specific areas of the brain, or to the biochemical analysis of the organic moods of patients suffering from mental illnesses they rarely ever get the chance to see. Others try to modify a subject's inappropriate behaviour using conditioning techniques, with or without regard for the specific biological substrates affecting this behaviour. Still others consider the unconscious contents of the verbal communication of isolated patients or those in groups, in an attempt to modify their personalities. There are also those who study the social evolution of the population of a given area, in order to devise detailed preventive programmes for mental disorders in a particular community. And even if they are less numerous today, some specialists still persist in trying, through their political activism, to change the state of a society which they consider to be alienating for the individual, and to eradicate mental illness through purely utopian ideals. All of these specialists consider themselves psychiatrists, even if their professional profiles are decidedly different.

A Sociological Priesthood

Priests, because of their sacramental calling, are endowed with an exceptional 'role' and 'status' which they share with the members of two other groups in the so-called sociological 'orders' that can be compared with the priesthood, i.e., those with political power and physicians. Indeed for many primitive peoples, physicians are confused with priests, to the extent that both are divine representatives, and hold the power over the life and death of the body and soul in their hands.

According to Gracia (1996), it is this sacerdotal sociological stereotype that gave birth to the *professions*. Thus the judiciary is a profession, as is the practice of medicine and as a corollary, psychiatry. On the other hand, carpentry, plumbing, gardening or financial management are *occupations*, or duties. It is only the so-called liberal professions, the bar, medicine, and so on, which are said to function according to a sacerdotal sociological stereotype. This bestows them with the power to create their own norms and the three consequent powers: social power, political power, and moral power.

As mentioned in chapter 25, the social body accepts the notion that those who exert duties are always motivated by interest—which is usually financial—but professionals (such as lawyers or priests) are expected to act out of *altruism*. The role they play within the social body is so important that it cannot be paid in money, which is why they do not receive formal payment for their services, but symbolic quantities charged with the notion of honour, or *honoraria*. Carr-Saunders and Wilson (1933, quoted in Gracia, 1996) already considered the dichotomy between *occupations* and the *liberal professions* or intellectual professions as artificial and socially harmful. It has since been suggested that in fact, the differences between *occupations* and *professions* are only of a motivational (or ethical) type in institutional (or social) terms.

Whatever the case may be, the shift from simple occupation to profession is highly valorised but very progressive. For Bullough (quoted by Gracia, 1996), medicine, which, even at the time of the ancient Siberian shaman, had a technical content, obtained university status in the Middle Ages, and only became a true profession toward the end of the 19th century, having developed a sufficiently scientific basis for its work to appear superior to that of irregular cures'. Bullough adds that, in the process of constituting itself as a profession, the occupational group tends to delegate certain, more mundane jobs to other groups or individuals, thus increasing division and differentiation within the same domain. As we shall see later, in the context of mental health activities, many occupational groups are in the process of trying to convert themselves into professions today.

A Qualified Sorcerer

The magical concept soon gave way to the medical concept of mental illness, but certain traces of ancient magical concepts have persisted in the accoutrements and activities of psychiatrists down the centuries. Let us recall, in the middle of the 19th century, particular figures such as Gall and Spurzhein with their doctrine of phrenology, or that of Messmer, the precursor of hypnosis. Moreover, it is easy to see the vast extent of magical perceptions that appear in certain ways of approaching mental illness today. Psychiatrists attached to asylums wore a special bonnet until quite recently, in some places, attributing to their esoteric powers. For the man in the street, we still have extraordinary powers, and it is rare to find someone who is not afraid of the psychiatrist revealing the deepest secrets of the soul, even among our own friends and acquaintances.

Behind most of the criticism and jokes about the psychiatrist's job, many uneducated people hide a magical idealisation: they are still quite prepared to marvel at modern shamans. It must be said, however, that this veil of admiration is largely responsible for the healing power of doctors in general, and of psychiatrists in particular.

What Should a Psychiatrist Be?

Monbour (1984), in trying to define the professional profile of psychiatrists, compared the different types of psychiatric practice and the various underlying ideologies of several mental health systems. In terms of the types of practice adhered to in all the countries studied (United States, Britain, Scandinavia, France, Benelux, Switzerland, Austria, Germany, and what was then the Soviet Union) a common tendency was found: that of fulfilling a wide range of functions, tending toward what the Americans call *comprehensiveness*. This refers to the idea that psychiatrists should be able to offer various kinds of services, regardless of the presenting mental problem, to whomever needs it. Psychiatrists are thus supposed to be able to diagnose and treat everything from organic disturbances, to psychoses, neuroses, mental retardation, and much more. Within this broad perspective, psychiatrists must apply a large number of somatic treatments, based on psychotherapy or sociotherapy or re-education, or must act in an advisory capacity for numerous organisations. They have to take responsibility for children, adolescents and adults from all socio-economic categories, regions and races; they also have to practise in hospitals, outpatient consultation units, institutions, re-education services, community mental health centres, and social institutions. This professional polymorphism is also inherent in the psychiatric sectors. It demands that a group of services and the necessary specialists take responsibility for a specific zone in the region.

Although there is overall agreement in these countries as to the 'global' attitude of the psychiatrist, there is considerable disagreement regarding how this should be is put into practice: for some, it is the way in which the individual psychiatrist operates; for others, it is conducted within the framework of the institution by highly qualified staff. In the United States, Canada, Britain, the Netherlands, and France, the view is that the psychiatrist should himself follow the principle of 'comprehensiveness'. The system followed in socialist countries, on the other hand, insists on psychiatry being sectorised. In this case, the psychiatrist usually practises in a regional community centre for mental health, offering global services, but with doctors and staff who are highly specialised in certain areas.

Monbour found that in all of the countries studied, there is a general tendency to separate psychiatry from neurology in the exercise of psychiatry. In countries like France, the Benelux countries, Germany, and the former Eastern Bloc countries, neurology and psychiatry used to be closely linked, but during the 1960s 'revolution' in France, there were separated. This was also true of Germany and the Netherlands, although it is still possible to specialise in both branches today. This possibility also exists in Austria and Belgium, but in reality the physician tends to specialise in one or the other.

Lambo (1982), for his part, said that if, in the developing countries, the psychiatrist has asserted himself and acquired political power like that of any other important branch of medicine, this is partly due to the fact that the psychiatrist has effectively acted in the role of 'doctor', and is seen and considered as a physician.

As we noted earlier, attitudes to the role of the psychiatrist in society and thus to the profile he should adopt, have changed profoundly in recent years.

For Langsley and Hollender (Langsley et al., 1988), if the psychiatrist has to be defined in terms of his action, it is also vital to decide which attitudes (in terms of their affective and cognitive connotations) and which skills he needs to possess or acquire. Considerable efforts have already been made to define these explicitly or implicitly. In the aftermath of increasing media interest in trials concerning the psychiatric malpractice, the public began to question the automatic assumption that anyone who presents himself as a competent specialist, was to be trusted at face value. Consumer organisations aroused public concern about the quality and safety of medical practice. Moreover, the rapid progress made in psychiatric treatment and the 'breakthroughs' in knowledge have not always been perfectly 'metabolised' by psychiatrists.

In response to public concern, ongoing medical education programmes were developed, as indispensable if psychiatrists were to continue practising their speciality after a certain period of time. However, no real guidelines exist yet defining the skills a psychiatrist is supposed to have. Traditionally, the psychiatrist considers himself competent if he fulfils the educational requirements of his country. But as we will see, these requirements vary enormously from one country to another. So it would be advisable to define what a psychiatrist is, listing the measurable and definable skills and knowledge which residents should have acquired by the end of training. Accordingly, Yager and Pasnau (Yager et al., 1979) defined the training objectives inherent in the curriculum of residents at the University of California in Los Angeles. The association of programme directors for psychiatry residents in the United States prepared another list. For his part, Thompson (1979) published a series of 800 objectives.

To define the objectives considered as desirable by a wide group of specialists, in 1980, Langsley and Hollender (Langsley et al., 1982) conducted a survey among 430 professors and 430 psychiatrists in clinical practice. The skills most often cited by both groups of psychiatrists referred to the ability to evaluate patients. They also referred to the ability to judge whether hospitalisation was necessary, to carry out diagnosis, assess the risks of suicide or criminal acts, to formulate the problems of patients presenting for consultation and the use of laboratory tests. In a sizeable proportion of responses, skills related to treatment were deemed to be important. Among the responses relating to the type of personality the psychiatrist should have, most referred to reliability, integrity, interest in patients, an understanding of the problems of transfer and counter-transfer, and objectivity.

In view of the evolution that the psychiatric profession had undergone in the 1980s as a result of biological psychiatry, new approaches to psychotherapy, and the systems of payment for services through various intermediary organisations, Langsley and Young (Langsley et al., 1988) repeated the study published by Langsley and Hollender (Langsley et al., 1982). The questions that elicited more than 50% agreement were those pertaining to evaluation, treatment, and the personality of the psychiatrist. Among the 25 questions which elicited 50% of agreement, 8 referred to evaluation, treatment and personality; diagnosis and treatment were thus the most important skills in the eyes of those surveyed, but differences did come to light in relation to the results obtained in 1980. Moreover, in the 1987 survey, the questions referring to the personality of the psychiatrist (knowledge of counter-transfer, personal idiosyncrasies and the capacity to show interest, tact and understanding) were listed higher. Treatment skills were still considered important, but in 1987 other skills appeared (crisis intervention and short-term psychotherapy); as for psychopharmacology, this was listed in 13th, as opposed to 8th, position.

Bureaucratisation of the Psychiatric Profession

Due partly to economic recession and the search for maximum efficiency in the health care system, the managed care movement was launched in an effort to cut costs, which had risen dramatically in recent years (but, to be honest, not only in psychiatry). No one questions the absolute need for this policy to curtail health expenditure, but it is equally clear that it has very often been conducted in such an inappropriate manner that the resistance it has met, especially among medical staff, has resulted in the system becoming less effective. Health centres have particularities that render them far more complex that any others. This is even more obvious in the case of psychiatric institutions; research carried out in the field of health sociology has demonstrated this for over thirty years. It is impossible to manage a hospital like a tool factory, and a support system like a supermarket network. In the case of psychiatry, like any other special institution (e.g., prisons), inappropriate management can not only cause it to function less effectively, but may also represent an institutional step backward, with unforeseen consequences, as described by Kernberg (1979).

The Executive Psychiatrist

Marcos says (Marcos et al., 1988), we are now seeing a clear trend toward the bureaucratisation of organisations specialising in mental hygiene. The norms of care are becoming specialised and balanced, quality controls are increasing, the activities of mental health specialists and administrators are better understood and are becoming more predictable, routine, repetitive, and programmed—all of which accounts for this bureaucratisation. According to Marcos true physicians need to be almost as expert in diagnosing the problems of organisation which hamper the smooth operation of services, as they are in diagnosing the state of their patients' health.

In today's *professional psychiatric bureaucracies*, the *operational base* is made up almost entirely of psychiatrists themselves. The specificity of their task is explained by their almost total independence in developing their activities, an independence that they defend jealously. Any control of quality in their personal work, which is particularly difficult in terms of the results of treatment, falls to their peers. Those in charge usually avoid any outside interference, and experience has shown the resistance which is very difficult to get beyond, resulting from these attempts. But as Marcos says

(Marcos et al., 1989), in the end those in charge cannot avoid resorting to the bureaucratic model. It offers a more comprehensive model of organisation than the non-bureaucratic alternatives. We expect psychiatrists in their executive role, to participate in the decision making process in planning and controlling services and in hiring the most appropriate staff. We expect psychiatrists who fulfil support roles, to be innovatory and to implement new knowledge and psychiatric techniques. Finally, and most important of all, executive psychiatrists need leadership qualities and to integrate the different sub-systems and components of the service".

Even in fields like research, the psychiatrist's skill as a bureaucrat is essential. Thus, according to Burke et al. (1986), the clinical researcher requires four basic characteristics: an essentially scientific orientation, a command of precise techniques, certain values and drives, and administrative skills. These authors thus indicate that even a small research assignment becomes a 'major enterprise'. The researcher has to become the effective manager of an entire series of tasks linked to the project, a whole group of specialists and assistants, and several local and national institutions. Administrators who manage other businesses receive specific training in schools specialised in business science or public administration. The efficient scientist also has to be able to show a high level of administrative skill, without the slightest former training. Moreover, efficient management entails much more than efficient administration. The researcher psychiatrist also has to motivate people and make sure they sustain their enthusiasm and curiosity.

What Will Tomorrow's Psychiatrist Be Like?

As Pichot (1982) has said, the essence of the psychiatrist is unique, and it would be inadvisable to train 'first-class' and 'second-class' specialists. Having said this, the methods adopted and the training dispensed should not be identical for industrialised countries, where there is more than one psychiatrist per 10,000 inhabitants, and some third World countries, where the proportion of psychiatrists is one for several million inhabitants.

Clearly, the same predictions cannot be made for different countries with distinct situations dependant upon very different socio-economic, political and sanitary conditions.

As regards the future professional profile, it seems that the number of psychiatrists will stabilise or decline in Western countries like the United States; the number of positions available will thus be greater and only the most viable will be filled. The number of psychiatrists will diminish in the public services, as it appears that newly qualified psychiatrists will tend to practice in the public sector on a part-time basis. As costs always have to be contained, hospitals will tend to take on specialists available for part-time work.

Private services will certainly increase, even if psychiatrists tend to be in competition here with less expensive mental health specialists. Competition, the managed care policy, the reduction in the number of psychiatrists, all of these elements will create a context in which the psychiatrist will be given greater participation in activities such as administration, advisory tasks, and teaching. Research efforts are also likely to slacken, due to worldwide reductions in budget allocation in this field, over recent years.

As a conclusion to the preceding paragraphs, several authors have stated that, in spite of the spectacular developments in psychiatry as a whole, resources are likely to diminish in the future. They thus emphasise the vital importance of developing the specific skills of the psychiatrist, and the need for research into the factors concerned in exercising the profession.

THEORETICAL AND PRACTICAL ORIENTATIONS OF CONTEMPORARY PSYCHIATRISTS

Theoretical Orientation

A number of works provide information on the theoretical orientation of psychiatrists in several countries, based on surveys of their attitudes toward the most important aspects of their profession. Overall, the biological model has made remarkable progress.

Representations of the Future of the Psychiatrist

Beitman et al. (1984), in a study of psychiatrists in Washington state, showed that in some areas of psychiatry that are important in their own right, there is tenuous interest and little consideration. This is the case for psychosomatics, psychogeriatrics, mental handicap, drug addiction, alcoholism, hospital work, and intermediary structures. As Fenton et al. (1984), pointed out, this absence of interest and information is prejudicial in view of the changes that have taken place in recent years on a number of levels: an increase in the number of psychiatrists, diversification of the practice settings and patients, an expansion of the field of psychiatry, and changes in its rapport with somatic medicine, as well as changes in the insurance system and the health care system as a whole. To this must be added the changes that Langsley et al. (1988) noted during the 1980s, and which have taken place directly on the therapeutic level: the breakthrough of biological psychiatry, multiplication of psychotherapeutic approaches, new emphasis on shorter treatment and crisis intervention, and the arrival of other professionals to the sphere of psychiatry. These changes obviously have repercussions in terms of training at all levels, but they also have an effect on psychiatrists' duties, including clinical work as such, and modify relationships with their environment: medicine, social services, sociopolitical organisations, and the social system as a whole.

In a recent study of Swiss psychiatrists (Guimón, Fischer et al., 1997; Guimón, Goerg et al., 1997), we examined the main themes that emerged from the many proposals made in response to our questions on priority commitments in psychiatry, training, current problems, and outlook for development. We deduced that several areas were considered nonpriority. This is true in the case of research and development (mentioned by only 12% of psychiatrists), evaluation of quality of care (14%), increase in prevention activity (9%), and relations with other other professionals who have been introduced into the psychotherapeutic field (8%). Even if a slightly higher number insisted on the need to redefine and improve relationships between psychiatry and somatic medicine (18%), or referred to the increasing problems linked to the economy and the costs of the health system (19%), present difficulties and their possible extension into the future seem to be low-profile concerns among Swiss psychiatrists. At least, they do not figure highly among the concerns they reported.

A very different role is attributed to psychotherapy in different countries. In socialist countries, instructive, suggestive psychotherapy is practised. Britain and certain Scandinavian countries place more importance on sociotherapy and re-education. In France, Belgium, Austria, and Germany, the situation is shifting; although traditionally suggestive psychotherapy has raised only mild interest, more interest has been shown in psychoanalysis in France, Germany, and, to a lesser extent, in Austria.

The theoretical orientation of psychiatrists has been substantially modified in the last 20 years. Whereas at the beginning of the 1970s dynamic psychiatry prevailed in most Western countries, in the 1980s and 1990s the advance of the biological model has been impressive. Spectacular advances in biological research, the presence of psychiatrists in the new short-stay units of the general hospital, and the scant efficacy of community approaches have led to a remedicalisation of the psychiatric profession.

Swiss psychiatry presents a number of differences, compared with the findings on other countries. Firstly, there is the important role of psychoanalytically oriented psychotherapy, in addition to psychoanalysis and other analytic approaches at the family, couple, and group levels. In the public as well as in the private sector, more than 80% of psychiatrists employ this therapy. The only other example of psychotherapy assuming such large proportions is in the Cypres study (Cypres, 1978), but this only covered psychiatrists working in the outpatient sector, and was extended to cover all forms of psychotherapy, as opposed to solely the psychoanalytic form. The same applies to the findings of Yager et al. (1978) for psychiatrists trained between 1956 and 1975 at UCLA's Neuropsychiatric Institute, which showed 86% of them practising dynamic psychotherapy. Individual psychotherapy was only practised by 25% of Connecticut psychiatrists (Redlich and Kelert, 1978). Of Spanish psychiatrists working in the public sector, 21% made use of dynamic psychotherapy, compared with 41% of those in the private sector (Guimón, 1990). Insofar as members of the Texas Society of Psychiatric Physicians were concerned (Kane et al., 1992b), only 39% conducted out individual psychotherapy. These studies also point to the change which came about in the 1980s, when there was something of a switch towards brief and support therapies and away from longer, mainly psychoanalytically oriented therapies.

The vast majority of Swiss psychiatrists (Guimón et al., 1997), as we said earlier, also use biological treatments (mixed treatments 94%, pharmacotherapy 70%). Comparable findings have been recorded in the studies by Yager et al., where they were used by 63% of psychiatrists; by Kane and Harper, where 59% practise it. Olfson et al. (1994) found that 62% of the members of the APA prescribed medication.

The Practice of Psychiatry

Some Data

Regarding the practice of psychiatry in the different countries of the world, its position within a health system undergoing major changes has become an increasingly important topic of debate at several levels. As the context of most of these studies is restricted, most of the work cited provides only partial answers. This debate is limited by the scarcity of studies on psychiatric practices as they are conducted in countries as a whole. Only national studies provide a basis for generalising the results and conclusions on the psychiatric profession, providing a clear idea of the different psychiatric practices. These, limited to a recent period, include, for the United States, studies by Fenton (Fenton et al., 1984), Olfson (Olfson et al., 1994, a et b), Sullivan (Sullivan et al., 1993), and Bodkin et al. (1995); for Spain, by Guimón (Azcunaga et al., 1986; Guimón et al., 1987, Guimón, 1990); for Australia, by Wright (Wright et al., 1993) and Murray (Murray et al., 1993); for Britain, Brook (1976, 1978, 1981, 1984); for Switzerland, Guimón (Guimón et al., 1996; Guimón, Fischer et al., 1997; Guimón, Goerg et al., 1997; Guimón, 2002); for the developing countries, Lenz (1984).

The United States is where the greatest number of studies has been conducted on the practice of psychiatry in all its aspects. Some information on psychiatrists' practices became available at the end of the 1960s and early 1970s, when the APA conducted several surveys on geographical distribution, professional activities, and the setting in which psychiatrists practised at that time. But the studies tended to be limited. It was thus impossible to define general trends indicating where psychiatrists practised and the settings in which their professional activities were carried out. The APA conducted its original surveys during a period of expansion in the profession; at that time, 1 out of 10 qualified graduates from the Medical School took up residency in psychiatry and one physician out of 13 was in psychiatry.

In a more global study, Cypres (1978) found that during the 1970s psychiatrists spent 86% of their office time in psychotherapy and 25% in pharmacotherapy. Redlich and Kelert (Redlich et al., 1978), in a studied conducted on psychiatrists' activities in southern Connecticut, showed that the main psychiatric therapies consisted of individual psychotherapy (25%), pharmacology (25%), group therapy (20%), and family therapy (15%). Roughly 40% of patients seen in psychotherapy by psychiatrists also received psychotropic medication.

Yager et al. (1979) questioned psychiatrists trained in the framework of the residents programme at the Neuropsychiatric Institute of UCLA between 1956 and 1975 on the subject of their professional activities. Virtually all of them led careers with very diversified activities. Less than 50% spent over half their working hours in private practice, and over 75% had contact with the Medical School. After 1966, the proportion of graduates involved in psychoanalytical training was lower than for graduates before this date. However, more were undergoing personal psychotherapy. The new graduates had more often studied a subspeciality, and were more involved in an administrative or consultancy post, or group or family treatment. As for the importance given to the different types of treatment used in their daily practice, they ranked first as very important or important dynamic psychotherapy (86%), pharmacotherapy (63%), couple and family therapy (43%) and psychoanalysis (34%), and considered as less important electroshock therapy, behaviour therapy, group therapy and environmental therapy.

Several years later, Fenton et al. (1984) compared psychiatric practices in the years 1979–1980 and data on practices in the years 1964–1965, to try to examine the way in which the profession had evolved. In 1979, the average number of hours a psychiatrist worked per week was up to 48, with a slight increase from 44 in 1965. The number of psychiatrists practising between 1 and 34 hours in general hospital units, treating patients in a state of crisis had risen. Those practising from 1 to 24 hours in university positions, care units for crisis patients at psychiatric hospitals, and outpatient services had also increased.

A comparison of the two surveys shows psychiatry as a far more diversified profession in 1979 than it was 15 years earlier. In 1979 in the United States, psychiatrists practised in far more varied settings, and with a greater number of professional activities than previously. The authors gave speculative explanations of this phenomenon, in relation to the health care system, number of psychiatrists, and certain specific economic factors.

On the other hand, from 1965 to 1979, the number of psychiatrists increased from 15,500 to 30,000, and the number of work hours was easily doubled. Easier access to community mental health services and the increasing number of non-physician specialists in mental health, gave rise to a net increase in competition among psychiatrists. The profession seems to have adapted to the new circumstances, but also to the increase in competition, during the last ten years in the United States, by diversifying its activities. When the circumstances are favourable to private practice and there is strong demand from mental health organisations, psychiatrists are far less inclined to commit themselves to the various programmes, and so in order to maintain the continual presence of psychiatrists, it is necessary to call on part-time staff. Therefore, psychiatrists often devote more time to administrative, consulting, and teaching tasks; this may explain the marked increase in all of these activities between 1965 and 1979.

In the following decade, Beitman et al. (1984) published a survey on the daily clinical practices of 334 psychiatrists in Washington state, in which 48% described themselves as analytical, 27% as dynamic, 14% as biological, 8% as cognitive and 3% as existential. Psychiatrists devoted at least 50% of their time to individual psychotherapy, particularly of a psychoanalytical orientation. Those who practised in small towns engaged in very little family or group therapy. Half of the patients received pharmacological treatment, and 38% treatment combining pharmacotherapy and psychotherapy.

The results of our survey in Switzerland (Guimón, Fischer et al., 1997) obtained the following distribution of the therapeutic profiles: cognitive-behavioural practice, 9%; psychoanalytical practice, 24%; biological practice, 29%; general practice, 25.5%.

The psychiatrists nevertheless appeared to be dissatisfied, even with such a wide range of activities, and some hoped to intervene in more peripheral areas. In one survey (Guimón et al., 1997), a number of Swiss psychiatrists replied that they would be interested in intervening in the following areas, in descending order of interest (the figures in brackets represent the mean of their evaluation from 1 to 4): victims of violence

(3.4), parent/child relationships (3.3), psychological problems among prisoners (3.3), chronic pain (3.1), risk behaviour (3.0), loss of independence in the elderly (3.0), educational or training problems (2.9), and problems of immigrants (2.9).

Data is available for Britain, provided in particular by Brook (Brook et al., 1987), giving information on the number of psychiatry residents, the reasons why they chose this speciality, where they practice after completing training, and why they chose one subspeciality or another. One of the most interesting findings from the 1707 responses to a questionnaire that Brook sent to psychiatric consultants in Britain concerned the question of their theoretical psychiatric orientation. Of those questioned, 65% stated they were eclectic, 30% psychodynamic, and 5% organic.

A survey we conducted in Spain (Azcunaga et al., 1986) looked at the social setting in which Spanish psychiatrists practised, and their clinical activities. This study revealed that among Spanish psychiatrists, there is a great preference for combined public and private practice. Only 5% of specialists worked in children's mental health centres, whereas 18% were engaged in adult mental health centres, indicating a growth in this type of assistance. On average, Spanish psychiatrists devoted 30 hours a week to activities related to the state health care services, and 11 hours in private practice. The general profile of the activities carried out in the public sector setting differed considerably from that of the private sector. According to our findings, psychopharmacological treatment was the type most often used, followed by dynamically oriented psychotherapies. Family therapies represented another therapeutic process that was used quite often by Spanish psychiatrists. Although 69% of psychiatrists never used individual psychoanalysis, 14% nevertheless used it very often. Psychosurgery was the least used therapy, and electroshock treatment, conditioning and dynamic group psychotherapy were not often used.

Lenz (1984) studied the number of psychiatrists present in developing countries, and their proportion per 100,000 inhabitants, as well as the characteristics of the different types of training. According to this study, psychiatrists in developing countries were very unevenly distributed over the different continents. In all the countries, psychiatrists devoted most of their time to treating patients, but a considerable part of their time was taken up by teaching, supervising other health specialists, and planning and managing the services for which they were responsible.

A major proportion of psychiatrists from all these regions are trained in developed countries, which gives cause for thought (Leon, 1982): first, many of them wind up emigrating to developed countries, which offer them very good working and salary conditions, but which means an enormous loss for their home countries; and secondly, the training in developed countries is not necessarily well adapted to the situation in their countries of origin, for ethnic, social, economic, and cultural reasons.

Differences between Countries

The tendency to use combined therapies was reported by Redlich et al. (1978), who showed that roughly 40% of patients treated with psychotherapy in Connecticut also received medication, which proved to be a more effective combination and one which, according to these authors, should be proposed as a supplementary model in psychiatric training. The work of Beitman (Beitman et al., 1984) on psychiatrists in Washington state was also conducted in view of redefining the training programme in accordance with future needs. They found that 38% of the patients treated by the psychiatrists questioned received combined therapy, principally psychotherapy plus medication. The prescription of medication does not appear to be a discriminating feature between non-psychoanalytical psychiatrists and psychoanalysts. Indeed, Kane (Kane et al., 1992a) found no difference in recourse to anxiolytics and antidepressants.

Several studies also suggest that the work of the psychiatrist is now broken down into a wider number of activities conducted in a larger number of work settings. This diversification is a clear reflection of the changes that have occurred in the modalities of practice, since the same findings emerge in the studies conducted by Fenton (Fenton et al., 1984), and Olfson (Olfson, Pincus, and Dial, 1994; Olfson, Pincus, and Sabshin, 1994), both among psychiatrists who finished training a long time ago, and for those who finished more recently. For Dorwart (Dorwart et al., 1992), this diversification is increasingly taking the form of subspecialities in psychiatry. Regarding Switzerland, our results lead us to think that the same phenomenon is occurring here, because the psychiatrists of this country are engaged in an average of 3.4 different activities, representing a higher proportion than in the United States.

Switzerland appears—when compared with other countries—to be characterised by a sharper separation between the public and private sectors and by a higher frequency of exclusive private practice: we noted 37% of psychiatrists involved in both the private and public sectors, 33% exclusively in the public sector, and 30% exclusively in the private sector. According to the study by Yager et al. (1979), three-quarters of the psychiatrists engaged in private practice regularly collaborate with the psychiatric services. And 59% of Spanish psychiatrists work both in the public and private sectors, 37% in the public sector only and just 4% in the private sector only (Guimón J. et al., 1987). The structure of psychiatric practices in Australia seems close to that of Switzerland in that 32% of psychiatrists are engaged in exclusively private practice.

As other studies have shown, even though in the United States the main activity of psychiatrists was made up of direct contact with patients, there was a strong tendency to increase other activities (supervision, consulting, teaching, and training), and the work of the 'average' psychiatrist was seen to be divided into a higher number of activities carried out in a higher number of work settings. Thus, the average number of settings in which psychiatrists worked increased from 1.7 in 1965 to 2.3 in 1979, and the range of different activities from 2 to 2.7, a trend confirmed by Dorwart (Dorwart et al., 1992). According to the study by Yager et al. (1979), three-quarters of the psychiatrists engaged in private practice collaborated with university psychiatric services.

Private and Public Psychiatry in Switzerland

A national survey of psychiatrists that we conducted in Switzerland showed that almost a third (30%) of Swiss psychiatrists work solely in private practice; a fifth (22%), in addition to their private practice, also act as supervisors or consultants for colleagues or institutions for a limited number of hours a week, and 15% have activities in the private and public sectors in more or less equal proportions. Thus, two-thirds of psychiatrists are engaged, either exclusively or partially, in private practice. Of those who work in institutions, 15% are in the ambulatory/outpatient sector, 12% in hospital services and 6% work in both.

Private psychiatrists refer to the psychological model much more often than psychiatrists working in the public sector (47%/29%), whilst distancing themselves from the eclectic model (34%/48%). Adherence to a medical/medical-psychological model (12%/16%) or to a social model (7%/7%) is not frequent in both cases. In their theoretical orientations (measured globally by the degree of information in different areas of psychiatry, the interests of psychiatrists in diverse fields, reading of reviews and scientific journals, and membership in learned societies and professional and social associations), private psychiatrists show a very great interest in psychoanalysis. However, they are less oriented towards biology, research, and social aspects of psychiatry than psychiatrists working in the public sector.

A considerable number of the private psychiatrists work solely in private practice (44%). The others (56%), who can be considered as having a mixed practice, either work as consultants or supervisors for a limited number of hours a week or combine private practice and work in the public sector. In their clinical work, psychiatrists having a mixed practice are found more often than those working solely in private in the psychoanalytical practice profile (34%/24%) and less often in the other profiles.

As far as adherence to theoretical models is concerned, there is no difference between these two categories of psychiatrists. However psychiatrists having a mixed practice are more psychoanalytically oriented (degree of information, interests, and so on) than psychiatrists working solely in the private sector. Thus, private psychiatrists with a psychoanalytical orientation and having a mixed practice occupy a very important position as theoretical and therapeutic guarantors for the principles of psychoanalysis. It constitutes the most sure means of perpetuating the pre-eminence of psychoanalytical practice, and of ensuring through theoretical and practical training the renewal of generations of psychoanalytically oriented psychiatrists.

Comparisons between Different Countries

Switzerland, compared with other countries, seems to be characterised by a more clear-cut separation between public and private and a high frequency of exclusively private practice. 37% of psychiatrists are both in the private and public sector, 33% exclusively in the public and 30% exclusively in the private. According to the previously cited study by Yager et al. in the United States, three-quarters of the psychiatrists established in private practice regularly collaborate with academic activities, and 59% of Spanish psychiatrists work both in the private and public sector, 37% exclusively in the public and only 4% exclusively in the private sector (Guimón et al., 1987). The structure of psychiatric practice in Australia is close to that of Switzerland, since 32% of psychiatrists are in exclusively private practice.

Private psychiatrists work less hours a week than psychiatrists in the public sector (mean number of hours: 44 versus 54 hours). However, they devote a higher percentage of their working time to clinical work (69% of their time versus 44%), and they spend much less time in meetings, teaching and research (6% versus 53%).

Psychiatrists mainly work with individuals, but this tendency is much stronger among private psychiatrists: 86% of their clinical activities involve individuals, compared with 64% only among psychiatrists working in the public sector. Work with couples and families (11% versus 25%) or with groups (2% versus 5%) represents a much smaller percentage of their clinical activities.

Lazarus (Lazarus et al., 1996) thinks that the system of managed care will redefine the traditional roles in health networks. Practitioners who are not physicians will take greater responsibility in caring for the patient. The tension observed between psychiatrists and non-medical therapists also exists between certain physicians and certain professional groups whose practice and skills are similar, for example, to those of residents, practitioner-nurses and chiropractors.

According to Fink (1993), 'dissension between psychiatrists is negative and an appearance of unity is decisive in reaching the prime objective, that of a non-discriminatory health coverage for the patient.' Psychiatrists must be united, not only among themselves, but also with the rest of the medical profession. To divide up into groups with political interests will only reinforce the pressure interested legislators place on exploiting the divergent interests of physicians.

Physicians must have a greater participation in management and be represented in a more adequate manner at the national political level. It is important, according to Creager (1993), to ensure the co-operation between providers and payers of services in certain fields such as utilisation review. In certain regions, 'the relationship between supervising psychiatrists and attending psychiatrists has deteriorated to a state of crisis. Relationships can, however, be improved if the two parties adhere to certain basic rules. Consulting psychiatrists must learn to communicate in an effective manner by offering objective therapeutic goals which can be evaluated in layman's language. They should not be defensive or feel that they are forced to deform facts to prove their ability. Attending psychiatrists must not become discourteous with their peers during telephone reviews. Psychiatrists must avoid dragging patients and their families into conflicts with managed-care companies and their employees, trying to prevent altercations arising on questions of insurance.'

According to Lazarus (1996), the question of managed care is probably that which most divides professionals in psychiatry. Over the last decades, the death of psychiatry has been predicted by those who think that it is impossible to solve the problems of the mentally ill. But, as Fink (1993) puts it, 'In the early days of psychiatry, when there were few effective treatments and psychiatrists often struggled simply to keep patients alive through asylum, there may have been some rationale for such dire predictions.' But not today after a decade which has seen the development of the most important progress in the history of psychiatry and which draws us closer to other medical specialities.... At the end of the day, we continue to bear witness to the process of restructuration of the health-care system, a restructuration which could easily lead us to become the objects of reform rather than its standard-bearer, if we do not act in a decisive manner, by using an infallible strategy in the days to come. The quickest means of losing our independence consists in ignoring or even rejecting (because we think them inoffensive) the economic and political forces which are remodelling the health-care system at every level.... This is not the time to get emotional, but rather to keep a level head'.

THE IMAGE OF PSYCHIATRY: CONSEQUENCES FOR THE IDENTITY OF PSYCHIATRISTS

A thorough reflection has to be made on the need to strengthen the professional identity of future psychiatrists in the course of their training. Lacking this, psychiatry as a medical speciality is at the risk of disappearing within the next two decades.

Indeed, the limits of the role of psychiatrists are becoming increasingly vague. In the 1970s, within the context of the community psychiatry movement, the different specialities of mental health have mixed and confused their various areas of activity. Consequently, in the course of the last two decades, psychiatrists have increasingly abandoned the practice of psychotherapy to the benefit of others professionals, especially psychologists. An exception has to be made in Switzerland where specialists' titles (as much in adult as in child psychiatry) are double specialisations in psychiatry and in psychotherapy. This is also the case in Germany. On the other hand, in some countries, psychologists have developed their biological knowledge and have also lobbied for the right to prescribe medicines. Because of this, a specific programme was created in the United States. Similarly, a new speciality was born in psychology departments, called Psychology of Health, which invaded an important sector of psychophysiological medicine, until then traditionally the domain of 'liaison' psychiatrists. Furthermore, general practitioners are increasingly becoming educated in psychiatry, and in some American universities, for example, they have tried to create a speciality in psychiatry for internists.

On the other hand, to the lack of definition of the role of psychiatrists are to be added two other factors that entail an aggravation of the identity crisis: confusion regarding the theoretical model, and the excessive size of the field.

Confusion about the Theoretical Model

If we observe the attitude of psychiatrists in a country, a region, or even simply within the framework of a treatment centre, we note that they have different ideas on matters with which they deal due to the size of the theoretical framework to which they have to refer. The development of a typology allows the definition of the main tendencies or models to which we referred above (chapters 1, 2).

As noted above, many studies provide insight into the theoretical orientation of psychiatrists in a number of countries, based on replies to questionnaires regarding their attitudes with respect to various important aspects of their profession.

In summary, we can assert that in the course of the last twenty years, the theoretical orientation of psychiatrists underwent deep modifications (Guimón, 1998). In the early 1970s, the psychodynamic model predominated in many leading countries, and orientations aimed at psycho-social action and the antipsychiatric movement reached their peak, while the progression of the biological model at the expense of the other models has become indisputable in the 1980s and 90s. Indeed, the huge progress made in biological research, the presence of psychiatrists in the new short-stay units of general hospitals and the ineffectiveness of community approach techniques, have entailed a 're-medicalisation' of the psychiatric profession. The new specialists, in the course of their years of postgraduate training in psychiatry, are beginning to receive a solid education in behavioural biology, a good knowledge of reliable procedures for the evaluation of descriptive psychopathology, the interpretation of complex diagnostic processes, and the handling of effective psychopharmacological substances. This does not preclude the fact that in Western countries, the vast majority of psychiatrists try to adopt an eclectic theoretical attitude, by including other models in their practice. But they are not always successful.

The Excessive Size of the Field

The excessive size of the theoretical framework the psychiatrists has to face obliges him to disperse his activities enormously and contributes to his identity crisis. This is even more visible when he has to practice in small localities, or in large cities' emergency services. He cannot then confine himself to one subspeciality. He must, on the contrary, be capable of setting aside the existence of a subjacent organic lesion in the psychopathological picture, of evaluating a patient's suicidal risk, of managing psychopharmacological proceedings in a flexible way, of using simple conditioning techniques, of detecting basic psychodynamic aspects in the patient's problems, and of intervening in the dynamics of the couple and of the family. Ocasionally, he must give his opinion on the psychomotor development problems of a child, and to carry out an assessment of a handicap or the degree of responsibility of a delinquent.

VICTIMS OF OUR OWN SUCCESS

Today's psychiatrists no longer encounter those perfect clinical pictures, so neatly described by the classic authors, now that the effective action of psychopharmacological products leads to the rapid disappearance of their symptomatology. Clinical reports, which used to be veritable novels, have become a body of data, programmed to be processed by computer. The psychiatrist's therapeutic skill is measured not in terms of the patient's recognition of the support and help offered, but by the shortness of his/her stay in hospital. Wounded by forays into sociology, returning now to the security of the hospital office after engaging on the frontlines of the community, direct contact with the patient is now delegated to the rest of the staff.

Having observed this evolution over the last 20 years, the author of these lines cannot help recalling the words of Pio Baroja (1965) spoken by the intrepid sailor Shanti Andia when, in retirement, he reflected on how the sailing ship had been replaced by the steamship:

> "I am sometimes preoccupied by the idea that one of my sons is tempted by the desire to become a sailor or an adventurer. But no, this is not what they want, and I'm happy to hear it... and yet.... Those superb masts! White sails, so white! Elegant frigates, their figureheads rising above the waves! Curved vessels, light frames! It saddens me to think that you'll disappear and I will see you no more! Yes, I'm glad my sons have no wish to become sailors... and... yet...."

And yet. The profession does not appear to be disappearing, as some have predicted. Progress in the fields not only of biology but also of sociology, point to a prodigious future for our speciality. Psychiatry today is indeed a victim of its own success. The future of psychiatry and the value of future psychiatrists will depend above all on the quality of the physicians who decide to choose this speciality, and the adaptation of their training syllabuses. But it is true that the profession must not restrict its field of action to the neurobiology of behaviour, conferring the more psychological aspects of mental suffering on non-physician specialists. The idiosyncrasy of the profession lies in its eclecticism in terms of theory, the capacity to develop work that is multifaceted in terms of practice, and in the curiosity and capacity to tolerate ambiguity and frustration in personal terms.

REFERENCES

Azcunaga, D., Sacanell, E., and Guimón, G. (1986). Perfil sociololaboral y actividades clínicas de los psiquiatras españoles: implicaciones para la formación de los residentes en psiquiatria. *Psiquis*, 242(86), 21–32.

Baroja, P. (1965): Las inquietudes de Shanti Andia, Obras completas, Biblioteca Nueva, Madrid.
Beitman, B. D., and Maxim, P. (1984). A survey of psychiatric practice: Implications for psychiatric training. *Journal of Psychiatric Education*, 8, 149–153.
Beitman, B. D., and Maxim, P. (1984). A survey of psychiatric practice: implications for psychiatric training. *The Journal of Psychiatric Education*, 8, 149–153.
Bodkin, J. A., Klitzman, R. L., and Pope, H. G. (1995). Treatment orientation and associated characteristics of North American academic psychiatrists. *The Journal of Nervous and Mental Disease*, 183 (12), 729–735.
Brook, P. (1976). Where do psychiatrists come from? The influence of United Kingdom medical schools on the choice of psychiatry as a career. *British Journal of Psychiatry*, 128, 313–317.
Brook, P. (1978). Consultant psychiatrists: who are they and where are they going? *Medical Education*, 12, 382–383.
Brook, P. (1981). The choice of career of consultants psychiatrists. *British Journal of Psychiatry*, 138, 32–328.
Brook, P. (1984). Consultant Psychiatrists: Their career choice and training. *Bulletin of the Royal College of Psychiatrists*, 8 (1), 2–5.
Brook, P., and Wakeford, R. (1987). Continuing medical education. A survey of consultant psychiatrists' attitudes and practices. *Bulletin of the Royal College of Psychiatrists*, 11, 38–42.
Burke, J. D., Pincus, H. A., and Pardes, H. (1986). The clinician researcher in psychiatry. *American Journal of Psychiatry*, 143, 968–976.
Creager, C. (1993). Managed care: hope amid the horror. *Professional Counselor* (February), 24–27.
Cypres, B. K. (1978). *Office Visits to Psychiatrists National Ambulatory Medical Care Survey. United States* 1975–76 (National Survey). Washington: Department of Health, Education and Welfare, 38 National Center for Health Statistics.
Dorwart, R. A., Chartock, L. R., Dial, T., et al. (1992). A national study of psychiatrists' professional activities. *American Journal of Psychiatry*, 149, 1499–1505.
Fenton, W. S., Leaf, P. J., Moran, N. L., and Tischler, G. L. (1984). Trends in psychiatric practice, 1965–1980. *American Journal of Psychiatry*, 141 (3), 346–351.
Fink, P. J. (1993). Psychiatrist's roles in managed care programs. *Hospital and Community Psychiatry*, 44 (723–724).
Gracia, D. (1996). El poder medico. In P. Ridruejo and A. Medina and J. L. Rubio (Eds.), *Psicología Médica*. Madrid: McGraw Hill Interamericana.
Guimón, J. (1990). Psiquiatras: *De brujos a burócratas*. Barcelona: Salvat Editores.
Guimón, J. (2002). *Los profesionales de la Salud mental: Tareas y vicisitudes*. Madrid: Core Academic.
Guimón, J. (1998). *La profession de psychiatre. Evolution et devenir*. Paris: Masson.
Guimón, J., Azcunaga, D., and Sacanell, E. (1987). Orientacion teórica de los psiquiatras espanoles. *Actas Luso-Espanolas de Neurologia, Psiquiatria y Ciencias Afines*, XV (2), 173–183.
Guimón, J., Azkunga, D., and Sacanell, E. (1987). Presencia en España del llamado sindrome del residente que comienza su formacion en psiquiatria. *Psiquis*, 8, 11–19.
Guimón, J., Fischer, W., Goerg, D., and Zbinden, E. (1996). Orientations théoriques des psychiatres suisses. *Annales Medico-Psychologiques*, 155 (3), 184–201.
Guimón, J., Fischer, W., Zbinden, E., and Goerg, D. (1997). Therapeutic practice profiles, work settings and activities of Swiss psychiatrists. *Archives Suisses de Neurologie et Psychiatrie*.
Guimón, J., Goerg, D., Fischer, W., and Zbinden, E. (1997). Pratique de la psychanalyse parmi les psychiatres suisses. *Médecine et Hygiène*, 55(2177), 1743–1746.

Kane, F. J., and Harper, R. G. (1992a). Psychotherapy: Past training and current practice. *General Hospital Psychiatry*, 14, 131–134.
Kane, F. J., and Harper, R. G. (1992b). Psychotherapy: Past Training and Current Practice. *General Hospital. Psychiatry*, 14, 131–134.
Kernberg, O. (1979). Regression in organizational leadership. *Psychiatry*, 42, 24–39.
Lambo, T. (1982). Psychiatrists. In M. Shepherd (Ed.), *Psychiatrists on psychiatry*. Cambridge: Cambridge University Press.
Langsley, D. G., and Hollender, M. H. (1982). The definition of a psychiatrist. *American Journal of Psychiatry*, 139 (1), 81–85.
Langsley, D. G., and Yager, J. (1988). The definition of a psychiatrist: eight years later. *American Journal of Psychiatry*, 145(4), 469–475.
Lazarus, A., et al. (1996). *Controversies in Managed Mental Health Care*. Washington, DC: American Psychiatric Press Inc.
Lenz, G. (1984). Postgraduate training in developing countries. A questionnaire study by the WPA secretariat. In J. J. Lopez Ibor and G. Lenz (Eds.), *Training and education in Psychiatry*. Vienna: Facultas.
Marcos, L. R., and Gil, R. M. (1989). The diagnosis of public mental health care bureaucracies. *British Journal of Psychiatry*, 155 (suppl.), 96–101.
Marcos, L. R., and Silver, R. A. (1988). Psychiatrist-executive management styles: Nature or nurture?. *American Journal of Psychiatry*, 145, 103–107.
Mombour, W. (1984). Comparison between different systems of psychiatric education. In J. J. Lopez Ibor and G. Lenz (Eds.), *Training and education in psychiatry*. Vienna: Facultas.
Murray, W., Parker, G., and Harris, M. (1993). Structural characteristics of Australian psychiatric practice. *Australian and New Zealand Journal Of Psychiatry*, 27, 298–305.
Olfson, M., Pincus, H., and Dial, T. H. (1994a). Professional practice patterns of U.S. psychiatrists. *American Journal of Psychiatry*, 151, 89–95.
Olfson, M., Pincus, H. A., and Sabshin, M. (1994b). Pharmacotherapy in outpatient psychiatric practice. *American Journal of Psychiatry*, 151, 580–585.
Pichot, P. (1982). Psychiatrists on psychiatry. In M. Shepherd (Ed.), *Psychiatrists on Psychiatry*. Cambridge: Cambridge University Press.
Redlich, F., and Kelert, S. R. (1978). Trends in American mental health. *American Journal of Psychiatry*, 135, 22–28.
Sullivan, M., Verhulst, J., Russo, J., and Roy-Byrne, P. (1993). Psychotherapy vs. pharmacotherapy: Are psychiatrists polarized? A survey for academic and clinical faculty. *American Journal of Psychotherapy*, 47 (3), 411–423.
Wright, M., Parker, G., and Harris, M. (1993). Structural characteristics of Australasian psychiatric practice. *Australian and New Zealand Journal of Psychiatry*, 27, 298–305.
Yager, J., Pasnau, R. O., and Lipschultz, S. (1978). Professional characteristics of psychiatric residents trained at the UCLA Neuropsychiatric Institute, 1956–1975. *The Journal of Psychiatric Education*, 3 (1), 72–85.
Yager, J., Pasnau, R. O., and Lipschulz, S. (1979). Professional characteristics of psychiatric residents trained at the UCLA Neuropsychiatric Institute, 1956–1975. *Rev. J. Psych.*, 3, 72–86.

27

The Therapeutic Team

TEAMWORK

One of the basic characteristics of interventions in community psychiatry is teamwork. A team is 'a small number of persons with complementary skills, committed to a common purpose for whose achievement they consider themselves mutually responsible, under the leadership of one of them' (Arrazola, et al.). The leaders use their power to obtain conformity, proposing incentives to moderate resistance and favouring negotiation to reach the objectives previously agreed upon with the rest of the team's members.

The team thus constituted incorporates all of the potential held by informal relationships and the force of group unity, and makes it possible to carry out many tasks that each member on his own would be unable to do individually. Teamwork provides an opportunity for personal and professional development, because every member contributes his competence while gaining in knowledge and skills. The discrepancies that arise in the group can be used to continue to explore issues in more depth.

The relationships among the members of therapeutic teams are complex, and can mobilise anxieties that sometimes cause major dysfunctions. To illustrate this, Fornari (2000) uses the parable of the hedgehogs that Freud took from Schopenhauer: 'To defend himself from the winter cold, the hedgehogs decided to get together to warm each other with their body heat; however, when they approached their fellows, they pricked themselves and so moved away again; when they moved away, they felt cold again, and once more approached each other to get warm, but they pricked themselves again and so again moved away, seeking alternatives to protect themselves from the cold and from prickles. This went on until, after various attempts, the hedgehogs found the right distance that enabled them to not prick each other, but to warm each other; that is, to protect themselves simultaneously from the cold, and from prickles'. This ambivalence in team relationships comes from the primary persecutory and depressive anxieties that are produced within the group.

THE IMPORTANCE OF SELF KNOWLEDGE

There are subjective aspects that each professional brings to a relationship (value judgements, mood states) which can influence the relationship with the patient, and which it is indispensable for the professional to control. The relationship with psychiatric patients produces a certain amount of anxiety, which sets into motion in the professional different neutralisation mechanisms that can lead to actions not aimed towards resolving the patients' problems, but rather to defend himself against the patient. The professional, due to inexperience or fear of not knowing how to respond appropriately, may maintain rigid or stereotypical attitudes, or project his own problems onto the patient, so that the relationship sometimes acquires an antitherapeutic character. Therefore, it is fundamental for teams and/or their individual components to be offered supervision. Frequently, such supervision leads to a demand for personal psychotherapy on the part of the professional.

Professionals can also acquire expertise in individual counselling and group and family work, enabling them, the context permitting, to function as therapists. This type of training is particularly important when the professional is operating in units that function under the principles of therapeutic communities, in which there is a certain amount of decentralised decision making, and work is carried out in teams. The professional should, in such contexts, become more a part of the mental patient's surroundings, be they social, family, or occupational, forming part of the multidisciplinary teams created to deal with these areas.

Indeed, with growing frequency, in these types of units the psychologists, nurses, and social workers lead different types of recreational, occupational, or more specifically psychotherapeutic groups.

It is important to clearly differentiate the genuinely psychotherapeutic activities from the rest. Indeed, psychotherapy requires specific training in which a university-level professional, specialised in a clinical field, studies a specific psychotherapeutic curriculum, which includes some kind of personal therapeutic and supervisory experience. Without these prerequisites, it is unethical to subject patients to delicate interventions, which can entail some risk.

Moreover, it is important to remember that, although the functions of the team's different members may become diffused, the working hierarchy must not be called into question, and each profession has specific functions, which should not be neglected.

THE TEAM COMPONENTS AS ATTACHMENT FIGURES

Psychiatric illness threatens the individual's security, and professionals can be temporary *attachment* figures who provide an affective holding environment similar to the maternal function described by Bion (1962). Through sympathetic listening, they help the patient to develop the *capacity to think* and to tolerate anxiety, using their own mental processes to hold and digest the patient's projections.

In children (Ainsworth 1978), different attitudes of *insecure attachment* (avoiding, ambivalent, and disorganised) have been described, which, when they interact with other vulnerability factors, can predispose them to psychiatric disorders. As we discussed earlier, some professionals experienced inadequate attachment in childhood, leading them to have a need for compulsive caring but very reluctant to seek professional help.

Normally, having discovered many times that the mother, and later, others survive his attacks, the child learns to have confidence that his love dominates his hate, and that his reparation activities are successful. This reduces his fears of persecution and retaliation by the bad mother whom he has attacked. But when external reality fails to refute the child's anxieties, for example, if the mother dies, or retires, or retaliates, then the depressive anxieties can be too heavy to be borne. The individual then abandons his failed reparation activities, and recurs instead to more primitive paranoid, manic, and obsessive defences.

Those who work in the 'caring' professions often, and inevitably, fail in their work with damaged and needy clients. If this failure sparks intolerable guilt and anxiety, these professionals (like infants) may regress to these primitive defences with the aim of maintaining their precarious self-esteem, and defend themselves from the retaliation they feel is coming to them for failing to obtain a cure.

In adults, there are three main styles of inadequate attachment—*dismissing*, *worried*, and *irresolute*—which can be assessed with semi-structured interviews. When they enter into contact with mental health services, those with a dismissing style may find it difficult to get involved in their treatment; the worriers may feel blocked or ambivalent about the help that is offered to them; the irresolute may have difficulty managing the painful feelings that treatment produces. However, those with childhood antecedents of *secure attachment* show themselves more open in talking about their symptoms, and tend to present better pharmacological compliance.

In psychiatric units, some situations can set off attachment behaviours in patients. They may, for example, feel excessive fear of leaving the hospital, and their symptoms may worsen when the time comes to do so. If one of the unit's professionals leaves, this can also produce, in patients who were attached to him or her, adverse reactions which can manifest themselves in the form of aggression, explosions of violence, or other ways, all inadequate attempts to keep that person from going away.

Many patients with antecedents of having suffered abuse provoke excessive attachment behaviours in professionals. However, hostile reactions from patients may lead professionals to experience intense countertransferences, and use, for example, inadequate holding measures. If they themselves had been subjected to abuse by their parents or educators, they may have a tendency to physically or sexually abuse their patients in a more or less open or hidden way (Gabbard, 1990).

Mental institutions themselves can become attachment figures for patients who did not experience a secure attachment in infancy. Attachment to professionals and institutions can sometimes persist for long after the patient has left them.

Professionals should provide patients with a secure base, an affective holding environment able to modulate their anxieties. It is more a matter of *being with* patients more than *doing things to* patients.

REGRESSION IN TEAMS

In seriously ill patients' psychoanalytical treatment process, especially psychotics, the professional first aims to induce a regression which will make it possible to take better care of the patient (Guimón, 1985) in order to then, through interaction, enable him to restructure his personality. However, it is well known that in this interaction, psychotic transference, due to the interplay of projective identifications, produces in the therapist a countertransference quite independent of his own personality.

Some situations created by different psychotic patients seem to be dominated by what has been termed 'projective counter-identifications' (Grinberg, 1962). Indeed, the therapist's role is that of receiving the patients' projections, elaborating them, and enabling them to be introjected once they are transformed. However, with psychotics the therapist is often compelled to act countertransferentially, as if moved by these nuclei deposited by the patient's projective identifications and which acquire, within the therapist, a life of their own, if he is not able to perceive them, elaborate them, and transform them.

The therapeutic team should represent, for the patient, an alter family, which enables him to have a 'corrective emotional experience' to remedy other experiences that may have been responsible for the origins of his illness. However, there are different difficulties within the therapeutic team, some stemming from reality elements (e.g., workplace stress, professional rivalries), others from projective identifications that the patients have deposited in their therapists. Due to a splitting phenomenon, therapists deposit in their patients all of the sick parts that they reject in themselves. In such a situation of denial, rarely does the team have sufficient flexibility to adapt to patients' varying needs.

As Racamier (1983) saw it, the therapeutic team can come to feel dissociated by these projections. The tension in working teams increases, and their members try, at all costs, to look as if they understand each other perfectly, to present themselves as an 'ideal family', a containing environment where patients can grow. This need that the therapeutic team members have to simulate that they function like a happy family can lead them to firmly maintain an anti-authoritarian, egalitarian ideal in which all of the team components are supposedly equal, denying their obvious differences in professional training and personality. In such situations, it is not infrequent for such pseudoegalitarianism to tend to spread to patients, who are theoretically considered able to assume the teams' responsibilities, although in practice, and in a hidden way, the therapeutic team acts as if the patients were incapable of doing so. In that case, what arises is, in the words of Sacks and Carpenter (Sacks et al., 1974), a *pseudo-therapeutic community*, which has a great deal to do with Winnicott's concept of the *false self* (Layland, 1981; Winnicott, 1971).

Winnicott redefined, in his book *Playing and Reality* (1971), the concept of the *good-enough mother*: one who actively adapts to the child's needs, an adaptation that gradually diminishes, according to the child's growing capacity to handle his adaptation failures, and to tolerate the results of frustration.

Layland (1981) stressed that one of the good-enough mother's qualities is her capacity to accept that the child has the right to transmit all of his needs, desires, phantasies and feelings to her, which he feels as good or bad, pleasant or unpleasant; but she also needs to not expect her child to deal with the more or less unconscious needs, desires, or feelings of the mother herself, which are inappropriate to the mother-child relationship, and for which she should seek satisfaction elsewhere. The example that Layland gives of this is the child's right to bring to his mother his own depressive feelings, and expect her to help him with them. It is not, however, the child's task to deal with a depressed mother. The good-enough mother, in Layland's terminology, is a *'loving mother'*.

Along these same lines, we could call a *'loving therapeutic team'* one that is able to take on the patients' needs and avoid making them deal with the team members' own difficulties. However, just as the function of the 'loving mother' is not, according to Winnicott, the only function of a good-enough mother, there are other functions that are demanded of a good-enough team: teaching appropriate reality management, self-care, care for others, and so on, some of which could be adscribed to the functions of a *'good-enough father'*, who has yet to be described.

The therapeutic team should, in addition, from a utopian viewpoint, try to create an imaginary space, one for preconsciousness, an *'illusion'* in Winnicott's sense of the word—which is, in reality, the space of creativity and psychoanalysis. However, it is self-evident that none of this is exactly simple.

In 1963, President John F. Kennedy of the United States offered a great deal of funding to psychiatric centres for creating new units inspired by the ideology of community psychiatry. Hundreds of centres of this kind then sprang up like mushrooms all across the country, with the aim of getting their hands on this economic aid. Since the 1970s, I have visited dozens of centres of this kind, in different areas of different countries. The typical image of an activities session in one of these programmes could be that of a young mental health worker, trying, with an expression of cheerful enthusiasm but clearly bored inside, to get a few defeated-looking chronic patients to form a band, docilely sawing away at some musical instruments. My feeling, in such situations, is sceptical. Between a costly set-up whose efficiency is merely that of a child-minder, and an exceptionally valuable therapeutic setting, the difference is the existence of a space for hope, and the presence of a good-enough therapeutic team.

RIVALRIES

Since the beginning of the community psychiatry movement, strong tensions and rivalries have arisen among the team members. Within a 'democratic' therapeutic setting that promoted the equality of its personnel (e.g., everyone conducted psychotherapy, everyone was involved in decisions about the patients' future), there were, however, obvious differences in training and status: salaries varied a great deal according to individuals' academic level; physicians continued to be the ones who were legally responsible for treatment, involuntary hospitalisation, and reports for legal trials and payment of interventions.

During the 1960s, the development of the community mental health system provoked an overload in the number of professionals, their respective roles became quite diffuse, and everyone was considered a 'therapist', with or without the proper training. Psychoanalysis was the favourite psychotherapeutic treatment in the 1960s, and the therapeutic model around which most of psychiatrists' training revolved. In the United States, therapists who were not physicians had no right to practice psychoanalysis, and in Europe the legal situation was similar. However, in the mid-1980s, a result of a judicial action on the part of the American Association of Psychologists, psychiatrists could not continue to monopolise the psychotherapeutic treatment of ambulatory patients. Thus, psychiatrists soon found themselves moving over to make room for non-medical therapists (Fink, 1996). In the meantime, the transition had already been made in Europe, without as much trauma.

In this context, major conflicts arose over the psychiatrists' desire to reserve for them the function of psychotherapy, excluding psychologists, social workers, psychiatric nurses, and occupational therapists, whose role in community mental health centres was, in their opinion, becoming too prominent. Enriquez (2000) points out that today, in such teams, every professional, from the psychoanalyst to the teacher, plays a therapeutic role, all believing that they have a right to 'function like "*influence machine*" (Tausk, 1933) who try to modify some behaviours of those "assisted", in different and contradictory ways. Some wielded more "influence than others, and even, when getting the patients to talk, try to show the preference that the patients have for them . . . ". The patients experience a contradictory situation, one that drives them insane, and they find themselves immersed in a process of fragmentation, since they are not supported in their experience by an organising law, but feeling directly in their psyches and their bodies the violence of the institution's fragmentation, incarnated by its members' rivalry and narcissistic self-affirmation'.

STRATEGIES FOR CHANGING FROM ONE ORIENTATION TO ANOTHER

In the process of constituting a community team, or in an attempt to change a team that functions according to a classic model into one using a new model, it is necessary to modify antitherapeutic attitudes learned from previous roles, and also to create less rigid ideas about each individual role. A fundamental part of this is to attain a common attitude regarding the understanding of psychiatric patients, which will enable the worker to take on new roles, and form more significant relationships within the framework of treatment. For such an effort to be successful, it is advisable for the team members to interact with patients, including them in some of the team's activities and organising social activities within the centre itself, or trips and excursions sponsored by the programme. However, relationships outside the centre are not advisable.

The modification of traditional professional roles to diminish their rigidity tends to meet resistance, especially among the more highly trained professionals, who prefer to work in a setting where their authority is recognised and praised. When the team works under ideal conditions, although the psychiatrist is the one ultimately responsible for diagnosis and prescribing medication, he has no more authority regarding treatment than any other member of the team, since these decisions are made between the team and the patient. However, power problems are often channelled into arguments about theoretical orientation: whether or not psychopharmaceuticals should be given; whether a behavioural, dynamic, or system approach should be used; individual versus group psychotherapy, and so on.

It is in the practice of psychotherapy where, as we have mentioned earlier, power problems most often arise among team members. There are frequent objections on the part of psychologists and psychiatrists to sharing any of their psychotherapeutic functions with nurses, whom they do not consider adequately trained for these functions. For their part, the nurses sometimes resist taking part in theoretical or supervisory programmes, especially if they are directed by the team's most highly trained professionals.

The supervisory group is especially useful when it is directed by a leader from outside of the programme, and when it does not become just another institutional ritual, as described in the previous chapter. A particular method of working is that of mentoring, under which each professional has an assigned mentor.

In any case, perhaps, and just as, for women, there is an ideal age for mothering a baby, therapeutic teams also have their time limits. Everyone knows that a psychotherapist working with psychotics has close theoretical and practical relationships with child psychoanalysis. Often, child psychoanalysts work enthusiastically with children for some years, and then tend to quickly abandon working with them directly and draw back to a more comfortable supervising position. A similar phenomenon can be seen among therapists specialised in psychotics.

The therapeutic team also has a time limit on its capacity for illusion. That is why, in our view, the staff of such units should never be long-term, but rather easily renewable, predominantly by new, young, enthusiast therapists. A young, uncultured mother often takes much better care of her longed-for baby than a psychology professor does of her own unplanned last-born child.

We could say that the instability of the changes suggested above would make teams vulnerable. But the vulnerability of community health care mechanisms is precisely, in my view, an unfortunate prerequisite for their success. Just as tolerance of ambivalence and frustration, and acceptance of resistance, are indispensable prerequisites in the personality and education of a psychoanalyst.

REFERENCES

Ainsworth, M. (1969). Object relations, dependency and attachment: a theoretical review of the mother–infant relationship. *Child Development, 40*, 969–1025.

Bion, W. R. (1962). *Learning from experience*. New York: Basic Books.

Enriquez, E. (2000). Le travail de la mort dans les institutions. In R. Kaës (Ed.), *L'institution et les institutions. Etudes psychanalytiques* (2nd ed.). Paris: Dunod.

Fink, P. J. (1996). Are psychiatrists replaceable? In A. Lazarus (Ed.), Controversies in managed Mental health care. Washington, D.C.: American Psychiatric Press.

Fornari, F. (2000). Pour une psychanalyse des institutions. In R. Kaës (Ed.), L'institution et les institutions. Etudes psychanalytiques (2nd ed.). Paris: Dunod.

Gabbard, G. O. (1990). Psychodynamic psychiatry in clinical practice. Washington, D.C.: American Psychiatric Press, Inc.

Grinberg, L. (1962). On a specific aspect of countertransference due to the patients projective identification. *International Journal of Psycho-Analysis*, 43, 436–440.

Guimón, J. (1985). El equipo suficientemente bueno. *Rev. Asoc. Esp. Neuropsiquiatr.*, 5, 501–505.

Layland, W. R. (1981). In search of a loving father. *International Journal of Psycho-Analysis*, 62, 125–225.

Racamier, P. C. (1983). *Le psychanalyste sans divan. La psychanalyse et les institutions de soins psychiatriques*. Paris: Payot.

Sacks, M. H., and Carpenter, W. T. (1974). The pseudo-therapeutic community: An examination of anti-therapeutic forces on psychiatric units. *Hospital and Community Psychiatry*, 25, 315–318.

Tausk, V. (1933). On the origin of the influencing machine in schizophrenia. *Psychoanalytic Quarterly*, 2(519–556).

Winnicott, D. W. (1971). *Playing and reality*. London: Tavistock.

28

The Professional in the Institution

When considering professionals' relationships with the mental health institutions where they work, the ideas of some psychosocial-analytical investigators are useful, so we shall review them in this chapter.

GROUPS, ORGANISATIONS, AND INSTITUTIONS

The point that different mental health units have in common, as is the case for all psychosocial entities (Petit et al., 1998), is that they are constituted by groups, composed of individuals who get to know each other from day to day, who meet, interact, and find each other in a state of interdependence that is not only functional—their work—but also psychological. Following Lapassade (1970, cited by Petit and Dubois, 1998), we can describe three levels in these health care units: groups (e.g., a mental health team); organisations (e.g., a psychiatric hospital); institutions (e.g., the department in a ministry that defines everything established by the laws on mental health which give the institution its legal force).

Group

Kaës (2000b) defines the *group* as a set of individuals who interact (e.g., with roles and statutes) and share certain norms in carrying out a task. He believes that every group has a type of relationship that, 'paradoxically, is a *non-relationship*', a '*non-individualisation*', which is the matrix or the base of every group, and persists in a variable manner throughout its life. He calls this type of relationship 'syncretic sociability', to differentiate it from 'interaction sociability', and refers to interaction as 'the figure of a Gestalt on the ground of "*syncretic sociability*".'

The individual is subjected to peer pressure to adopt opinions and behaviours in keeping with the group norms (*conformism*). But conformism is not always so coercive: the individual can value his belonging to the group and conform to its norms with the aim of achieving a personal objective, such as satisfying his need for affective relationships.

In addition, groups generate a certain team spirit that enables the individual to defend himself more efficiently against organisational pressures. Individuals can use the systems of roles and institutionalised norms within the organisation to reinforce their defence mechanisms against anxiety (Jacques, 1955).

Group affiliation also provides its members with a certain security, which is consolidated by the fact that its members experience 'together and simultaneously the same process of identity access' (Sainsaulieu, 1977, cited by Petit and Dubois, 1998).

Organisation

Those espousing the trend towards 'scientific organisation of work' believed that organisations function like machinery, whose cogs are perfectly adjusted to one another; however, they ignored the affective factors stemming from the relationships among their members. Contrariwise, the so-called 'human relations' theorists, enriched by the neo-human relations school (McGregor, 1974; Maslow, 1943; Herzberg, 1971, cited by Petit and Dubois, 1998) showed that organisations originate a series of satisfactions and dissatisfactions.

In an organisation, the individuals, groups, settings, and services that it comprises are articulated in an interdependence that is necessary for meeting the common objective of producing goods and services. Any modification of one element leads to modifications in all the others. Work can be a source of personal growth and realisation when the organisation functions according to the idea of a 'happy family'.

Institution

An institution (which can be both a group or an organisation) is defined as a set of norms applied in a social system, which define what is and is not legitimate in this system (Mendras, 1979, cited by Petit and Dubois, 1998). To sum up the difference between an organisation and an institution, Petit and Dubois (1998) use the example of education, which is, *par excellence*, an institution, i.e., 'a set of ideas, beliefs and rules of conduct proposed to, and frequently imposed on, the individuals of a certain society'. However, a primary school group, a secondary school, a university, a ministry of education, are all organisations, which both rely on the institution of education, while also providing it with a concrete basis of existence.

Kaës (2000b) points out that the concept of the institution has been employed with a wide variety of meanings, and that he uses it to refer to the set of rules, regulations, and activities grouped around social values and functions. Although the institution could also be defined as an organisation, in the sense of a hierarchical arrangement of the functions that are generally carried out inside a building, an area, or a certain space, he used the word organisation, exclusively, with the latter connotation.

According to Kaës, every organisation has a tendency to maintain the same structure as the problem that it is trying to solve or for which it was created. 'Thus, he says 'a hospital winds up having, as an organisation, the same characteristics as the patients (isolation, sensory deprivation, communication deficits, etc.). Our psychiatric organisations, our therapies, our theories, and our techniques also have the same structures as the phenomena that we are trying to confront. They have become organisations; therefore they carry out the same function of maintaining and controlling: a tendency towards bureaucratisation.... The technical staff or administrative team of a hospital also have a tendency to structure themselves like organizations.... Jacques has said that institutions serve as a defence against psychotic anxieties. This is a limited statement, and it would be more accurate to say that institutions and organisations are depositories of syncretic sociability, or the psychotic part, and that would be a good explanation for their tendency towards bureaucratisation and resistance to change'.

THE INSTITUTIONAL DYNAMICS

When acting as a consultant for a mental health organisation, it is indispensable to first diagnoses the organisational systems as a whole, and the subsystems that they comprise (Petit and Dubois, 1998): the real working groups, the departments or services, particular hierarchy, the top management and mid-level executives, and so on. Specifically, a diagnosis of this kind consists of asking questions about the organisation's functioning: How are decisions made? How are objectives and plans drawn up? How do professionals and working groups communicate? What is the state of the relations among groups? How are conflicts solved?

The Socio-Analytical Method of Studying Mental Health Institutions

Using the socio-analytical method, the consultant lives with the organisation as a whole, a 'professional' relationship that excludes any kind of private or privileged link with the organisation's members or groups, and imposes on the consultant confidentiality with regard to the outside world, unless there is an explicit agreement with the organisational system regarding the publication of certain results of his research. In addition, the socio-analytical procedure refers to psychoanalytical ideas to clarify certain phenomena: the ambivalence of professionals, who are simultaneously attracted by change and discouraged by the fact of having to change certain behaviours; positive transference, through which the professionals project on the consultant their desire for change; negative transference, through which they project onto the consultant hidden feelings of hostility—indeed, their resistance to change. Dubost proposed that these resistances constitute defence mechanisms against anxiety which can be analysed and overcome through a method called *perlaboration or interpretative elaboration* (equivalent to *working through* in psychoanalysis): a consultant with training in group methods calls the group's attention to interpreations that concern facts known by all of them, regarding the nature of the resistance that are obstacles to progress. The consultant, says Kaës (2000a), 'should take advantage of all the opportunities that arise over the course of meetings to clarify "here and now" the meaning of feelings (fear, guilty, mistrust) that provoke changes which are simultaneously perceived as necessary and threatening to the group'.

Psychosociological references (Petit and Dubois, 1998) came out of the work of Jacques, based on that of Bion (1965) and Lewin who, on the frontier of psychoanalysis and psychosociology, studied the development of unconscious processes within small groups. Later, Rapoport, at the Tavistock Institute, with his 'action-research' procedure, tried to apply these concepts to persons who find themselves in problematical situations (Rapoport, 1973, cited by Petit and Dubois, 1998).

Psychoanalytical References

Kaës (2000a) pointed out that 'we still do not have the means necessary to establish a psychoanalytical theory of the institution, beginning with the constitution of its object.' Jacques's first reflections on the matter arose in the context of a research project of Britain's first Labour government after World War II. Defining institutions from a socio-analytical viewpoint, Jacques differentiated two concepts: *social structures*, which are the set of roles played by the persons in an executive hierarchy, and the manner in which they are distributed; and *cultural mechanism*, which are the rules, taboos, and habits that form the structure of a given institution (Fornari, 2000).

The model of Melania Klein's school considered institutions to be defence mechanisms against primary persecutory and depressive anxiety. The ideas of *container* (Bion, 1959) and the containing function (Kaës) have led to a reflection on the need to find a place (supervision or intervision) in which the anxieties and intrapsychological and intersubjective conflicts present in the institution can be updated, listened to, and thought out. Anzieu's work on the *ego-skin* and psychological covers have led to research on group and institutional covers (Anzieu, 1985).

The psychoanalytical viewpoint also bears in mind the characeristic '*climate*' of each institution: its history and structure, the nature and difficulties involved in its principal work, the unconscious infrastructure which organises satisfaction-seeking relationships (Kaës, 2000b). In this sense, the 'family' comes up as a constant reference point, a favourite example that even justifies and legitimises resorting to analysis (Vidal, 2000).

Kaës points out that institutions inflict various types of narcissistic wounds on professionals: they must realise that the institution was not made for 'each one of them personally, like Providence'; on the other hand, they must admit that their psychological life is not 'exclusively focused on their personal unconscious... their unconscious does not belong to them, but rather to the institutions to which they are underpinned and which depend on this underpinning.' However, he adds, 'institutions are not immortal. The order they impose is not immovable, the values they proclaim are contradictory and deny that on which they are based.'

INSTITUTIONAL DIAGNOSIS

The application of findings on institutional organisation to the study of patients' therapeutic settings has notably enriched our understanding of the *habitat* where mental illness evolves (Guimón, 1989; Guimón et al., 1989). Some authors, such as Gruenberg (1968), state that 'the needs of psychiatric epidemiology will not be satisfied merely by the classification of mental disorders. We should be able to classify data on the environment ('conditions') in which the disorders manifest themselves or do not manifest themselves'.

In 'diagnosing' the organisational situation, it is necessary to study the intragroup and intergroup dynamics, paying special attention to the organisation chart. This makes it possible to evaluate the degree of bureaucratisation, and the size of the gap between the levels of integration and the levels of syncretic sociability (Kaës). Once a general intervention strategy has been established, group dynamics techniques are used to confront organisational problems. Many therapists in psychiatric institutes have the basic abilities to collaborate in understanding the organisation itself, after undergoing specific training. However, as Bleger warns (Bleger, 2000), mental health professionals should take great care not to transfer the difficulties of psychiatric hospitals to general hospitals, and those of these two to other organisations (e.g., industrial, educational).

INSTITUTIONAL PATHOLOGY

According to Kaës (1996), the group psychological apparatus should ideally possess the capacity to articulate the strength and meaning of the interaction among its members, to ensure the existence of a 'symbolisation space that shelters, administers, and transforms the meaningless drive elements that immobilise common psychological formations'. Pinel (Pinel, 1996) suggests that the alteration phenomena (*deliaison*) of institutional ties are made manifest by a lack of this group economic regulation, both due to a lack or an excess of investment, and are the result of the lack of this skill, cited by Kaës for group psychic functioning. To understand these movements of *deliaison* and *reliaison* in institutions, Thom's catastrophe theory (1989) offers an interpretation of the dissociations, in terms of morphological accidents, and the reconstruction of the underlying catastrophic dynamics.

Kaës (2000a) refers to the existence in institutions of 'paranoid anxieties, the fear of the unknown or of a new situation... the fear occurs in the face of the unknown that each person carries inside in the form of no-person or no-identity (or of *syncretic ego*)... It is not only newness that provokes fear, it is also the unknown that exists inside of the known.'

In caring institutions, different defence mechanisms can be seen (hypertrophic memory, rituals) and dysfunctional symptoms (attack against thoughts, exclusion of some professionals, immobilisation), which we shall examine below.

Hypertrophic Memory

Correale (1996) described a phenomenon that other authors (Kaës et al., 1988; Bion, 1970; Douglas, 1986, quoted by Correale, 1996) had analysed previously, and which often occurs in institutions, especially when they are entering into advanced phases of their development, in which institutionalisation processes are important. It involves the fact that there are certain events which 'have a tendency to becomes fixed and almost petrified into a collective heritage of memories, following rigid and hard to modify modalities.'

These are collective memories, almost always of relational events from a distant past, which are always told in the same, repetitive way, as if to prove a hypothesis or affirmation for which they must be the proof. Correale (1996) affirms that they are true *'retrospective hallucinations'*, since these memories present, on the one hand, great vividness and clarify, a form of hyperclarity; but, on the other, they seem to not be susceptible to an evolution or an interpretation different to the ones already incorporated into the memory itself. The fundamental objective of these memories is the *evacuation* (Bion, 1965 and 1967) of something to free the group, although it may be only partially or incompletely, from its harmful effects.

In this context, we can also consider the ghosts of the *'founding fathers'*, which Enriquez (Enriquez, 2000) describes graphically: 'In such settings roams that ghost of the first founders, and of the mythical aura that surrounds them, thus enabling the institution to function. These ghosts have a number of functions: 1) to express that in primordial times, at the origin, there existed a cohesive team, without internal problems, since it was motivated by a consistent project, resulting in the appearance of guilt feelings among new members, who are not able to find themselves worthy of such ancestors; 2) maintain the power of the founders, who are still present in the institution; 3) keep the group from questioning the initial project, because if it were examined carefully, it would reveal the faults and inconsistencies that it presented from the first, and which are the origin of the current difficulties; 4) promote stories, legends, counter-truths, mad rumours that testify, on the one hand, to the underlying presence of an unbearable primal scene reproduced with dramatic trappings, and on the other, the perpetuation of a series of different "*crimes*" that were committed silently and which, once evoked, appear laughable as events, but which have served to give a tragic air to the whole of institutional life.'

Pseudo-Egalitarianism

Caring institutions (and psychiatric ones even more so) live under the utopia of an *'egalitarian'* ideology. Every one of the workers can be a therapist. The idea of 'co-operation among equals' is presented, according to Enriquez (2000) as a necessity which is, however, immediately denied: 'every specialist can succumb to the desire of thinking that the patient's progress is due only to the specific technique that he/she uses, and that the action of others is nothing but an obstacle. Jealousy and rivalry are going to come up in everything concerning these techniques, and confirming who is the "owner" of the patient'.

Group Rituals

Correale (1996) highlights institutions' general tendency to preserve ritual moments and group habits, consecrated over time into true ceremonies. These are habits and behaviours that have become stratified over the course of time, and have often lost their origins in a distant past; they can be interpreted as a 'kind of obsessive pathology of the institution, with regard to its strict needs for preservation and self-preservation'. For example, institutions try to resolve conflicts between professionals by creating group clinical casework sessions, and obligatory team meetings (Enriquez, 2000); however, the interventions of some profesionals (e.g., the psychoanalysts) tend to carry more institutional weight than others (e.g., the teachers); those of the more senior members (the *founders*) than of newer ones. Finally, the meetings called 'talk about problems' become an empty ritual. 'The professionals talk, but the really important questions are rarely tackled because, if they were, they could originate conflicts that would put everyone's security and identity in danger'.

Pinel (1996) points out that the 'many meetings organised in institutions to solve issues or conflict do nothing more than reinforce paranoid or psychologically empty experiences. These meetings, repetitive and sterile, are limited to organising the next meetings for analysis or regulation; they do not more than reinforce the process of entropy. The only 'advantage' that professionals get out of going to so many meetings is avoiding relating with the patients'.

Attacks against Thoughts and Immobilisation

The professional has an ambivalent relationship with the institution, because he finds himself trapped between the desire to satisfy his own ends, and the renunciation necessary to team functioning. This relationship with the institution mobilises negative affects, such as hatred, and above all, envy. The professional can find himself suffering from a true 'psychological thought paralysis' (Pinel, 1996), through which 'his personal thoughts that stray from the common discourse are attacked and destroyed'.

According to Pinel (1996), caring institutions reveal their fragility by the recurrence of dysfunctional episodes that mark the course of their history. These crises can proceed from an excess or a lack of investment (*'institutional usury'*), which render the institution unable to carry out 'its essential functions as a defence system against primitive anxieties. Anxiety, whether dull or massive, spread into every part of the institution' (Jacques, 1955). All of these processes are sources of anxiety for professionals, who fear possible aggressions on the part of the institution against their security and survival. Deroche used the term *'umbrella myth'* to describe the tendency to evoke some chance event in the history of the institution, such as the omission of a formality due to accident or ignorance, with catastrophic consequences inflated by the imagination. Although the professional is aware that, except for extreme cases, his job is not at risk, the umbrella myth enables him to create a rational basis for a set of precautions and protection rites: multiplication of forms, duplicates, authorising signatures from hierarchical superiors, references to regulations, and so on.

The Exclusion of Some Professionals

In any case, all of this produces suffering in the professional (Pinel, 1996), which becomes manifest in the appearance of scapegoats or episodes involving the *ritual sacrifice* of a colleague. Pinel points out that 'the sacrifice can take the form of a clear exclusion, of underhanded manoeuvres that lead a professional to resign (or cause a patient to drop out of treatment), but more often with the appearance of psychological or somatic symptoms in certain persons, who become the symptom-bearers of the whole group.' Often, envious attacks against the idealised institution or one of its members are seen, which can come from the professionals, the administrators, or the patients. Unconscious alliances are formed which result in perverse actions destroying the most elaborate ties, and creativity (Klein, 1968).

Utilisation of Patients on the Part of Professionals

Enriquez (2000) points out that the relationship that professionals maintain with their clients is moulded according to the relationship that they have with the institution: 'Since they can find themselves trapped by repetition, opaque secrets, guilt and rivalry, then can fall into the temptation of utilising their patients to express their narcissistic needs, and to solidify a continually threatened identity'. At times they devote themselves only to discussing 'analytical theories, educational practices, legal problems, without mentioning their patients, their specific suffering, and the relationship that the therapeutic team should establish with them'. If by chance the patients are mentioned, it is to usurp their voices, presenting themselves as the patients' spokesmen, since these people, with their anxiety and their violence, have nowhere to express themselves directly in a collective space, where their words would be expected, and heeded.

REFERENCES

Anzieu, D. (1985). *Le Moi-peau*. Paris: Dunod-Coll Psychismes.
Bion, W. (1959). *Experiences in Groups and other papers*. New York: Basic Books.
Bion, W. R. (1965). *Recherche sur les petits groupes*. Paris: Presses Universitaires Françaises.
Bleger, J. (2000). Le groupe comme institution et le groupe dans les institutions. In R. Kaës (Ed.), *L'institution et les institutions. Etudes psychanalytiques* (2nd ed.). Paris: Dunod.
Correale, A. (1996). L'hypertrophie de la mémoire en tant que forme de patholgie institutionnelle. In R. Kaës (Ed.), *Souffrance et psychopathologie des liens institutionnels*. Paris: Dunod.
Enriquez, E. (2000). Le travail de la mort dans les institutions. In R. Kaës (Ed.), *L'institution et les institutions. Etudes psychanalytiques* (2nd ed.). Paris: Dunod.
Guimón, J. (1989). The biases of psychiatric diagnosis. In J. Guimon, G. E. Berrios, and J. E. Mezzich (Eds.), Psychiatric Diagnosis (Vol. 155). London: *British Journal of Psychiatry*.
Guimón, J., Mezzich, J. E., and Berrios, G. E. (Eds.). (1989). *Diagnóstico en psiquiatría*. Barcelone: Salvat Editores.
Kaës, R. (2000a). Préface à la nouvelle édition. In R. Kaës (Ed.), *L'institution et les institutions. Etudes psychanalytiques*. (2nd ed.). Paris: Dunod.
Kaës, R. (2000b). Psychanalyse, institution. In R. Kaës (Ed.), *L'institution et les institutions. Etudes psychanalytiques*. (2nd ed.). Paris: Dunod.
Kaës, R. (Ed.). (1996). *Souffrance et Psychopathologie des liens institutionnels*. Paris: Dunod.
Lewin, K., Lippitt, R., & White, R. (1939). Patterns of aggressive behavior in experimentally created "social climates". *Journal of Social Psychology, 10*, 271–299.
Petit, F., and Dubois, M. (1998). *Introduction à la Psychosociologie des organizations* (3rd ed.). Paris: Ed. Dunod.
Pinel, J. P. (1996). La déliaison patholgique des liens institutionnels dans les institutions de soins et de réeducation. In R. Kaës (Ed.), *Souffrance et Psychopathologie des liens institutionnels*. Paris: Dunod.
Vidal, J. P. (2000). Le familialisme dans l'aproche analytique de 'institution. In R. Kaës (Ed.), *L'institution et les institutions. Etudes psychanalytiques* (2nd ed.). Paris: Dunod.

29

The *Burn-Out* Syndrome

Over recent years many authors have described symptoms of depression and dejection among mental health professionals. They have described a 'burn-out' syndrome consisting of a low level of self-satisfaction and high levels of emotional tiredness and 'depersonalisation'.

STRESS AND *BURN-OUT* IN MENTAL HEALTH PROFESSIONALS

Mental health professionals are not free of prejudice against their patients. This, in turn, favours the appearance of *'burn-out syndrome'* (discouragement and even depression), which can have very detrimental effects on the patients themselves.

Definition of *Burn-Out* Syndrome

Discussing the 'burned-out psychiatrist', Freudenberger (1974) referred to young men and women who were highly idealistic, devoted to social causes, working to the point of virtual collapse with difficult patients—such as drug addicts—and feeling demoralised because many of their clients were not getting much better. Early descriptions of burn-out syndrome outlined the presence of three central factors (Maslach et al., 1986): emotional exhaustion, lack of personal accomplishment and depersonalisation (later re-conceptualised as *'cynicism'*). Other authors spoke about a combination of certain symptoms such as physical tiredness, emotional exhaustion, irritability, and intellectual fatigue. Over recent years many authors have added to this picture the presence of symptoms of depression and dejection, a low level of self-satisfaction and high levels of emotional fatigue.

Causes

As for the aetiology, some authors have attributed the syndrome to the existence of a previous psychopathology and others to the stress produced by the environment, including the physical risk.

Do Professionals with a Pre-Existing Psychical Pathology Choose This Speciality?

It is commonplace to refer more or less seriously to the dubious psychological health of mental health professionals, but research into the possibility of its veracity (including those statistics pointing to the existence of a higher suicide rate among psychiatrists) is not conclusive. Those who admit that there is a higher incidence of mental disorders among psychiatrists believe that these disorders may pre-exist in subjects who choose this profession, or that the work itself could be the cause. In the second case, there has been considerable discussion as to whether the work itself is particularly stressful or if psychiatric illnesses could be 'transmitted' through phenomena in which the psychoanalytical mechanism of projective identification would play an important role. Neither of these explanations is sufficient in itself to explain a hitherto unproven phenomenon.

Do Symptoms Depend on the Stress Produced by Work?

Other researchers claim that symptoms could depend on dissatisfaction with work (Guimón, 2002). In contrast, some papers found no connection between dissatisfaction at work and symptoms attributed to this syndrome: for example, psychiatrists both in public and in private practice considered themselves very efficient or relatively efficient, and none made a lesser appraisal of their work. Professionals from the private sector showed the most confidence in their work (32% considered themselves very efficient, versus 24% in the public sector).

In relation to these data, it should be recalled that, when community mental health teams were created, it was thought that the attraction would be such that most brilliant psychiatrists would move from psychiatric hospitals to these centres (Guimón et al., 1976). However, satisfaction with work in community centres was soon observed to be lower than previously expected. In the first place, the standard of staff training in new techniques (group and family psychotherapy, crisis management, etc.) was minimal, and most workers in community mental health centres kept to traditional forms of individual psychotherapy treatment. On the other hand, therapeutic goals were unclear and difficult to define, and this contributed to an increase in red tape. The most highly qualified staff, such as psychiatrists and psychologists, spent less time working directly with patients than the rest of the staff at the centres. A second problem was a frequently tense working environment, which contributed to undermining teamwork and affecting the quality of service offered. Confusion and mistrust abounded among professionals and paraprofessionals, and there were serious problems of communication, with important contradictions. The main problem in this sense was that a supposedly horizontal structure within the community was in fact highly hierarchical because of differences in qualifications and salaries.

Over recent decades, important cultural changes have occurred: a greater focus on profits on the part of providers of services has led to an emphasis on accountability, and the demand for immediate success. The number of hours that psychiatrists work has increased and the workplace has become increasingly technological with work often being performed as a solitary endeavour. Pursuit of adequate financial rewards and of personal advancement has largely replaced commitment to social causes and complaints about work overload and 'time famine' increased. Recent research emphasised the perception on the part of professionals that efforts to help others have been ineffective, that the task is endless, that the personal payoffs for their work have not been forthcoming. Managed care pressures increased their impression that it is impossible to provide the treatment that best serves their patients' needs. Feelings of anger, disillusionment and resentment ensue with interpersonal problems and family difficulties further complicating the situation.

Another depressing factor for professionals is the potential danger involved in their profession. According to Dubin et al. (1996), aggression against psychiatrists is pandemic to such a degree that some studies have found that between 20 and 74% (average: 42%) of psychiatrists and psychotherapists who responded to questions had been attacked at some time during their career.

Attacks in private consulting rooms are more of a danger because of isolation, lack of other personnel, and the possible absence of medication in patients. This means that the professional is more vulnerable than on the ward of a psychiatric hospital. Dubin et al. (1988) found that aggression with firearms or knives was less frequent than aggression without weapons or with other objects (32% versus 59%). Experienced psychiatrists were just as likely to suffer from aggression as inexperienced ones. Of those attacked by patients, 59% continued to treat their aggressors. Attacks without weapons or with objects had more serious consequences than aggression with a knife or firearm, but the authors pointed out the curious fact that in their data psychiatrists who had been murdered or who declined to reply to the survey or who were unable to, were not included. Only 36% of psychiatrists who had been attacked had believed beforehand that the patient was potentially violent, and hardly any special preventive measures were taken. In fact, only 23% had any kind of safety measures installed in their outside consulting rooms, since this type of measure is usually only available in psychiatric hospitals and other public centres.

Excessive Expectations

A great many of the conscious choices made by mental health professionals are based on idealism. However, these ideals also have unconscious determinants that can contribute to generating defensive institutional processes.

Roberts (1994) provides examples from her experience as a supervisor of dynamically oriented institutions, where she observed serious relational difficulties among some professional groups; for example, between nurses and psychotherapists. One of these centres (Fairlea Manor) was one of the few hospitals where there was a psychoanalitically-based therapeutic programme, and some therapists had gone to work there because they passionately believed in this approach. They wanted to ignore the fact that the environment had changed drastically since the 1940s, when patients could stay at the centre indefinitely if necessary, whereas now, insurance companies are demanding that the length of stay be held to a minimum. Many professionals were still in analytical treatment as part of their training, and had a deep need to believe in its efficacy. They felt that the survival of their speciality was threatened by the decline in psychoanalytical psychotherapy in psychiatric institutions, and they had set for themselves the *impossible task* of proving that they could cure any mental illness, no matter how serious, with this technique. This led to a splitting of the doubts that they had, which they projected onto the rest of the centre's personnel. This splitting also involved their rage towards those patients who 'refused to get better', and they accused the hospital of not providing the resources—especially, unlimited time—that they believed would enable them to carry out their *impossible self-assigned task*. They wound up basing their search for self-esteem on showing disdain towards the other professionals, who were trying to achieve a superficial improvement in the patients.

This disdain, even hatred, of external reality is typical of the *'basic assumptions'* group functioning mode (Bion, 1943), in which the task that the group is trying to carried out involves seeking to satisfy its members' internal needs more than the work for which it was created. It is associated with an absence of scientific curiosity regarding group efficacy, and an inability to think, to learn from experience, or to adapt to change (Bion, 1962).

Another of Roberts' examples is that of a residential unit for children who were separated from their families for their own safety, whose aim was to prepare the children to return to family life, whether with their biological parents or adoptive ones. According to its personnel, no parent was good enough to take care of a child, so that nearly all of the discharges were traumatic.

The impossible self-assigned task, in this case, seems to be to provide the children with the 'ideal parents' that they never had. The unresolved problems of the centre's personnel (several had been in such centres themselves, or came from broken homes) led them to identify excessively with the children, and believe that everything good and useful was within the organisation, and everything harmful and dangerous was in the outside world. Many teams and organisations are created as alternatives to other, more traditional ones, often by someone discontent with previous personal or professional experiences in other contexts. However, an identity based on being an alternative, better according to ethical or humanitarian criteria, tends to smother internal debate. Any questioning within the group is considered a betrayal of the new proposal. Inevitably, problems arise when the alternative approach turns out to be fallible. Working with chronic schizophrenics or with abused children or heroin addicts is intrinsically difficult, and success is never as great as one hopes. The alternative approach is based on a risk hypothesis, according to which, by merely changing certain conditions, extraordinary success will be achieved.

Dealing with Patients

'Insanity is contagious': this cliché has been repeated *ad nauseum*, and the idea is that those who deal with mental patients wind up getting tired of them, and that professionals have as many prejudices about their patients as the general public does. But what are the characteristics of patients that feed professionals' prejudices about them?.

Eker and Oner (Eker et al., 1999), in a study of fifth-year medical students, found that the severity and aggression of a patient's behaviour was related to worse acceptance. They also found, in the responses from various categories of professionals, that the characteristics that contributed to a perception of treatment difficulties were: psychosis, severe pathology, suicidal-depressive behaviour, and violent agitation. Those who were perceived as improving less and who had a poor prognosis were considered particularly difficult.

On the other hand, there is a real risk of physical aggression in the context of working with psychiatric patients. Kaës (2000) points out that professionals can be both physically and psychically attacked by their patients, but they are also the object of attacks against the tie that binds them (Bion, 1962) through suicide attempts, criminal acts, and acting-out, which place them in a situation in which they feel destroyed in their action and in their being.

Attacks against Creativity

Some creative activities of certain professionals, although they are to a large extent the result of the institution's overall creativity, are not accepted by the institutional climate prevailing at a given time. Professionals then think that these creative activities cannot be carried out because the institution has other projects, without realising that they are the real actors, and that the institution is nothing more than what they do. Professionals wind up carrying them out surreptitiously, and, as Enriquez (2000) puts it, 'they feel guilt every time that they are creative, since they have the feeling of transgressing against the sacred values to which they adhere.... Occasionally, they ignore the rules and act in a way other than the predictable one, but without daring to say it, for fear of being negatively evaluated....; they then begin to act in secret...., fearing that the truth about their actions will come to light, and that others will become their persecutors....; patients perceive the contradictions between intentions and actions, and they feel like part of a generalised lie, with which the therapists always make them accomplices'.

Prejudices against Mental Patients

Mental health professionals, mainly psychiatrists, are subject to the same prejudices and discrimination as the patients they serve, on the grounds of their own allegedly fragile mental health, ineffectualness or even their authoritarian, 'bad cop' practices (Guimón, 2001). A number of research papers discuss the variables related to these negative attitudes (Guimón et al., 1999).

On the other hand, mental health professionals are not free of prejudice against their patients. This, in turn, favors the appearance of 'burn-out syndrome' (discouragement and even depression) which can have very detrimental effects on the patients themselves (Guimón, 2002). Finally, families of dependent psychiatric patients experience a serious burden that frequently leads to psychological disturbances among them.

PREVENTION AND TREATMENT OF THE BURN-OUT SYNDROME

In 1982, in a study of a sample of psychiatrists, psychologists and social workers, Roberts reached the conclusion that we still have no indication that allows us to make a correct forecast of the likelihood of appearance of symptoms described in the burn-out syndrome. As to treatment for this problem when it arises, different approaches have been upheld.

Interventions Involving Professionals

When working with clients who are burned out, authors stress the importance of modifying the discrepancy between unrealistic expectations and results through cognitive-behavioural intervention or other approaches based on self-help psychology or alternative psychodynamic models (Pines et al., 1981). Cognitive approaches focus on the positive aspects of work, trying to avoid professional stress factors which are not always in the foreground and seeking to adjust client expectations of what work can provide in terms of fulfillment. Advice is given to strengthen the support network and to diversify social and recreational life.

Psychoanalytic authors believe that people choose an occupation that enables them to replicate significant childhood experiences so efforts are made to determine why a burned-out professional chose a particular career. Dynamic-existential theoreticians further contend that people attempt to find existential significance through their work so intervention seeks to make clear how feelings of failure relate to burn-out and what changes should be introduced.

Roberts (1994) proposed that the usual means of dealing with stress is sufficient to control the symptoms. Schkolnik (1985) studied the relationship between dissatisfaction at work, burn-out syndrome and so-called 'maintainence behaviour for professional carers' prevention techniques among 61 workers in mental health centres in Ohio, and he proved their effectiveness. Brarley (1985) proposed counselling based on psychoanalytical and organisational teaching. Ray (1982) proposed an individual approach to stress management—he described it as *'holistic'*—to fight burn-out syndrome in mental health professionals. Jayaratne et al. (1984) stated that any action destined to reduce stress at work should be specific to each environment.

The Need for Interventions on Families

Psychiatric patients are a heavy burden for members of their family (Eker, 1989). In fact, several authors have pointed out the stress that results from caring for the mentally ill. Severe cases can be difficult to manage even under the best hospital conditions and, in any case, chronically ill patients or those who are getting worse, are problematical for those who live with them, and even professionals may prefer not to work with them. Thus, we can observe that people under these circumstances present increased use of psychotropic medication considerably. This was the case for 30% of subjects who cared for patients with Alzheimer's, and 20% for those involved with other disorders, both figures being pointedly higher than those of the general population (13%).

Research carried out in Geneva (Gognalons-Nicolet et al., 1999) examined the health burden (somatic aspects, anxiety and depression) of caregivers (self-help groups, family and patient associations, etc.). A number of factors were found to be important in the emergence of these problems, such as the increased numbers of the elderly in the population and the commitment of families (especially women) to caring for them during chronic or terminal illness. Three psychopathological tendencies (extracted from the Derogatis scale, 1974) showed that 30% of the population surveyed, aged 50 to 75, gave help to family members, neighbours or friends. In a gender breakdown, 5.7% of men and 11.9% of women do so in a regular and intensive manner. Thus, 55% of women were helping family members, and 42% helped neighbours or friends; 72% of men mainly helped their families, and only 22% helped neighbours or friends. Half of all subjects spent more than one hour a day on such activities, whereas the other half spent somewhat less time. Out of 59 individuals, 41 reported that this responsibility was not a problem in terms of their own health; 18 found this responsibility a burden, especially those helping people with certain types of illness (chronic and/or mental).

Feelings of being burdened were associated with depression and with somatic illness, but not with anxiety. Psychopathological tendencies were greater for women. For caregivers feeling burdened, the differences between men and women diminished, but the severity of psychopathological tendencies increased notably for men.

In conclusion, the authors stressed that even if home care decreased the cost of mental health care, it adds to the family's burden, so that alternative modes of residential care should be considered.

Bungener (1999) conducted a survey among 1844 members of a family association in order to evaluate the burden of care on the family and other non-professional volunteers. The survey revealed that non-autonomous patients, regardless of age, remain most frequently in the home environment. The majority of those who live with mental patients presented serious psychosocial problems. Twenty-one percent of families admitted that it was a situation they did not choose, and 17% said they felt subjected to it (this feeling sometimes lasted for decades). Twenty-eight percent reported negative effects on their professional life. Most often, we observed a reduction in the work schedule, early retirement, and even an end to professional life. Conversely, an increase in the work schedule, although less frequent, was justified by the rising financial burden of caring for the patient. It is the professional lives of mothers and spouses (despite their low number) that are the most affected. Fathers remain most often shielded. The same can be observed for social activities, although on a larger scale. Nine-hundred and seven people (51% of those surveyed) complained of a reduction in their social activities and subsequent isolation. The frequency of repercussions on siblings is also very high (72%). Families tended to withdraw into themselves or develop pathologies perceptible only in terms of effects and symptoms. Health problems were described by 522 mothers and by 358 fathers. But it is most often spouses who see themselves as the most at risk since 63 out of 95 spouses mentioned health problems. Cohabitation is also the source of aggressive behaviour (more often verbal than physical or material) on the part of the patient and directed at his/her family and vice versa.

THE PSYCHOLOGICAL PROBLEMS OF PSYCHIATRIC RESIDENTS

Planning the training of future psychiatrists, should not be restricted to questions of theoretical courses or clinical practice. The personal life of resident must also be taken into consideration, in view of the fact that students in our speciality abandon their studies more often than in others, and that residents beginning their psychiatry speciality are often found to have emotional problems. Considerable effort has gone into studying the reasons for abandoning this speciality, and into the detection and prevention or treatment of the psychological problems that may arise during residency and may affect the decision to abandon the course.

Reasons for Abandoning the Speciality

One of the the most serious and earliest works published on this subject was that of Garfinkel et al. (1974); they looked at the reasons why 14% of residents who had begun their residency in Toronto, dropped out before completing training, representing a far higher percentage than that of their colleagues in other specialities.

As a whole, there was a high degree of similarity in age and academic results during medical studies between those who had dropped out and their colleagues. Their marks at the beginning of residency and at the end of the first year were the same, but as from the second year, the marks were below those obtained by residents who continued their studies. They tended to be divided into two groups: those who dropped out after two years or more of training (often with poor assessment on the part of their teachers), and those who dropped out after one year (generally with good assessments). In both groups, the majority had carried out their first year of residency in a traditional psychiatric hospital. Indeed 82.1% of those who had dropped out, had spent their first year of training in a large psychiatric hospital, compared to 51.1% of those who did not drop out.

According to the study's authors, the high dropout rate during residency, partly concerns doctors who are perfectly competent but who quickly realise their incapacity to become psychiatrists. When they persevere along this course, their results get steadily worse, and they show signs of maladjustment. The dropping out of these doctors can be interpreted positively. All the specialised courses in medicine, particularly those with a more specific vocational commitment, such as psychiatry, should allow for the possibility of switching specialities, in spite of the undeniable administrative problems this entails.

Nevertheless, the existence of the other group of doctors who abandon the speciality after a year of study, who still consider themselves capable of completing their studies, and who receive good or very good marks from their professors, is far more disquieting. For Garfinkel et al. (1974), the explanation may be as follows: in traditional psychiatric hospitals, the resident sees his very identity as a doctor called into question and this may induce him/her to abandon the speciality.

Like other authors before them, they suggest that the first year of residency be carried out in a regional hospital centre rather than in a psychiatric hospital. Other methods have also been proposed to help the resident to adapt, such as integration into groups (Sadok et al., 1969) or extending the tutorial system to allow the resident to discuss his/her personal or professional difficulties.

The 'Beginning Psychiatry Training Syndrome'

Merklin (Merklin et al., 1967) described, 35 years ago, the syndrome of the resident at the beginning of psychiatric training (which he called *'beginning psychiatry training syndrome'*) in first-year residents in psychiatry who presented neurotic, psychosomatic and behaviour disorders. In his view, this picture develops in three phases. The first, a *prodromic* phase, is characterised by a change in attitude towards patients, colleagues and professors, and during which interns tend to be more concerned about the physical problems of their patients than by their psychological problems. The second phase is characterised by the appearance of a particular *symptomatology*, such as anxiety, depression and/or psychosomatic symptoms. A third phase of *resolution*, is characterised by becoming aware of the previous phases, a change in attitudes to patients, colleagues and professors and renewed interest in questions of a psychological nature.

Several authors have subsequently confirmed the existence of personality changes (Miller, 1969; Pasnau et al., 1971; Shershow et al., 1976; Brent, 1981), and emotional disorders (Ford, 1981; Russel et al., 1975, 1977; Taintor et al., 1982) among psychiatry residents, particularly in the United States, but also in other countries, such as Canada (Falconer et al., 1984). In a study we carried out in Spain (Guimón et al., 1987), roughly half the residents seemed to have personally experienced signs of various phases of the syndrome, and 42% reported having experienced the prodromic phase, although to a lesser degree. As regards what is referred to as the *reaction* phase, a similar percentage recognised having suffered depressive and psychosomatic symptoms. Anxiety seemed to have been particularly felt, as 75% reported having experienced it (36% slight, 27% moderate, 11% marked). Finally, 56% of interns had experienced the *resolution* phase (14% intensely). Although 51% of interns had not heard of this syndrome, 66% reported reactions fitting this description in their colleagues. It must be added that in some, minor syndromes were present, that three residents reported a suicide, one reported an attempt at self-mutilation, and two reported the decision to abandon the speciality.

Some authors, despite having noted the same difficulties, advise against adopting an alarmist attitude. Thus Taintor et al. (1982), in a survey conducted among all the residents in the United States completing their studies in 1975, studied the impact of certain factors specific to the residency, on the personal or professional training of the future psychiatrist. The results demonstrate the high level of stress, present in numerous aspects of the residency course but they also emphasise the positive role of these difficulties in terms of personal development.

Suicide

Sometimes, however, very serious problems have been manifested, such as psychotic decompensation and suicide (Pasnau et al., 1975). Even though some authors have reported (Kelly, 1973) that the level of suicide was probably the same as for residents in other specialities, corresponding to the average for this age range, the four suicides reported during the year studied by Pasnau represent the highest level among all the specialities.

Some studies (Pasnau et al., 1975; Rebal, 1982), have attempted to distinguish the symptoms which might help to identify residents at risk. In their study, Pasnau et al. examined the clinical history of five residents in psychiatry who had committed suicide, in a wide metropolitan sector over a period of 11 years.

Although it was not possible to define a precise reason or reliable precursory sign, the different cases presented strong similarities, such as the serious repercussions of a psychopathology; it was possible to distinguish matrimonial problems, the absence of close personal relationships, alcohol or drug abuse, frequent previous demands for psychotherapy treatment. As for the possible causes, they stressed the marked effect of personal, institutional and relationship problems and recommended improving the residents programme by, for example, assigning a tutor to each resident and facilitating their access to psychotherapy. Rebal (1982) studied transcripts of the interviews of four psychiatry residents who had later committed suicide, and a random selection of 110 others that took place when the candidate applied for the course. The four residents, 2 men and 2 women, committed suicide 18 to 60 months after beginning residency training, and only two had completed training. The author proposed a psychiatric analysis which showed positive results in 3 of the 4 subjects who committed suicide as opposed to only 5 out of the 110 subjects chosen at random (significant difference of 0.0001).

Whatever the case, the emotional problems of residents in psychiatry had attracted sufficient attention to warrant a working group being set up by the American Association of Directors of Residency Programmes in psychiatry.

Aetiological Factors of Psychological Disturbances

Among the aetiological factors put forward, the most notable is the resident's previous individual characteristics (Bucher et al., 1969). Russell et al. (1975, 1977) underline the fact that contrary to expectations, women, doctors with foreign qualifications, and members of minorities show no higher risk. They compared the answers to questionnaires given to 2860 residents in psychiatry with those of 288 residents presenting emotional problems. They noted no differentiation between the two groups in terms of sex, race, holding a foreign degree, or having begun a residency in other programmes. There were twice as many single people among residents with problems as in the reference group; in the case of marriage, divorce, separation or matrimonial problems were three times higher. They also experienced more problems than those who had started training in psychiatry after having practised medicine in other specialities.

Another likely cause of emotional disorder was the fear of a possible personal pathology and the lack of a common culture between the different psychiatric institutions. Also mentioned were the stressful atmosphere at work during the first year (Brenneis, 1973; Taintor et al., 1982). Rockwell (1973) thinks that having to supervise the work of nurses with more experience than oneself may also give rise to emotional difficulties in the resident.

A further element cited as possibly causing problems is the identity crisis experienced by residents (Gilmore et al., 1980) faced with the different theoretical models in psychiatry. Likewise, Skodol (Skodol et al., 1981) studied the degree of satisfaction expressed by residents with regard to their role, their theoretical orientation (organic, behaviourist, or psychodynamic), their technical skills, and need for control. He concludes that forming a positive professional identity, as expressed by the residents' level of role satisfaction, was more closely linked to the idea of having acquired technical skills than by adhering to any particular theoretical orientation.

In the study we conducted in Spain (Guimón et al., 1987), residents were asked to indicate the degree of importance they attached to different factors described as possible causes of beginning psychiatry training syndrome. Over half the residents interviewed thought that all factors were of some importance, with one exception. For 66%, the opinion of members of the family of the profession of psychiatrists is an insignificant factor. Other factors considered by over 40% of residents as negligible, included the opinions of other residents, medical students or professors in other specialities, the psychiatric profession and rivalry with other residents in psychiatry. On the other hand, for over 90%, the existence of several conflicting theories and the ambiguity of their content, as well as having to assume responsibility for psychological treatment for the first time, were significant factors.

Preventive Measures

Several authors have proposed measures to improve psychosocial support for residents, (Berg et al., 1980; Yager, 1974; Hales, 1980; Garrard et al., 1983), through the use of intervention techniques, notably involving participation in group psychotherapy activities (Sadok et al., 1969; Lomax et al., 1983; Willenbring et al., 1983; Lomax et al., 1983; Salvendy et al., 1983).

Some authors have drawn attention to the importance of the problems of adjustment experienced by residents with foreign degrees in the United States, but other authors fail to confirm this. Thus, Mc Dermott et al. (1975) conducted a study to identify and resolve the emotional and cognitive problems of psychiatry residents holding degrees from medical faculties outside the United States, and who make up a third of the psychiatry residents of this country.

Sadock (1969) described a group psychotherapy programme for residents enabling them to understand the emotional problems which can be created by becoming aware of the limitations of psychiatric knowledge. He considered the experience as a way of facilitating the transition between the first and second years of residency. 80% of residents who responded to our survey in Spain, felt it would be useful to participate in training experiences in which they could discuss phenomena such as beginning psychiatry training syndrome. Questioned as to which type of experience seemed to be the most interesting, almost half opted for a weekly tutorial session with staff on the teaching team.

REFERENCES

Berg, J. K., and Garrard, J. (1980). Psychosocial support in residency training programs. *Journal of Medical Education*, 55, 851–857.

Bion, W., and Rickman, J. (1943). Intra-group tensions in therapy. *Lancet*, 678–681.

Bion, W. R. (1962). *Learning from experience*. New York: Basic Books.

Brenneis, C. B. (1973). Current strains for mental health trainees. *American Journal of Psychiatry*, 130, 41–45.

Brent, D. A. (1981). The residency as a developmental process. *F. Med. Educ.*, 56, 417–422.

Bucher, R., and Stelking, S. (1969). Implications of prior socialization for residency programs in Psychiatry. *Archives of General Psychiatry*, 20, 395–402.

Bungener, M. (1999). Reduction in costs but increased family burden. In J. Guimón and N. Sartorius (Eds.), *Manage or perish*. New York: Kluwer Academic/Plenum Publishers.

Derogatis, L. R., Lipman, R. S., Rick, K., Uhlenhuth, E. H., & Covi, L. (1974). The Hopkins Sympton Checklist (HSCL). In P. Pichot (Ed.), *Modern problems in Pharmaco Psychiatry*. Basel: Karger.

Dubin, W. R. (1996). Can providers and payers collaborate? In A. Lazarus (Ed.), *Controversies in managed mental health care*. Washington, D.C.: American Psychiatric Press.

Eker, D., and Oner, B. (1999). Attitudes toward mental illness among the general public and professionals, Social representations and change. In J. Guimón, W. Fischer, N. Sartorius (Eds.), *The image of madness*. Basel: Karger.

Enriquez, E. (2000). Le travail de la mort dans les institutions. In R. Kaës (Ed.), *L'institution et les institutions. Etudes psychanalytiques* (2nd ed.). Paris: Dunod.

Falconer, C., and Leichner, P. (1984). The 'beginning psychiatry training syndrome' among psychiatric residents in Canada. *The Journal of Psychiatric Education*, 8, 169–178.

Ford, C. V. (1981). Emotional distress in residents and interns. Paper presented at the *American Psychiatric Association Meeting*, May 15, 1981, New Orleans.

Garrard, J., and Berg, J. K. (1983). Psychosocial support of residents in psychiatric programs: A national survey. *Journal of Psychiatric Education*, 7, 251–262.
Gilmore, M., and Perry, S. (1980). The psychiatry internship and the development of professional identity. *American Journal of Psychiatry*, 137.
Gognalons-Nicolet, M., and Bardet-Blochet, A. (1999). Social networks and health burden on care givers. In J. Guimón and N. Sartorius (Eds.), *Manage or perish?* New York: Kluwer Academic/Plenum Press.
Guimón, J. (2002). *Los profesionales de la Salud mental: Tareas y vicisitudes.* Madrid: Core Academic.
Guimón, J. (2001). *Inequity and madness. Psychosocial and human rights issues.* New York: Kluwer Academic.
Guimón, J. (2002). *Los prejuicios contra la Psiquiatría* (Vol. 5). Madrid: Core Academic.
Guimón, J., Azkunaga, D., and Sacanell, E. (1987). Presencia en España del llamado sindrome del residente que comienza su formacion en psiquiatria. *Psiquis*, VIII, 11–19.
Guimón, J., Fischer, W., and Sartorius, N. (1999). *The image of madness.* Basel: Karger.
Guimón, J., and Rojas Marcos, L. (1976). Psiquiatria de comunidad: una visión crítica. *Archives of Neurobiology*, 39, 77–99.
Kaës, R. (2000). Psychanalyse, institution. In R. Kaës (Ed.), L'institution et les institutions. *Etudes psychanalytiques* (2nd ed.). Paris: Dunod.
Kelly, W. (1973). Suicide and psychiatric education. *Psychiatry*, 130 (463–468).
Lomax, J. W., and Webb, L. J. (1983). Differential utility of a national training laboratory experiential conferences for psychiatric residents. *Journal of Psychiatric Education*, 7, 274–287.
Maslach, C., and Jackson, S. E. (1986). MBI: *Maslach Burn-out Inventory*. Palo Alto: University of California: Consulting Psychology Press.
Merklin, L., and Little, R. (1967). The beginning psychiatry training syndrome. American *Journal of Psychiatry*, 124(2), 97–101.
Miller, A. A. (1969). Professional developments in psychiatric residents. *Archives of General Psychiatry*, 20, 385–395.
Pasnau, R., and Russel, A. (1975). Psychiatric resident suicide: An analysis of five cases. *American Journal of Psychiatry*, 132, 402–406.
Pasnau, R. O., and Bayley, S. (1971). Personality changes in the first year of psychiatric residency training. *American Journal of Psychiatry*, 128, 111–115.
Pines, A., Aronson, E., and Kafry, D. (1981). *Burn-out: From tedium to personal growth.* New York: Free Press.
Rebal, R. F. (1982). Identification of the psychiatric resident at risk for suicide. *Journal of Psychiatric Education*, 6, 160–165.
Roberts, V. Z. (1994). The self-assigned impossible task. In A. Obholzer and V. Z. Roberts (Eds.), *The unconscious at work.* New York: Routledge.
Rockwell, M. (1973). Psychiatric residents' disease: social system contributions to resident's emotional problems. *International Journal of Psychiatry*, 19, 226–229.
Russel, A., Pasnau, R. O., and Traintor, Z. C. (1975). Emotional problems of residents in psychiatry. *American Journal of Psychiatry*, 132, 263–267.
Russel, A., Pasnau, R. O., and Traintor, Z. C. (1977). The emotionally disturbed psychiatric resident. *American Journal of Psychiatry*, 134, 59–62.
Sadok, B. J., and Kaplan, H. I. (1969). Group psychotherapy with psychiatric residents. *International Journal of Group Psychotherapy*, 19, 475–486.
Salvendy, J. T., and Stewart, M. F. (1983). Periodic T-groups for psychiatric residents. *Journal of Psychiatric Education*, 7, 287–296.
Schkolnick, J. (1985). Career sustaining behaviors, burnout and job satisfaction in mental health workers. *Dissertation Abstract International*, *45*(11–B).

Shershow, J. C., and Sanodnik, I. (1976). Regression in the service of residency education. *Archives of General Psychiatry*, 33, 1266–1270.

Skodol, A. E., and Maxmen, J. S. (1981). Role satisfaction among psychiatric residents. *Comprehensive Psychiatry*, 22, 174–178.

Taintor, Z., Morphy, M., and Seiden, A. M. (1982). Emotional problems in psychiatric residency training: Recommendations for their reduction. *Psychiatric Quarterly*, 54, 157–162.

Willenbring, M. L., and Spensley, J. (1983). The support group in psychiatric residency: How can we best help our residents? *Journal of Psychiatric Education*, 7, 724–787.

Yager, J. (1974). A survival guide for psychiatric residents. *Archives of General Psychiatry*, 30, 494–499.

30

Training Tomorrow's Mental Health Workers

MOTIVATIONS AND SKILLS

The ideology of interns in psychiatry is affected by the nature of their training and practical activities. Human beings tend to devise belief systems to justify their acts. This explains why the ideological attitudes adopted will differ according to the psychiatrist's various activities. Thus, it is quite normal that applying electroshock treatment in a hospital does not have the same influence on an intern as does practising psychoanalysis in an outpatient clinic.

Therefore, it is necessary to bear in mind that the institutional path and the activities of students in postgraduate training are of particular importance in reinforcing the intern's identity as a psychiatrist. On the strength of this argument, it is clearly important to begin training with activities similar to those of other physicians, such as liaison psychiatry, later introducing interns to a large number of seriously mentally ill patients, as for example in a short-stay unit (Beitman et al., 1984).

The criteria for designing these curricula must be based not only on the views of professors and interns, but on other parameters as well, one of these being guidelines on what helps to train psychiatrists in clinical practice, so that the content of the syllabus can be consistent with the activities described (Amat, et al., 1984).

As we saw earlier, tomorrow's psychiatrists will not only have to be experts in the techniques of diagnosis and treatment of the mentally ill; they will also need solid administrative skills. Their profile will correspond more closely with that of other physicians. Indeed, psychiatrists have tended in the past to differ from their colleagues in terms of particular psychosociological characteristics. Rogow (1970), in his classic work, described them as almost always male, middle class, more often separated or divorced than their physician colleagues and more often atheist or agnostic. Their cultural level, evaluated on the basis of their reading habits, was also higher, their political orientation frankly progressive, and their interest in the economic aspects of their profession less marked than in other physicians.

As might be expected, the psychiatrists presenting these personal characteristics differed from other medical students in their motives for choosing their specialisation. Their conscious motives included a desire to help people with mental suffering and a general interest in mental health issues. Various unconscious motives were also found. Thus, as one study (Ford, 1981) stated: 'The earliest factor motivating male subjects toward psychiatry, is identification and objects related to the Oedipal and pre-Oedipal years. Among these, the most common does seem to be identification with the mother and the maternal image.'

Other studies have indicated as more or less unconscious motives, the emotional problems that future psychiatrists hoped to be able to get rid of through their training and professional activities.

The indications today are that the individual characteristics and motives of physicians opting for psychiatry have changed, becoming more like those of physicians in other specialities. Likewise, the psychiatrist's profile differs less and less from that of others. So it seems obvious that training programmes for future psychiatrists should adapt to this evolution. The following pages will be devoted to examining various points of view as to what to teach future psychiatrists.

However, we must also bear in mind that, as well as the traditional training objectives, the present era of managed care demands specific knowledge. The professional image of the psychiatrist is undergoing a profound change. Forced to lead therapeutic teams, manage medical care and research programmes as well as supervising budgets, they devote more and more time to management tasks, and so need certain administrative skills. Although specific training is not yet compulsory for psychiatrists to become administrators, certain specialised courses are strongly recommended. Psychiatrists will also be asked to act in emergency psychiatry, consultation-liaison psychiatry, crisis intervention, combined psychotherapy and pharmacotherapy treatment, short-term psychotherapy support, group psychotherapy and supervision. Curricula for postgraduate students should be designed to give interns an opportunity to develop their knowledge in these areas.

TRAINING PROGRAMMES

Training programmes for psychiatrists vary according to factors such as the level of development and the sociopolitical context. Developing countries need as many psychiatrists as possible with varied skills, (clinician, researcher, epidemiologist, administrator, teacher and leader) and specialised abilities in particular fields, while there is perhaps less need for psychogeriatrics, for instance, than in other countries. Furthermore, it is vital for them to have more experience in administration.

There is also a need for more training centres; most African psychiatrists, for instance, are trained in developed countries, where the training they receive is not necessarily adapted to the type of practice they go on to later. In the Latin American countries, until the end of World War II, psychiatric training was usually conducted on the basis of a very personal master/disciple relationship involving no structured programme, or else through courses in other countries (mostly Spain and the United States). Since the 1960s, the flow of students leaving to study in other countries has diminished with the setting up of specialised, two-to-four-year courses, usually in line with the American model. In countries from the former Soviet Union, programmes still follow Russian training guidelines—under which physicians specialised in psychiatry through daily practice in the centres where they would later work; some did, however, follow an *ordinatura*, or an *aspirantura*—although most of them are now adapting their requirements to those proposed by the European Union.

In the EU countries, the treaty of Rome laid down the requirement of a four-year specialisation in psychiatry. In France, training has been conducted along two parallel lines: either in the form of an internship in officially recognised hospitals, after obtaining a state examination, or as periods of practical training carried out in psychiatric establishments followed by a final examination. Attempts are underway to unify the system. In Germany, the future specialist could receive psychiatric training by specialising for at least four years, one of which is devoted to neurology, or by training in neuropsychiatry, specialising in neurology for three years and in psychiatry for three years. In Spain a unified, standardised programme has been in existence since 1978. In Britain, specialised training in psychiatry takes place in psychiatric hospitals, in the psychiatric wards of general hospitals (the number of beds ranging from 40 to 150) and in university hospital services (less common). The Royal College of Psychiatrists determines which hospitals are authorised to provide training, laying down guidelines for accreditation in the different centres. Under the British system, future psychiatrists work for roughly a year as *senior house officers*, and then apply to become *registrars*; it is at this moment that they sit a final exam, after which they may apply for a post as *senior registrar*. After an advanced training course lasting from two to four years, the senior registrar may apply for a post of *consultant*. Overall, training in Britain takes two to three years longer than in the United States. All of the European programmes are at present being adapted to EU requirements.

The system that has had the most influence on the others is that of the United States. Right after World War II, the U.S. Congress founded the National Institute of Mental Health (NIMH), with a mandate for overseeing assistance, teaching and research; university psychiatric departments also witnessed an enormous development. In 1951 and 1952, a new training model was established. The typical American programme is more structured than European programmes; the resident is considered as a student in training rather than as a doctor on a practical training placement. On the other hand, residents benefit from friendlier, more relaxed relationships with their superiors than do their European counterparts. Great importance was attributed to psychoanalysis in the programme, but in combination with other subjects, it has developed into what is known as *dynamic psychiatry* recently. From the 1960s onward, the arrival of community psychiatry changed training programmes, extending psychiatry beyond its usual scope of knowledge and competence. Recent progress in biological psychiatry and diagnosis is in the process of modifying training, and more attention is now focused on these fields. At the end of residency the student has to pass a comprehensive oral and written exam to be granted the title of *psychiatric specialist* by the American Board of Psychiatry and Neurology, a private organisation with no real legal powers. Up to now, less than half of psychiatrists have passed the exam, as opposed to 95% of other physicians for their respective specialities.

In Switzerland, training lasts six years (five, until recently). This must be carried out in different hospital units and outpatient services authorised as training establishments by the Fédération des Médecins Helvétiques (FMH). The assistant doctors receive theoretical training in analytical, cognitive-behavioural and systemic psychotherapy, and are required to conduct supervision of the patients in their charge applying one of these techniques. Doctors must present a thesis and are granted the double diploma of psychiatrist and psychotherapist.

Psychotherapy Training

In the United States, as we have just said, a truly *dynamic psychiatry* has developed. This trend allowed the resident to become an adroit and sensitive psychotherapist, capable of judging human behaviour objectively and intuitively thanks to understanding of the concept of transfer and counter-transfer. The patient is thus understood from the point of view of his or her development. This approach also motivates the future psychiatrist to work with colleagues from other disciplines in psychiatric consultation. Although psychoanalysis is less important today in the United States, dynamic psychiatry has continued to exert an influence on psychiatrists, and the majority of training programmes offer supervision in analytical psychotherapy and full courses in dynamic psychiatry.

After a period of crisis, dynamic psychiatry went on to gain new ground in the training of psychiatrists in western countries. In Germany, psychotherapy and somatic medicine are taught in medical schools; in France, post-1968 reforms increased the number of psychoanalysts in universities, but they are now decreasing in visibility. In Switzerland, Sweden and Holland, psychoanalysts have formed an integral part of the university scene for many years. In Eastern European countries, renewed interest is being shown in dynamic psychiatric after years of lethargy.

What Do Tomorrow's Psychiatrists Need to be Taught?

In view of the profound changes taking place in psychiatry, it is of the utmost importance to design training programmes that give psychiatrists access to the skills they require; it is essential to define the knowledge they will need to focus on, the skills which will be demanded of them and the attitudes they should adopt.

All the sectors concerned have made great efforts, explicitly or implicitly, to target the educational objectives in psychiatric training. Resident training programmes are generally designed by psychiatric specialists of high professional and academic standing, but who are not necessarily the most in touch with the realities of everyday clinical practice.

The Directors of Teaching Units

However, there are at least two reasons why it is important to consider the opinions and views of the directors of teaching units on the programmes: 1) because they know to what extent the different points are likely to be put into practice; 2) because the personality and orientation of the training staff will influence the resident.

When future psychiatrists begin a residency programme, a large part of their identity—within which the professional identity as a doctor plays a considerable role—has already been defined. It has often been said, however, that the effect of extending this period of dependence on their supervisors is to maintain the resident in a sort of prolonged adolescence. In what

Erikson (1960) has referred to as a *psychosocial moratorium*, psychiatric residents are required to question their identity as a doctor, in order to adapt to their new identity as a psychiatrist. In this process, the type of activity engaged in during residency, the cognitive information received and the construction of their personality through contact with their supervisors, will play a fundamental role, through the more or less unconscious processes of identification. Indeed, psychiatrists' therapeutic and ideological orientation of the psychiatrist is partly developed during their residency period, and becomes increasingly like that of their professors.

Thirty years ago, Brown (1972) said that society expects the psychiatrist to specialise in 10 fields: 1) individual psychotherapy; 2) group psychotherapy; 3) crisis intervention; 4) intra-hospital treatment of patients; 5) teaching and supervision of residents in psychiatry and medicine; 6) advice to physician colleagues in clinical and specialised disciplines, both in hospital and in outpatient services; 7) advisory services to community and national health organisations; 8) participation in teaching programmes for general practitioners, professors, police services, nursing auxiliaries, nurses, and behavioural therapists; 9) psychiatry in the service of the courts; and 10) counselling activities in associations. Apart from general knowledge, a psychiatrist is expected to have specific understanding in three areas: 1) child psychiatry, 2) gerontopsychiatry, and 3) alcoholism and drug addiction.

Twenty years ago, the following objectives were proposed by group of Spanish psychiatry professors (Amat et al., 1984): 1) to serve the individual and the community through mental health care, applying the resources of psychiatry within the overall framework of public health; 2) to adapt to currents of thought in psychiatry and affiliated sciences; 3) to apply knowledge, psychiatric techniques and affiliated sciences to clinical activities and to predict, diagnose, give a prognosis, treat and re-educate; 4) to recognise motives and attitudes that influence the exercise of one's profession and to manage these positively; 5) to contribute to mental health training for psychiatrists, general practitioners, health specialists, and other members of the community; 6) to participate in setting up the best provision for health assistance, within the community, in the field of psychiatry, and to alter negative public attitudes, promoting the development of an appropriate health policy; 7) to collect, interpret and apply relevant information, and to participate in research projects; 8) to maintain a critical standpoint in regard to their own activity, to be able to gauge and modify this if necessary.

During the last decades, less interest has been devoted to these issues, even though the radical changes in the profession would justify a deep reflection.

The Consumers' Perspective

As indicated by Greden and Casariego (Greden et al., 1975), it is important to understand the feelings of residents toward psychiatric activities, firstly because they are the prime consumers of psychiatric teaching and their views can provide information about the type of product offered today by medical schools; secondly, residents represent a significant proportion of specialists and seem to be more flexible than psychiatrists already in practise; thirdly, because residents are the future guides to the profession which they will later change. Various studies on what residents consider important in their psychiatric training reveal changes over the course of time, consistent with the views of teachers, as has already been noted here.

However, while it is important to understand the views of teaching units directors in regard to the programmes, it is no less important to consider those of the consumers of this educational product, i.e., the residents themselves. The opinions of residents in psychiatry are very different from those of practising psychiatrists or those of their professors. Their views on training programmes also undergo changes, as we have already seen, in the course of their residency and not only through the phenomenon of identification with their professors.

Indeed, practice alters ideology. Timmons (1963) devised an ingenious experiment showing how the human being tends to invent beliefs to justify his or her acts. Transposed to the field of psychiatric ideology, this tendency might explain the way in which different ideological ideas are adopted depending on the type of activity engaged in by the psychiatrist. Thus, it follows that, as we said earlier, the regular practice of electroshock treatment in a closed institution will not have the same influence on those who set up the treatment as the use of psychoanalytical therapies in outpatient clinics.

Similarly, in a survey on Spanish psychiatrists, we were able to observe that psychiatrists working in the hospital setting, regional hospitals, or psychiatric hospitals, those who work in care units for alcoholics or drug addicts, or in outpatient public services largely opted for the medical model. On the other hand, those who worked in mental health centres stated a preference for the psychological model. The social model is marginal, having most impact among psychiatrists working in psychiatric hospitals.

Lidz (1970) contended 30 years ago that students should be offered a training programme that is radically different to what is currently available, leaving a number of aspects considered as significant in medical training, in the background. He seriously suggested creating semi-autonomous psychiatry schools in the future. Brown (1972), on the contrary, considers, like most authors, that medical studies must be completed before specialising in psychiatry.

The attitudes of residents and their professors regarding the various ideological models in psychiatry increasingly converge during residency. Comparing the attitudes of residents to different therapies throughout their residency, Willmuth and Spiner (Willmuth et al., 1978) saw an increase in their confidence in sociotherapy, whereas their confidence in psychotherapy diminished and their confidence in somatotherapy remained unchanged.

Thus, it is important to consider that the routes followed and activities planned as part of the residency course play an important part in forming the identity of the resident as a psychiatrist. Leading on from this idea, we have stressed the value of the first activities in residency being similar to those of other doctors, such as liaison psychiatry, and of placing residents in contact with a large number of seriously mentally ill patients in a short stay unit at a later stage.

Whatever the case, the view of residents themselves as to what should be taught to future specialists in psychiatry, lacks the time perspective. This is why the criteria used in designing programmes should include not only the views of the teachers and the taught but other parameters as well. One of these is a description as to what a psychiatrist really does in clinical practice (see chapter 26 of this book), so that the contents of the programme are able to achieve the intrinsic aims of the activities described.

Specific Issues

Three decades ago, Melges (1972) had already called attention to the fact that is important for physicians specialising in psychiatry to be aware of research in clinical practice. To this end, he called for thorough training in methods for evaluating the subjective alterations in an individual over the course of several years. This recommendation becomes nowadays of the utmost importance.

The New Programme in Geneva

The Department of Psychiatry is one of the 12 departments of the University Hospitals of Geneva, and is the only public psychiatric service in the Canton of Geneva (400,000 inhabitants) offering inpatient and outpatient services. No private facilities exist for psychiatric inpatients, but 200 private psychiatrists work in the canton on an outpatient basis, and 100 residents work in the Department. A high proportion of residents are foreigners, and they do not stay in Geneva when they finish their residency.

Educational Objectives

The two separated postgraduate training programmes in 'Psychiatry and Psychotherapy' for adult and child psychiatrists have been under scrutiny in Switzerland over the past 10 years, and a new adult psychiatry training programme was put into practice in 1996. In order to adapt this programme to Geneva's Department of Psychiatry, and in recognition of the fact that a knowledge of the psychiatrist's daily practice is essential in the formulation of appropriate training objectives, we made a survey of the psychiatric ideology (Guimón et al., 1998) and clinical practices (Guimón et al., 1997) (see chapter 26 of this book).

Swiss psychiatrists appeared to have relatively weak biological training whereas. On the contrary, Switzerland appeared to be one of the countries in the world where psychoanalytically-oriented psychotherapies are most widely used. A large number of correlations were obtained amongst all the variables studied, rising to some enlightening insights into ways in which training programmes might be improved.

A New Postgraduate Programme

A certain number of hospital services are accredited in Switzerland to give full training, and others to provide a one-to-two year element of the training (e.g., psychogeriatrics, substance abuse). One year of research is allowed during this period, and another year is spent in a medical service other than that of psychiatry. The psychotherapy component of the programme is taught through lectures and supervisions carried out by trained outside psychotherapists. Psychoanalysis used to be the exclusive orientation of psychotherapeutic training.

With modifications of the syllabus, the length of the specialisation programme has been transformed from six years into five (Guimón, 2000). The components of the theoretical courses have been standardised with a greater emphasis in the diagnoses and biological therapy issues. The psychotherapy element has been better defined. In fact, after one year of general psychotherapeutic teaching, students have the choice between three main orientations: psychodynamic, cognitive-behavioural, and systemic. Insofar as the application of these modifications in Geneva is concerned, the programme has been concentrated more on adult psychiatry, and an emphasis placed on biological issues. Consultant supervisors in psychotherapy, with an orientation different from that of the psychoanalytical, have been hired (Guimón, 2001).

The Training of the Psychiatrist Manager

The number of doctors in key positions in the present system of medical care throughout the world is insufficient. The American Medical Association (A.M.A.) has estimated that only 2% of doctors in the United States devote most of their time to management (Roback et al., 1994). In a survey carried out in 1986 (Schenke, 1986) of 848 doctors identified as administrators, fewer than 14% had qualifications other than their medical degree (M.D.), and only 1% had a masters in business administration (M.B.A.). Nevertheless, a more recent survey (Lloyd et al., 1994) showed an increase in the numbers of doctors studying for an M.B.A. As Lazarus (1995) has said, there is no doubt that with the new system of managed care, administrators with poor clinical experience will take responsibility for supervision, and there will be a real need for doctor-managers.

Many clinicians today are seeking to pursue careers outside the clinic for a variety of reasons (Crane, 1988), including disenchantment; increasing third party interference; growing fears of committing an act of negligence; and personal and financial considerations, such as competition with other doctors, irregular working hours, health problems, age and retirement. In an A.M.A. report (1993), practising doctors who are attracted by the challenge of leadership generally experience less stress and anxiety at the point of making the transition.

For Marcos (Marcos et al., 1988) and Silver (Silver et al., 1989), psychiatrists have the potential to become excellent managers because of their varied training and clinical experience. Penzer (1989) also notes that psychotherapists have many similar attributes to those of a good administrator: for example, they can tolerate ambiguity and make difficult decisions, they use timely judgement to resolve complex problems, they work with individuals who are preoccupied and angry and they can fathom resistance to change. Because of their mental health training, psychotherapists are ideally placed to access administrative posts, whereas clinicians may lack some of the interpersonal skills needed to become efficient managers.

Doctors with management qualifications earn 7% more than those without these qualifications (Mangan, 1993). A business graduate is generally expected to bring greater economic return on training investment than a medical graduate (Weeks et al., 1994). However, at the start of their careers as doctor-managers, the rewards may not outweigh the possible benefits of a strong clinical practice. Increasing the administrative salary of doctors with the revenues of the clinical practice may limit the cost of placing a doctor in an administrative post.

There are nevertheless a number of reasons (Silver et al., 1989) why it may be difficult to recruit psychiatrists for management: fear of abandoning the practice, a lack of administrative know-how, a level of uncertainty about relationships with administrators who are not doctors, and the lack of doctor-executive role models for medical students. Regarding the latter (Lazarus, 1995), medical students are rarely in contact with head physicians during their studies, since the emphasis in training is upon individual patient care rather than on managing medical systems and patient populations. Furthermore, the rare opportunities medical students do have to meet doctor-managers (such as deans and department heads) are often considered as outside their main interests or even undervalued.

Changing careers may be stimulating, but it does involve certain risks (Lazarus et al., 1996). To climb the management ladder, for example, it may be necessary to change jobs frequently, job security may be threatened, and apart from a few exceptions, psychiatrists who are employed by managed care organisations ultimately work under administrators who are not doctors, which may cause tension. In fact, doctors receive training medical schools and as interns, whereas managers are principally trained in university business schools; they tend to have different value systems (toward the sick, for example); and they usually differ in psychological make-up (more introverted physicians and more extroverted administrators). Psychiatrists demoralised by the fact that the managed care system has eroded their autonomy, gain no more autonomy working for a managed care organisation. Lazarus sums up the biggest challenge to doctor-managers not in terms of whether they can master the job, but in their ability to develop fruitful and collegiate relationships with managers who are not doctors.

Whatever the case, a career in medical management (Lazarus et al., 1996) is not a haphazard affair. Management training does not necessarily entail taking an advanced degree. The teaching requirements may be fulfilled by selective lectures, workshops and seminars on management training. Many universities offer courses of this type. Supplementary training can also be dispensed in the form of seminars offered by various professional organisations.

Some psychiatrists who work in managed care organisations have previous official training in university business schools, public health or public administration institutes. Vavala (1994) insists that the M.B.A. is the best university degree for training future doctor-managers. The typical business studies curriculum includes elements like marketing, finance, accountancy, statistics, economics, planning strategy, human resource management, and business ethics and law. The differences compared with health-oriented master's level courses are minimal, as most of the required conditions are practically identical (Vavala, 1994).

WHAT PSYCHOTHERAPY SHOULD THE PSYCHIATRISTS DO?

The psychiatrist cannot abdicate his therapeutic function. Our view is that only psychoanalysis is able to provide the human being with a sufficiently valid frame of reference for the psychiatrist to act in a psychotherapeutic manner. But over the last decades, the application of Freudian theories to psychiatry has given rise to a 'decaffeinated' version of psychoanalysis, referred to as *dynamic psychiatry*, which is probably the only way in which psychoanalysis can play a relevant role in the future of mental health.

Psychiatrists must first have training in dynamic psychiatry to enable them to evaluate certain factors of the personality of the patient, such as his or her ego fortress, the nature of unconscious conflict and the defence mechanisms, and the structures of the superego. They must also be able to assess family relationships, transference models, and what has been called the *internal objects relationships*.

The psychiatrist must be capable, secondly, even if he only treats patients with medication, of 'containing' (in the Bionian sense) the superabundant suffering of his patients. Indeed, over 70% of hospitalised patients are diagnosed under Axis II. In addition, as we saw in the previous chapter, the frequency of characteristic resistance to medication and 'negative placebo' effects require a dynamic approach.

Finally, the psychiatrist must be able to offer his patients psychotherapy treatment if this proves necessary. Most psychiatric patients are not psychoanalysable, but there are a number of diagnoses for which psychoanalysis continues to be the priority indication. For certain patients, cognitive-behavioural or systematic techniques are indicated. For the majority, finally, an *'eclectic'* (or *syncretic*) psychotherapeutic approach would be the most appropriate choice. Indeed, therapists, whatever their theoretical orientation, have an extremely important function in the success of psychotherapy: that of providing an appropriate space in which the patient can set down his or her preoccupations, desires and anxieties. A 'containing space', where all these things can be developed, and then gathered up again by the patient, once they are modified. This containing space responds to the patient's expectations of emotional contact and cognitive information, and leads him or her towards a passive learning experience. From this point on, the patient is prepared through communication and interaction to accept the conceptual framework of the therapist, and the therapist's views on the world, human beings, the causes of the patient's disturbances, and the means of recovery. This is an active learning process, in which the clinician attempts to modify the patient's perceptions, feelings, cognition and behaviour.

Most of the reticence in psychiatry today towards the psychoanalyst comes from the psychoanalysts' own reluctance to submit their theory and practice to scientific scrutiny. Even if the roles attributed to psychotherapy vary greatly from one country to another, there is. As we said above, a distinct resurgence of interest in psychoanalytical techniques in certain Western and Eastern European countries. The European Psychotherapy Association and a European Association of Psychoanalytical Psychotherapy have been created, bringing together psychotherapists of all tendencies. Psychoanalytical psychotherapy appears to be the most popular of these tendencies, and psychiatrists are the most numerous and influential of its members.

REFERENCES

A. M. A. (1993). Leaving *the bedside: The search for a nonclinical medical career*. Chicago: American Medical Association.

Amat, E., Carbonel, C., Cervera, S., et al. (1984). The educational objectives of medical psychology and psychiatry in pregraduate and postgraduate medical curriculum. In J. J. Lopez-Ibor and G. Lenz (Eds.), *Training and education in psychiatry*. Vienna: Facultas-Verlag.

Amat, E., Carbonell, C., Cervera, S., et al. (1984). Recent developments of the training in psychiatry in Spain and Portugal. In J. J. Lopez-Ibor and G. Lenz (Eds.), *Training and education in psychiatry*. Vienna: Facultas-Verlag.

Beitman, B. D., and Maxim, P. (1984). A survey of psychiatric practice: implications for psychiatric training. *The Journal of Psychiatric Education*, 8, 149–153.

Crane, M. (1988). Thinking about leaving practice? Read this first. *Medical Economics* (August), 132–136.

Erikson, E. H. (1960). The problem of Ego identity. In M. Stein, A. H. Vidich, and D. M. White (Eds.), *Identity and anxiety*. New York: The Free Press.

Ford, C. V. (1981). *Emotional distress in residents and interns*. Paper presented at the American Psychiatric Association Meeting, May 15, 1981, New Orleans.

Greden, J. F., and Casariego, J. I. (1975). Controversies in psychiatric education: A survey of resident's attitudes. *Psychiatry*, 132, 3.

Guimón, J. (2000). New forms of psychiatric education: The Geneva Experience. European *Journal of Psychiatry*, 14 (1), 52–60.

Guimón, J. (2001). Scope and limitations of psychonalysis in clinical psychiatry. In *Challenges of psychoanalysis in the 21st century*. New York: Kluwer Academic.

Guimón, J., Fischer, W., Zbinden, E., and Goerg, D. (1997). Therapeutic practice profiles, work settings and activities of Swiss psychiatrists. *Archives Suisses de Neurologie et Psychiatrie*.

Guimón, J., Fischer, W., Zbinden, E., and Goerg, D. (1998). Therapeutic practice profiles, theoretical models and representations of the psychiatry of Swiss psychiatrists. *Archives Suisses de Neurologie et Psychiatrie*, A paraître.

Lazarus, A. (1995). The psychiatrist-executive: New role, new economics. *Psychiatric Annals,* 25, 494–499.
Lazarus, A., et al. (1996). *Controversies in managed mental health care.* Washington, D.C.: American Psychiatric Press.
Lidz, T. (1970). Towards schools of psychiatry: *Training tomorrow's psychiatrist.* Yale University Press.
Lloyd, J. S., and Lyons, M. F. (1994). The physician executive 'arrives'—a new generation prepares for the future. *Physician Exec.,* 20(7), 31–36.
Mangan, D. (1993). Lured by the promise of a new career? Read this first. *Medical Economics* (November 22), 159–169.
Marcos, L. R., and Silver, R. A. (1988). Psychiatrist-executive management styles: Nature or nurture? *American Journal of Psychiatry,* 145, 103–107.
Melges, F. T. (1972). Integrating Psychiatric Research with clinical training. *Journal of Nervous and Mental Disease,* 153, 3.
Penzer, W. N. (1989). Clinician turned administrators: drawing upon clinical experience for managerial expertise. *Administration and Policy in Mental Health,* 17, 105–109.
Roback, G., Randolph, L., Seidman, B., et al. (1994). *Physician characteristics and distribution in the U.S.* Chicago: American Medical Association.
Rogow, A. (1970). *The psychiatrists.* New York: Putnam's Sons.
Schenke, R. S. (1986). Administration. New Physician, 35, 44–45.
Silver, M. A., and Marcos, L. R. (1989). The making of the psychiatrist-executive. *American Journal of Psychiatry,* 146, 29–34.
Vavala, D. (1994). A matter of degree: the trend toward physician executives' pursuing master's degrees. *Physician Exec.,* 20 (7), 31–36.
Weeks, W. B., Wallace, A. E., Wallace, M. M., et al. (1994). A comparison of the educational costs and incomes of physicians and other professionals. *New England Journal of Medicine,* 330, 1280–1286.
Willmuth, L. E., and Spinner, N. (1978). Changing therapeutic ideologies: First-year psychiatric residents. *Psychiatric Education,* 2, 178–184.

31

Training of Non-Psychiatrist Professionals

THE TRAINING OF GENERAL PRACTIONERS IN THE PSYCHIATRIC ASPECTS OF PRIMARY CARE

The High Prevalence of Mental Health Problems in Primary Care

Despite the fact that the first psychoanalysts who were interested in psychosomatic medicine (including Ferenczi, Alexander, Dunbar, Balint) had already accentuated the importance of psychological factors in health care, mental health aspects of health care continue to be neglected. The importance of these problems, however, was not unknown to them. Thus, as early as 1964, Taylor and Chauve in Britain had reported that 33% of the population suffered from psychiatric symptoms for which they received no treatment, and that 8.1% of the population was treated for psychiatric disorders by general practitioners, whereas 0.44% of the population received treatment in psychiatric outpatient services and only 0.19% were admitted to psychiatric hospitals.

Nevertheless, years were to go by before the high prevalence and low detection rate of these disorders was to be studied more extensively. As we said earlier, the significant Epidemiological Catchment Area (ECA) project carried out in the United States over a six-month period, showed that at least 19.1% of the population suffered from some diagnosed mental disorder according to DSM III-R criteria. Other studies showed that between one-third and one-fifth of patients consulting general practitioners presented psychiatric symptoms. Nevertheless, general practitioners' expertise in identifying psychiatric disorders does not, unfortunately, appear to be sufficient, with an estimated detection rate of 60% detection. General practitioners refer an excessive number of patients to psychiatrists, and when they do try to treat psychiatric patients themselves, they tend to use principally psychotropic medication (which is not always adequate) and vitamins.

Among the most frequently encountered psychological disorders are depression, anxiety disorder, and disorders linked to the consumption of alcohol and somatic illness. As frequently in developed as in developing countries, most patients who present a well-defined psychological disorder seek help for complaints similar to those associated with physical illnesses. Mental problems therefore, represent a major public health problem, and they are not sufficiently treated. We must develop programmes for the public and for targeted care-providers on the detection and management of psychological problems in primary care, which must be underlined at all levels of medical training and taught by specialists in mental health. We must develop research on how to improve detection of these disorders, on the transformation of the structural organisation of health services, and on techniques of treatment and prevention of disabilities.

The links between primary care services and mental health vary according to the countries concerned. In the British model of 'derivation', general practitioners are the first recourse of patients with psychological complaints, and refer them to psychiatrists. The 'substitution' model proposes that family doctors and other professional networks (e.g., educational, social services) or laypersons (support systems) take charge of care. Psychologists and psychiatrists provide temporary support to primary care physicians until they can be replaced by well-trained general practitioners. The third model is that of collaboration between general practitioners and psychiatrists, working in proximity but at different locations, which fosters the risk of becoming a model of derivation. In the fourth model, real 'mental health in primary intervention', the mental health team works at the same location as the general practitioner.

Whatever the relationship between primary care medicine and psychiatry, it is clear that in the future general practitioners will act (as is already the case in some countries such as the Netherlands and Britain) as the gatekeepers of the system and will be the first recourse not only for physical complaints, but for psychological or social problems, unless they arise in an emergency situation.

In the United States, HMOs are increasingly prevalent. For example, in Seattle, Washington, they insure 385,000 inhabitants, with 29 clinics for primary care and five specialised clinics. This system furnishes care by capitation, and the physicians are employees of the system. Under this system, the patient must be sent to the specialist by the general practitioner.

In contrast to the widespread belief according to which mental illness encountered in primary care medicine is of minor significance, these cases effectively show that it is a major public health concern, which is being insufficiently addressed. Therefore, mental health must be an integral part of primary care, and there is a great need for the acquisition of a dynamic attitude on the part of general practitioners.

Classical psychiatric practice has little value for general practitioners. Patients who go to general practitioners with mental problems have frequently suffered numerous losses and frustrations and by the time they consult the GP, they have already been overcome by very primitive anxieties. They often present bodily dysfunction which forms the basis of their decreasingly ability to personally deal with contention. A good doctor can implement contention, and a health organisation that does not provide contention will promote disintegrating effects. The basic job of the mental health team in primary intervention consists of backing up the 'family doctor' in helping the integration of the body and its disturbances (Guimón, 1996), by dealing with phantasies arising from the unconscious. Institutions, social and moral norms, and the culture also possess a function to promote contention. Most often, our job consists of helping patients not to further inflict damage on themselves, something which administrators find hard to believe.

The predominance of patients' somaticising their illness when they consult general practitioners is explained by the medical establishment's wish to act as biological 'apostles', which favours the expression of anxiety and patient conflicts in a physical form. The initial task when working with these patients consists in de-contextualising the physical manifestations of conflicts in order to then confront them more directly on both the inner and interpersonal levels.

Using the model of psychoanalytical interpretation, we apply biological, psychological or psychosocial techniques.

Training in Psychiatry for Swiss Generalists

The Swiss system seems to be *'good enough'* (in Winnicott's sense of the term, 1971) since certain elements lead us to think that the psychiatric training of general practitioners and internists in Switzerland is more intensive than in other countries. This is not surprising, since training in medical psychology is very important in the education of medical students at most Swiss medical schools. In a study carried out in Zurich on medical students, it was found that the vast majority of them considered psychiatry an important field of training for non-psychiatric physicians. In fact, physicians—especially general practitioners and internists—are very interested in psychiatry. An opinion poll carried out with internists practising in the Canton of Geneva showed that an important number of general practitioners and internists elected to undertake voluntary training in psychiatry during their medical studies (Goerg et al., 1996). Similarly, a high number of GPs and internists undertook postgraduate training in psychiatry. For example, in Geneva, more than half (51%) of GPs and more than one-third of internists had under- or postgraduate training. Similarly, more than half of internists and GPs took part in training groups for psychological problems and interpersonal relations. Approximately 30% of these physicians participated in Balint groups, either in courses whose objective was to improve the diagnosis of certain illnesses or in programmes including personal psychotherapies, or as part of programmes offered by organisations such as the Psychosomatic Association of Paris. Thus, 75% of 3rd year students and 88% of 6th year students considered psychiatry to be important; 40% of them believed psychiatry to be as scientifically grounded as other medical disciplines.

Medical students surveyed in Geneva regarding psychiatric training were relatively satisfied with their educational background in most of the areas they considered to be important.

In an opinion poll about the education and abilities that a general practitioner should have concerning psychiatry, the most rated were:

1. the doctor–patient relationship (ability to discuss problems with their patients, to be familiar with the dynamics of the doctor-patient relationship);
2. the detection of the principal psychiatric problems, with their elements of risk (differential diagnosis, psychopharmacological, referral to the psychiatrist, risk of suicide and necessity for hospitalisation);
3. the understanding of a set of complaints with psychosocial, somatic elements linked to stress, emotional aspects for patients with chronic or terminal illness, alcoholism, drug abuse, etc., which imply a knowledge of the social resources from which the patient may benefit.

Even if the aforesaid priorities did not always coincide with those proposed by the professors of psychiatry, they were taken into account at the time of establishing the objectives. The fact that the students considered certain common problems to be insufficiently taught, moved us to concentrate the programme on disorders frequently encountered in general practice.

A classic, discipline- and lecture-based approach existing in our Medical School was replaced by a new educational model that has been put into practice during the last four years with the help of a newly created Unit of Development and Research in Medical Education, directed by a newly appointed professor, Christine Vu. The aim of the new programme was to integrate the teaching of basic, clinical and psychosocial sciences with an orientation towards community health care, through active, self-directed learning based on extended practice.

The first-year curriculum uses a classical approach, with lectures on topics in physics, chemistry, statistics, anatomy, biology, embryology, physiology, organisation of the central nervous system, and a 28-hour introduction to psychosocial medicine.

The curriculum for the combined second and third years consists of 11 four-week learning units (among them one on the Biological Basis of Behaviour), four two-week learning units to foster multisystem integration and a 27-month Clinical Skills programme in small groups. Students are also offered a thorough community-based learning experience.

The fourth and fifth years begin with 12-week small-group sessions, comprising topics on the main medical branches including psychiatry and designed to facilitate knowledge of mechanisms underlying common clinical syndromes. There is afterwards a 1-year rotation of 11 practice-based clinical internships with a duration of eight, four or three weeks. The internship in psychiatry lasts four weeks and consists in problem solving, case-based sessions emphasising self-directed learning. A standard week includes four 2-hour sessions of case-based discussions, 17 hours of self-directed learning, three seminars on non-psychiatric topics, six hours of medical visits, two afternoons of patient admissions, and daily morning rounds.

The sixth year consists of 10 consecutive months of full-time activity in some elective subjects.

The students have expressed satisfaction with the clinical pertinence of what they learn in the basic medical sciences. The new small group, problem-based learning approach encouraged the participation of many students who had previously not enrolled in the traditional curriculum. On the part of the tutors, the contacts between clinicians and basic scientists were reinforced, thus increasing interdisciplinary work and the understanding of some patterns of interpersonal and group dynamics .

As outlined in an internal report, the integration of the psychological and psychosocial aspects of the 'vignettes' has been less successful than that of basic and clinical sciences in the second- and third-year curriculum. Even when problems contained aspects concerning psychological issues, the students and the tutors tended to put the emphasis on basic medical sciences and clinical aspects, rather than on psychological or psychosocial issues. The explanation for this probably lies in the fact that the choice of vignettes for the pre-clinical period was carried out in a group discussion with the rest of the faculty of the other departments, and our educational objectives could not be adequately maintained. In fact, the representatives of the other medical branches insisted on our taking responsibility for the biological basis of behaviour, to the exclusion of the psychological aspects of illness —which had been the main component of our prior teaching activities. The result was that very skilled teachers, more oriented towards the transmission of knowledge of patient-doctor interaction and the physical expression of emotional conflict, desisted from taking part in this teaching and were replaced by teachers of psychiatric neurosciences who, although equally skilled in their own area, did not have the expertise necessary to assure the other set of objectives.

In the clinical period, students were very satisfied with the clinical exposure they had to the main psychiatric syndromes. However, we realised that they had, in fact, been exposed to syndromes they would rarely see in their general medical practice. Mild anxiety or depressive disorders and other frequent psychological disturbances were not prevalent in the population to which the students had access. This consideration is now being brought to bear on the need to expand the population with whom they will have contact to medical rather than psychiatric populations, in the guise of psychiatrists having special skills in the detection and treatment of these kinds of mild, frequent syndromes.

OTHER NON-MEDICAL PROFESSIONALS

Psychologists

Psychologists' mental health training varies from one country to another; some demand years of schooling, whereas others foresee no kind of formal education.

In Spain, there are some individual training programmes that are more or less complete. In addition, a ministerial order created a training programme for psychologists in public mental health centres (known by its Spanish initials as the PIR), with a curriculum similar to that of medical residents; however, it has, unfortunately, not been developed as much as it should. In France, a report for reforming the national psychiatric system, *De la Psychiatrie à la Santé Mental* (From Psychiatry to Mental Health) (Piel and Roelandt, 2001), proposed eliminating psychiatric hospitals, increasing sectorisation, bringing treatment closer to patients, changing the laws, and adapting professional training to practical developments in the field.

The report pointed out the need for psychiatrists-in-training to acquire experience in different kinds of psychiatric units, and not just in university departments; to train them in all of the different developmental life stages; to improve continuing education; and provide complementary training in public health and team management.

For clinical psychologists, internships are essential, and the report cites the positive Spanish experience of creating a framework for psychology interns, including a competitive examination to select them followed by two years of on-site hospital training.

Training in public health, according to this report, is also essential. Its authors recommend that to establish therapeutic guidelines, patients be sent to the psychologist by a psychiatrist in order to rule out somatic disorders, and for reimbursement.

Nurses and Social Workers

The experience of World War II confirmed the need to elaborate a massive training plan for these professionals, due to the human suffering caused by mental illnesses. In 1946, the first post-war United States Congress approved the National Mental Health Law, which stipulated the establishment of the National Institute of Mental Health to implement the programmes authorised by that law.

The first psychiatric nursing school in the United States was founded in 1870 in Waverly, Massachussets, although this kind of training did not become common practice in the United States until 1946–1960. Peplau's *Interpersonal Relations in Nursing*, published in 1952, had a deep impact on the management and content of psychiatric nursing and mental health curricula, and provided a theoretical framework for practice and research in this field.

In most European countries there are various professional categories which, logically, involve different degrees and levels of training. For the most highly qualified nursing personnel, there are two formulas, according to their training systems: a general degree followed by post-graduate specialisation in psychiatry, as is the case in Belgium, Italy, or Norway; or working directly towards a specialist degree, as in Britain, Germany, or Portugal.

In France, until 1958, there was not a standard curriculum for psychiatric nurses' training, and each psychiatric hospital trained its personnel according to its own criteria, resulting in a wide variety of levels. However, since the social laws of 1936, personnel could get away from the tradition of being more guards than therapists, and they had better access to professional competence. However, it was not until 1958 that the situation of French psychiatric hospital personnel was generally comparable to that of today's psychiatric nurses in Spain. With the decrees of 1956 and 1958, the regulations concerning psychiatric nursing changed, and in 1970 certain aspects of training were significantly reformed.

The report *De la Psychiatrie à la Santé Mental* (Piel and Roelandt, 2001) recommends integrating their specialised training into the university system, including specific classes on social representations and their relationship with the community if a psychotherapeutic practice was to be included, with complementary training modules.

Another interesting approach to training psychiatric nurses came from Britain. Generally, British nurses enjoy a great deal of autonomy. The teaching of psychiatric nursing in Britain is structured around very consistent general guidelines. The curriculum, based on studying human relations, stresses the relationship between mental health and mental illness.

In the Spanish region of Catalonia, the country's first school for specialised nursing was created in 1930. In 1967, Spain created a speciality in psychiatry for general nurses. The first course organised officially by the Department of Health was held at the University of Navarre. Three years later, the Schools of Specialisation were created by decree, in Madrid, Barcelona, and Seville, and later (1978) in Valladolid; they also disappeared by decree in 1986, and since then there is no possibility of studying a speciality in psychiatric nursing.

To evaluate the introduction of clinical practice guidelines in nursing and other professions allied to medicine eighteen studies were reviewed (Thomas et al., 2002). The conclusion was that there is some evidence that guideline-driven care is effective in changing the process and outcome of care provided by professions allied to medicine.

Social workers' training should be accentuated, because the development of mental health depends largely on innovations in their practice. They should have more mobility in networking, and be able to assume case management functions. If they conduct psychotherapy, it should be under conditions similar to those of psychologists. The mental health training of physical therapists should also be improved.

Professionals coming from other branches of the social sciences should be introduced to psychotherapy with serious, well-supervised programmes. Administration and management personnel could also benefit from internships and specific training. Medical secretaries should have appropriate mental health training, as well.

Host families who accept the challenge of living with others suffering from mental disorders provide an important alternative to hospitalisation, offering their homes as hospices, and these families should receive training adapted to their needs, be granted an appropriate status, and properly assessed.

For all health professionals, there should be a common core curriculum in health and social studies, with complementary training in mental health, enabling them to recognise the work of 'mental health facilitators', and so on, in those who already show these skills. Every five years, they should do 1–3 month internships.

Artists have always shown a special ability to listen and to become integrated into social life, so that they should be made co-participants as paid social actors (Piel and Roelandt, 2001).

Collaboration between Mental Health Professionals

To assess the effects of interventions designed to improve nurse-doctor collaboration, a Cochrane review of three trials was conducted, with interventions consisting mainly of daily, structured, team ward rounds, in which nurses, doctors and other professionals made care decisions jointly. The reviewers' conclusion was that increasing collaboration improved outcomes of importance to patients and to health care managers. These gains were moderate, and affected health care processes rather than outcomes (Zwarenstein and Bryant, 2002).

Effective collaboration between health and social care professionals is frequently unsatisfactory. A series of procedures have bee proposed to improve it among them 'inter-professional education' (IPE) whose results have been reviewed in a Cochrane study (Zwarenstein, et al., 2002) comparing it to an educational programme in which the same professions were taught separately. Unfortunately, among the 89 reports reviewed, none of them had the methodological rigour needed to begin to truly understand the impact of IPE on professional practice and health care outcomes.

REFERENCES

Goerg, D., Fischer, W., Zbinden, E., and Guimón, J. (1996). Opinions des médecins sur les contenus psychologiques et psychiatriques dans la formation médicale pré-graduée. *Medecine et Hygiene*, 54, 1768–1772.

Piel, E., & Roelandt, L. (2001). *De la Psychiatrie à la santé mental. Informe al Ministerio de Sanidad sobre la situación de la Salud Mental en Francia*. Paris: Unpublished repport.

Thomas, L., Cullum, N., Rousseau, et al. (2002). Guidelines in professions allied to medicine. *The Cochrane Library* (1), 2002.

Winnicott, D. W. (1971). *Playing and Reality*. Londres: Tavistock.

Zwarenstein, M., Reeves, S., Barr, H., et al. (2002a). Interprofessional education: effects on professional practice and health care outcomes. *The Cochrane Library* (1).

Zwarenstein, M., & Bryant, W. (2002b). Interventions to promote collaboration between nurses and doctors. *The Cochrane Library*(1).

Index